THE LOVERS' GUIDE ENCYCLOPEDIA

ADVISORY COMMITTEE FOR THE LOVERS' GUIDE ENCYCLOPEDIA

Professor Milton Diamond, Professor of Anatomy and Reproductive Biology, sex educator and researcher, University of Hawaii, John A Burns School of Medicine, Pacific Centre for Sex and Society; author of *Sexwatching*. Consulted on 'Sex and Culture' and commented on the general text.

Hazel Slavin, Principal lecturer in Health Studies, South Bank University, London; sex therapist. Consulted on 'Sexual Attraction', 'Making Love', 'Sexual Practices' and 'Sexuality', and commented on the general text.

Professor Michael Adler, Professor of Genitourinary Medicine (Sexually Transmitted Diseases), University College London Medical School, and author of *The ABC of Sexually Transmitted Diseases* and over 200 papers and articles on STDs and AIDS. Consulted on 'Health and Hygiene'.

Dr Lars-Gosta Dahlof, Associate Professor in Psychology and Sexology, Goteborg University, Sweden; main author in Sexology for Swedish National Encyclopedia. Consulted on 'Sexual Attraction' and 'Sexual Practices'.

Harriett Gilbert, writer and broadcaster; author of *A Woman's History of Sex* and editor of *The Sexual Imagination*. Consulted on 'Sex and Culture'.

Tricia Kreitman, psychosexual counsellor, advice columnist for *MIZZ* and *Chat* magazines, director of Brook Advisory Centres. Consulted on 'Growth and Change' and 'Sexual Learning'.

Dr Diana Mansour, Medical Adviser/Lecturer, Margaret Pyke Family Planning Centre, London. Consulted on 'Conception to Childbirth', 'Contraception' and the Dictionary of Sex and Sexual Terms.

Dr Tuppy Owens, author of *Planet Sex* and *The Sex Maniac's Diary*, and Administrator for the Outsiders Group for the disabled. Consulted on 'Sex and Disability', 'Sexual Practices' and 'Sex and Culture'.

Dr Fran Reader, Consultant in Reproductive and Sexual Health Care, Ipswich Hospital. Consulted on 'Anatomy of Sex', 'Growth and Change', 'Sexual Intercourse' and the Dictionary of Sex and Sexual Terms.

Ryo Tanaka, Director of Human Sexuality, Centre for Education and Culture, Gifu City, Japan. Consulted on 'Sexuality'.

Kaye Wellings, AIDS Public Health in Europe, London School of Hygiene and Tropical Medicine. Consulted on 'Making Love'.

Simon Wilson, Tate Gallery, London, author of books on modern art and on Aubrey Beardsley and Egon Schiele. Consulted on 'Sex and Culture'.

Support also came from:

Vivienne Evans, Deputy Chief Executive, TACADE (The Advisory Council on Alcohol and Drug Education).

Prof Dr Erwin J Haberle, President of German Society for Social-Scientific Sex Research and Secretary General, European Federation of Sexology.

Dr Dinant Haslinghius, The Netherlands Institute of Social Sexological Research, The Hague.

Dr Meera Kishen, Abacus Centre, Liverpool.

Dr Prakash Kothari, sexologist, Bombay.

Dr Nathaniel McConaghy, Prince of Wales Hospital, Randwick, New South Wales, Australia.

Ellen Visser, Staffworker on Disability and Sexuality and Gehandicaptenraad (National Council for the Disabled), Utrecht, Netherlands.

Morgan Williams, SPOD (The Association to Aid the Sexual and Personal Relationships of People with a Disability)

Dr Kenneth Zucker, Child and Family Studies Centre, Clarke Institute of Psychiatry, Toronto, Canada.

The Editor wishes to thank the above for their invaluable help, advice and support in the writing of this book. However, the opinions expressed here are her own or those of the credited authors.

THE LOVERS' GUIDE ENCYCLOPEDIA

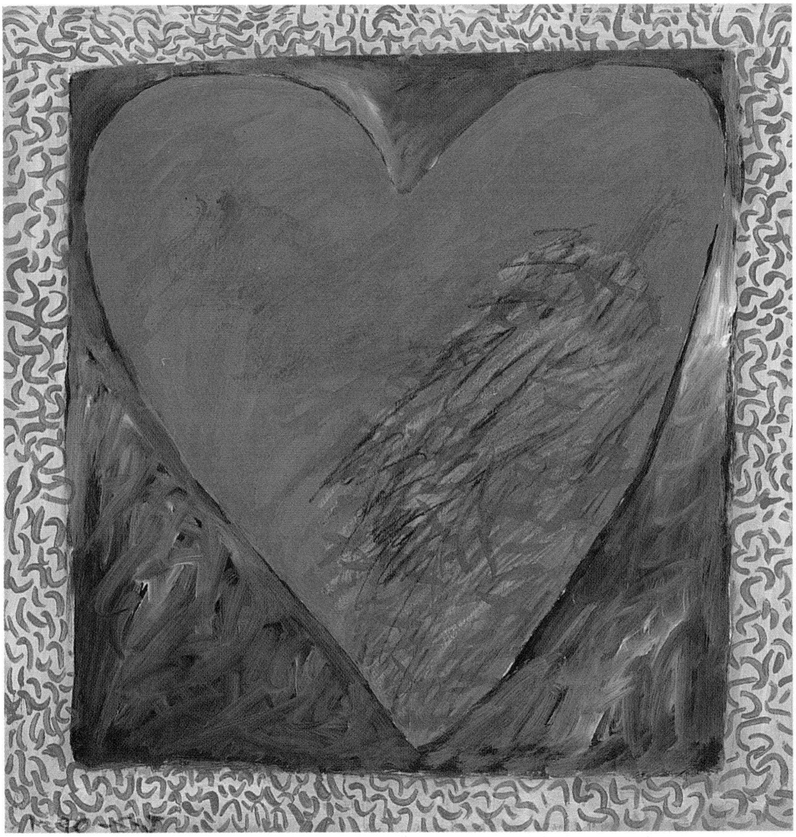

Consultant Editor
DOREEN E MASSEY

BLOOMSBURY

THE LOVERS' GUIDE ENCYCLOPEDIA

The Lovers' Guide is a trademark of Lifetime Vision Limited

The Lovers' Guide Encyclopedia
first published 1996 by
Bloomsbury Publishing Plc, 38 Soho Square, London W1V 5DF

This paperback edition published 1997

For copyright © in individual illustrations and photographs see picture credit list page 248

Consultant Editor: Doreen E Massey
Project Director: Robert Page
Writer and Researcher: Olivia Preston
Author of 'Sex and You': Elizabeth Fenwick
Author of 'Sex Through the Ages': Reay Tannahill
Picture Editor and Researcher: Liz Boggis
Art Direction: Simon Jennings
Designer: Glen Breeds
Additional Research: Zoe Lyall

A CIP catalogue record for this book is available from the British Library

ISBN: 0 7475 3260 5

Edited, designed and typeset by Book Creation Services, London
Typeset in FRANKLIN GOTHIC EXTRA CONDENSED, Friz Quadrata,
Garamond Condensed Optima.
Printed in Hong Kong

CONTENTS

INTRODUCTION

By
Doreen E. Massey

Sexual information has long been inhibited by myths and taboos. Reliable, comprehensive and up-to-date information is now needed more than ever as individuals increasingly take charge of their personal lives.

The key change in the 1990s, following the growth of literacy and the expansion of education, is the explosion in communications. People are today far more aware of a vast diversity in sexual practices and attitudes than ever before. Increased information brings great benefits. As a leading churchman has said, far better the risks associated with free discussion of sex than the much greater risks that come from ignorance.

The nature of sexual partnerships has evolved in recent years. Sexual partnerships between people of different racial, cultural and age groups have increased, although marriage is becoming less common and divorce rates are higher than ever. Particularly in western countries, women have asserted their right to sexual pleasure and resisted exploitation. Gay men and lesbians have demanded positive recognition. Sexual harassment and abuse have become the subjects of public debate, and are challenged openly and often successfully.

The latter part of this century has also seen the rise of the pandemic HIV and AIDS which has had a profound impact on sexual awareness and forced people to develop their capacity for understanding.

These and other phenomena have brought about the redefinition and reconsideration of our attitudes to – and practice of – sex and sexuality, in all of their physical and emotional aspects.

The Lovers' Guide Encyclopedia addresses all of these issues in a non-judgmental way. It aims to provide adults with a wealth of sexual information in an accessible and clear manner. A valuable reference book, it will also help readers to redefine their assumptions and open their minds to new possibilities.

The Lovers' Guide previous productions have had an enormous impact on social history, virtually world-wide, because of their honesty and frankness. They have helped to break down many prevailing taboos about sexual matters and have thereby removed much of the guilt many once associated with sex. The responses of both the general public and experts to **The Lovers' Guide Videos** were overwhelmingly positive. People appreciated being encouraged to explore sexuality and sexual techniques which they offered. Many were reassured that their own desires and practices were shared by others and were, at long last, being discussed openly.

The over-riding aim of the **Lovers' Guide** team has always been to improve people's sex lives, encouraging the view that sex is a natural activity to be enjoyed and need not involve guilt, fear or danger. **The Lovers' Guide Encyclopedia** continues, and builds on, this tradition.

My own experience in sex education, with both young people and adults, leads me also to believe that ignorance and fear are dangerous. We teach people to cross roads safely, to read, to write and to swim. Yet so often, we neglect to teach them anything about sexual behaviour. The notion that, as long as people are kept in ignorance about sex, they will be kept from promiscuity has been shown to be thoroughly false and misguided. Research has clearly shown that the better informed people are about sex, and able to discuss sex in a knowledgeable way, the more responsible is their behaviour. It allows them to engage in safer sexual activity, to give and receive greater pleasure, thereby acheiving greater fulfilment.

Throughout most of the world, there are concerns about the high incidence of teenage pregnancies, abortions and sexually transmitted diseases, including HIV, AIDS and chlamydia. The most effective weapon we have to deal with such issues is to educate people, giving them knowledge of the facts, the available choices and the responsibilities that they have as sexual beings. Advice columnists, clinics and voluntary organizations working in the sexual health all report increasing public demand for more extensive information and reliable advice. Sadly, the way sex is represented in the media is often sensationalist, inaccurate and exploitative. Young people describe sex education in schools as inadequate, regarding it as 'too little, too late'. Many parents say they do not know how to talk to their children about sex.

A fundamental aim of this book therefore has been to deal with these concerns. It has four sections, which are designed to help the reader to identify her or his interests easily. The first section is concerned with facts, a body of information which forms the basis for the sexual attitudes, feelings and practices examined in Part 2. Part 3 encourages the reader to explore his or her own sexuality, offering advice and challenges. Part 4 discusses sex and its relationship with society, recognising that sexual attitudes and behaviour are closely linked to, and influenced by, their social context. Part 5 provides a comprehensive dictionary of sexual terminology.

We are all sexual beings who are influenced by a variety of circumstances on a global, local and intimate level. **The Lovers' Guide Encyclopedia** provides a wealth of insights into human sexual behaviour, enabling the reader to make her or his own informed choices.

1

SEXUAL FACTS

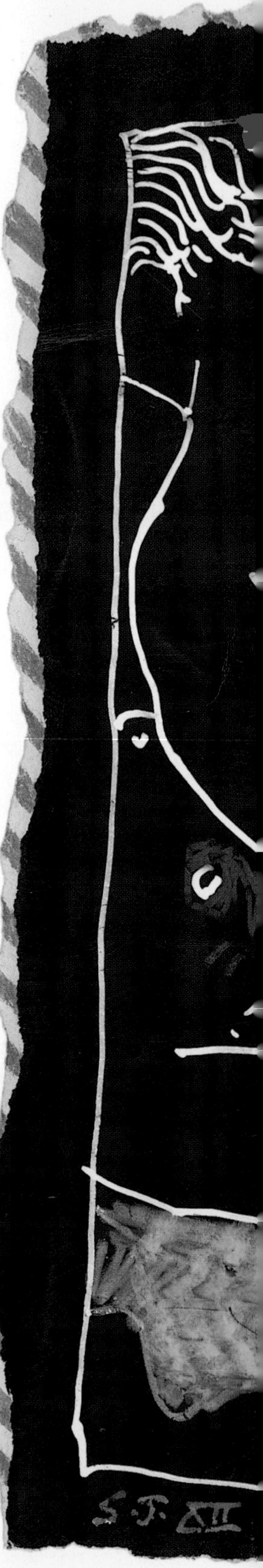

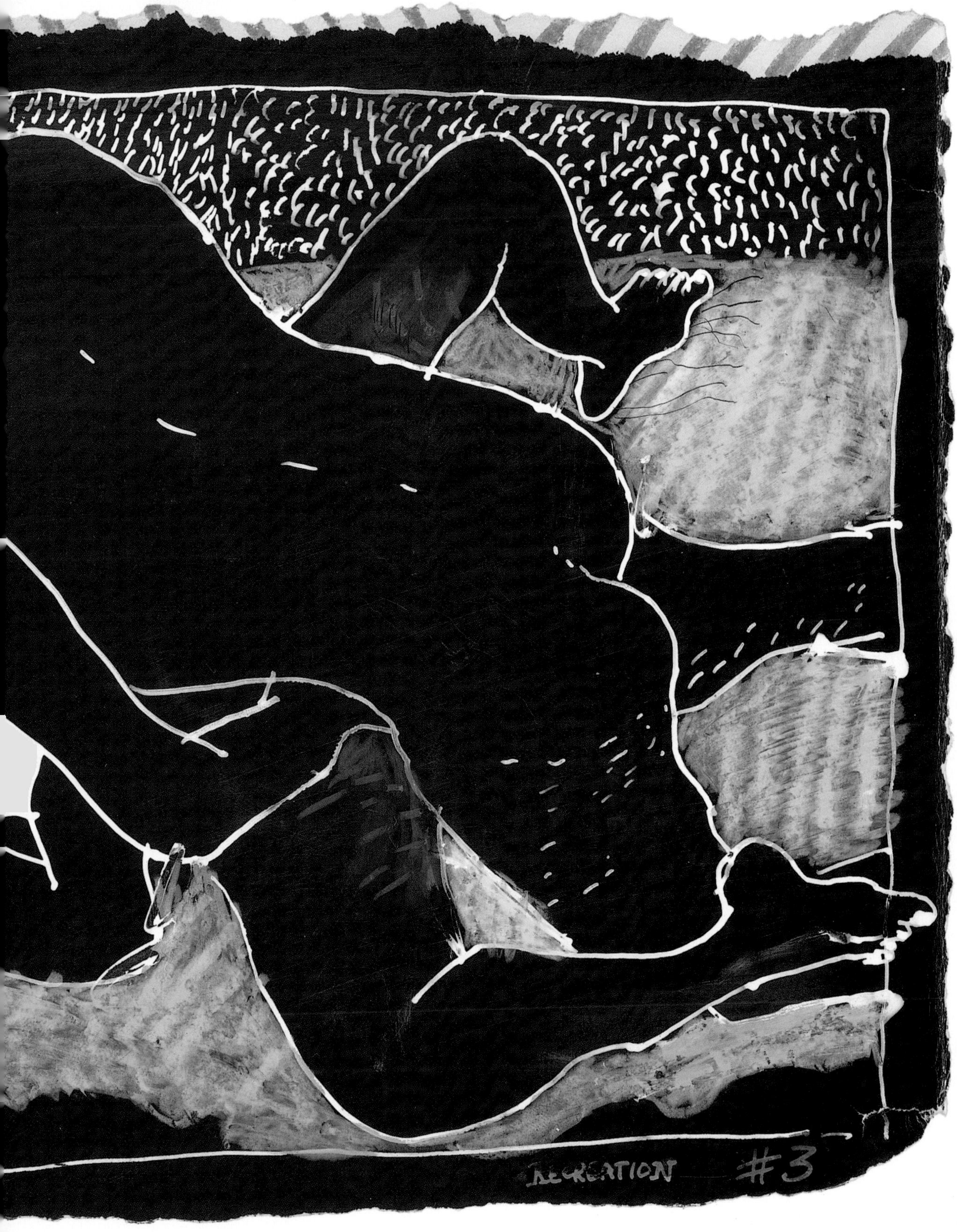
RECREATION #3

FEMALE ANATOMY

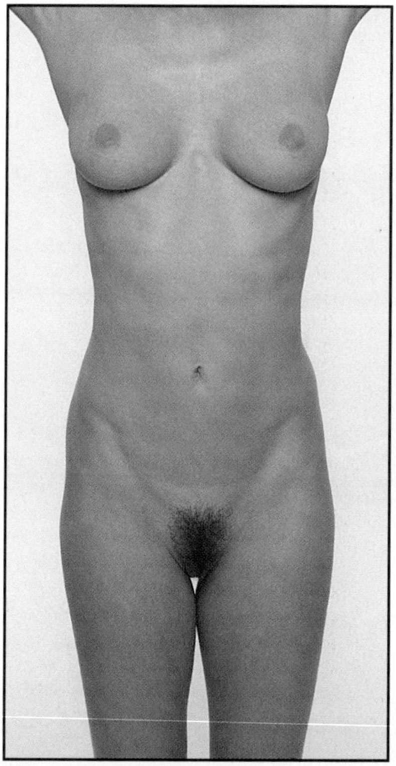

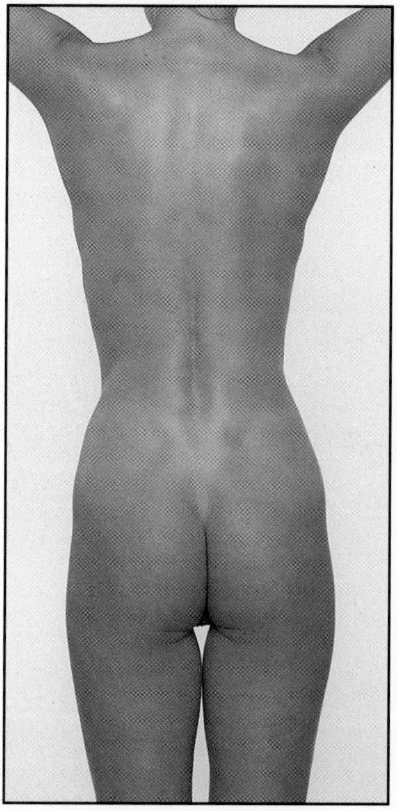

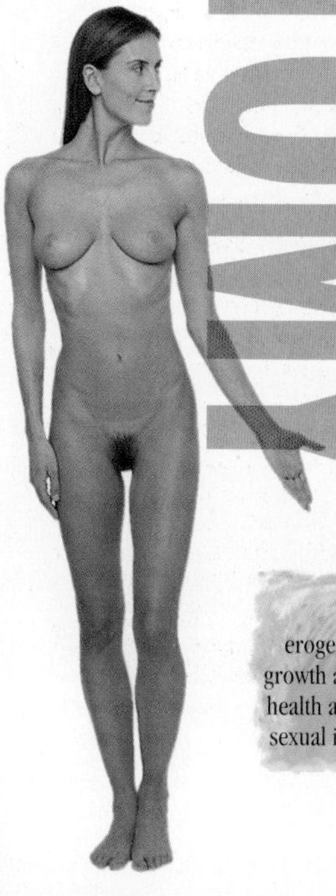

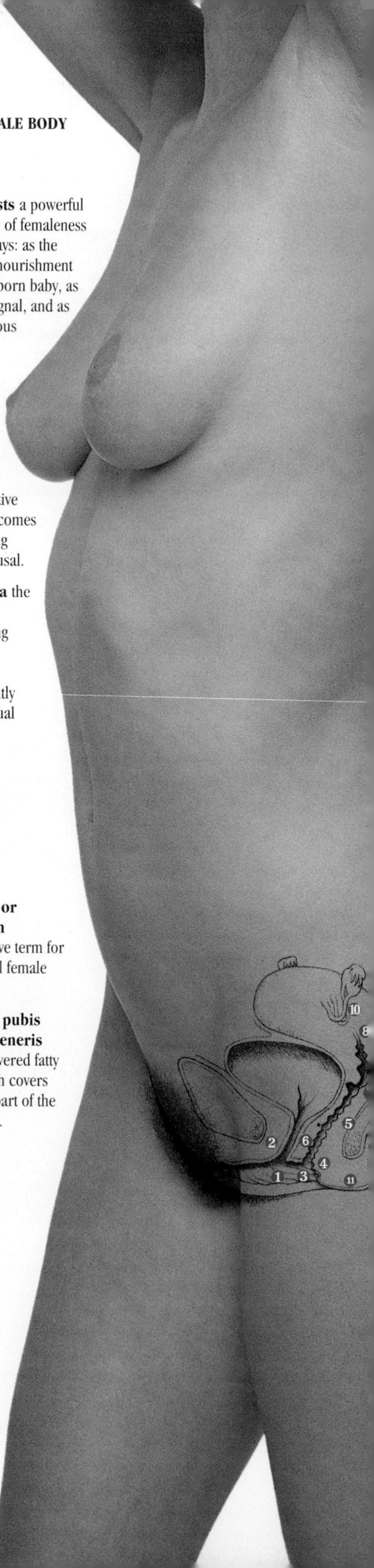

THE FEMALE BODY

The breasts a powerful expression of femaleness in three ways: as the source of nourishment for a new-born baby, as a sexual signal, and as an erogenous zone.

The nipple the tip of the breast, and the most sensitive part. It becomes erect during sexual arousal.

The areola the dark area surrounding the nipple, which swells slightly during sexual arousal.

The vulva or pudendum the collective term for the external female genitalia.

The mons pubis or mons veneris the hair-covered fatty tissue which covers the upper part of the pubic bone.

See also:
erogenous zones
growth and change
health and hygiene
sexual intercourse

SEXUAL ANATOMY

❶ **The vestibule** the term sometimes used to refer to the area between the labia minora in which the vaginal opening and the urethral opening are situated.

❷ **The urethra** the tube through which urine is passed out of the body from the bladder. It lies just in front of and above the vaginal opening.

❸ **The fourchette** the point where the labia minora join (the delicate area of skin at the very back of the vaginal opening).

❹ **The hymen** the thin membrane which in childhood partially covers the opening to the vagina.

❺ **The vagina** the passage which leads in from the vulva to the cervix.

❻ **The G-spot** a small area of highly sensitive tissue situated inside the front of the vagina behind the pubic bone. It is thought to be the female equivalent of the prostate in the male, although it may not be present in all females.

❼ **The cervix** the neck of the uterus.

❽ **The uterus or womb** the organ in which a fertilized ovum develops into a baby. It is about the size of a small pear (upside down), and lies between the bladder and the rectum where it is held in place by various ligaments.

❾ **The ovaries** the organs which produce the female sexual hormones oestrogen and progesterone and the reproductive gametes, the ova. They are equivalent to the testes in the male.

❿ **The ovarian or fallopian tubes** the tubes which connect the ovaries to the uterus, in which fertilization occurs.

The perineum the area of skin and underlying fibrous and muscle tissue between the vagina and the anus.

The rectum the last part of the intestine, leading to the anus.

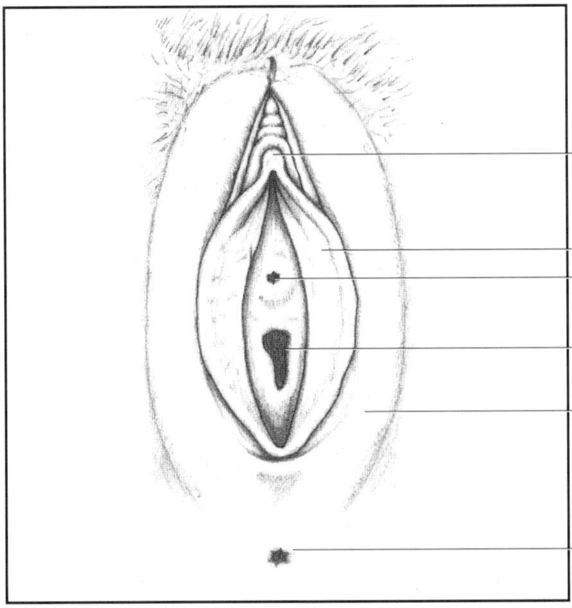

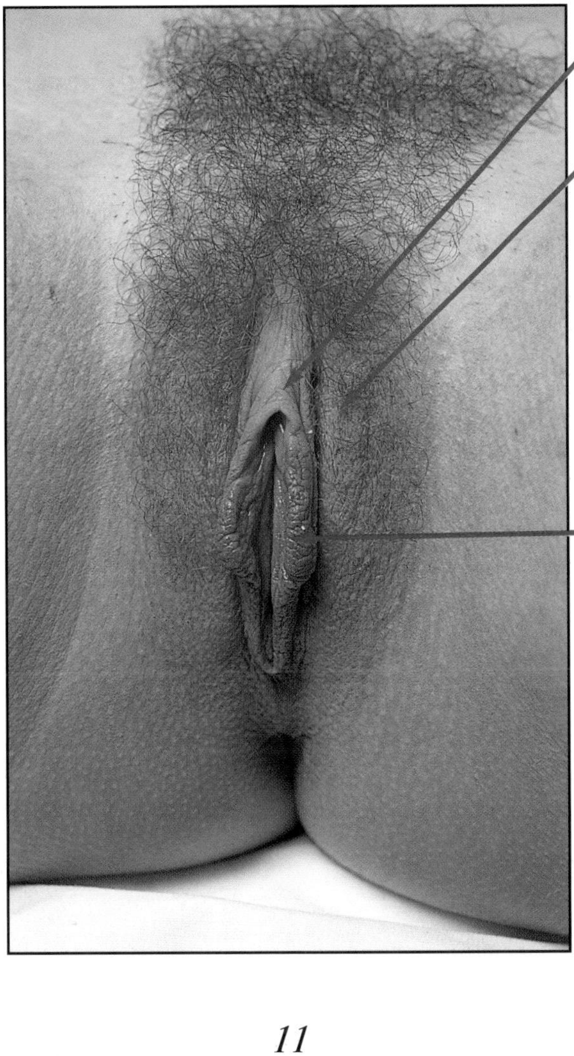

THE VULVA

The clitoris the female equivalent of the penis, and the most sensitive and erotic part of the female genitalia.

The labia majora or outer labia the two 'lips' which surround the vaginal opening, usually lying close together to protect it. Anatomically they are equivalent to the scrotum in the male. At the front they join at the mons pubis; at the back they join at the perineum. They are plump enough to act as a cushion during intercourse. They contain sweat- and odour-producing glands, which keep the smooth inner part moistened and give the vulva its highly individual sexual odour.

The labia minora or inner labia the smaller, hairless 'lips' or folds of skin within the outer labia, immediately around the vaginal opening. At the front they join to form the hood of the clitoris and at the back they form the fourchette. They contain sebaceous glands on their outer side and sweat glands on the inner parts which help with lubrication. During sexual arousal they become engorged with blood (in a similar manner to the penis), which makes them darken in colour and swell to about two or three times their normal size.

BREASTS

In most societies the breasts are seen as a powerful expression of femaleness. Humans are unique among mammals in that the breasts seem to serve not one but several purposes: as well as producing the milk for the new-born offspring, they have taken on secondary roles which are purely sexual, particularly in Western society.

The breasts as a sexual signal
FACT: no other mammal has large (as opposed to flat) breasts constantly throughout adult life. In every other mammal the breasts remain flat except during pregnancy.

The best-known explanation for this is that proposed by Dr Desmond Morris. He suggests that the breasts developed in this way as part of the evolutionary process, when humans started to have sexual intercourse face-to-face. In this way, the breasts mimic the shape of the buttocks which were the primary sexual signal in man's distant ancestors, the apes.

This role is emphasized by the 'sex flush' which occurs during intercourse in some women, and which centres on the breasts.

Breasts and milk production
The breasts are made up of fatty tissue which contains thousands of tiny milk-producing glands known as alveoli, with ducts leading to the nipple. These structures are supported by a network of connective tissue, which also maintains the shape and firmness of the breasts.

The changes in hormone production in the course of pregnancy cause a number of changes in the breasts. Within the first three weeks of pregnancy the woman may notice some increased sensitivity, but it is not until the fifth month that the first milk is produced. At this stage a difference in size becomes noticeable and the areolae grow darker and more prominent.

STRUCTURE OF THE BREAST

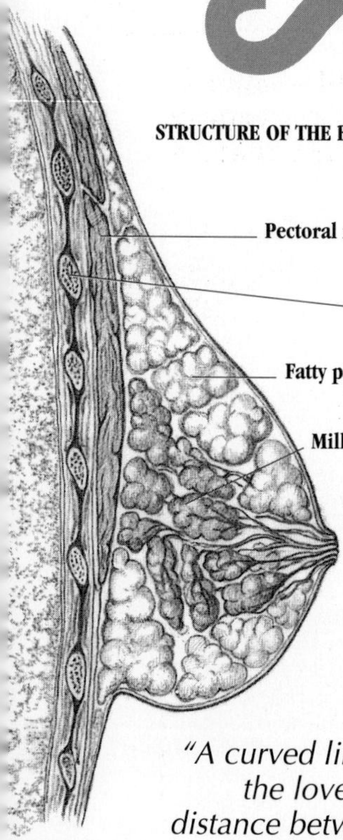

"A curved line is the loveliest distance between two points."
MAE WEST

Bras are designed and worn for more than their functional qualities – they emphasise the sexual attraction of the breasts, as this advertisement shows.

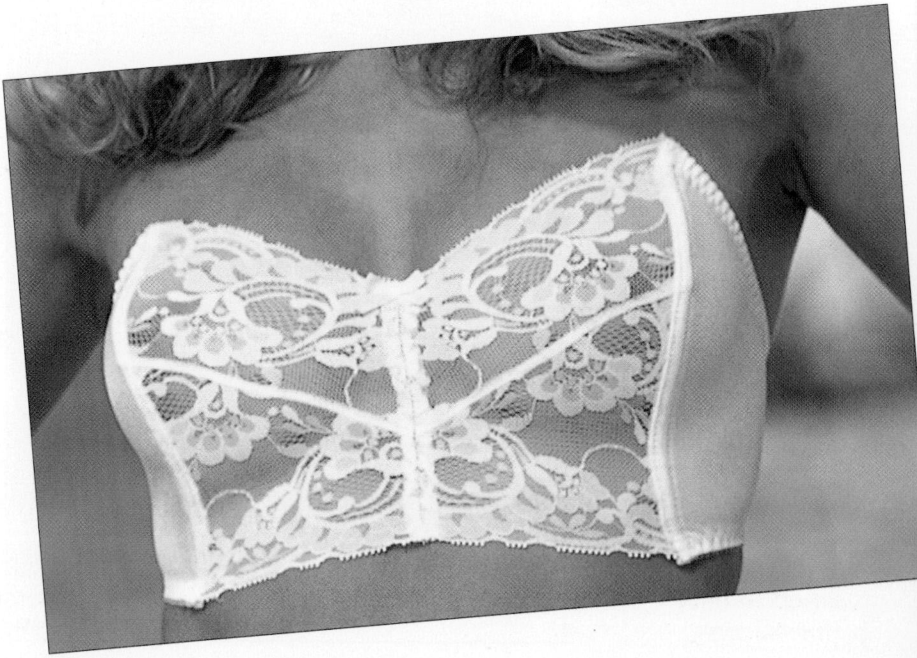

See also:
growth and change
sexual attraction
sexual intercourse

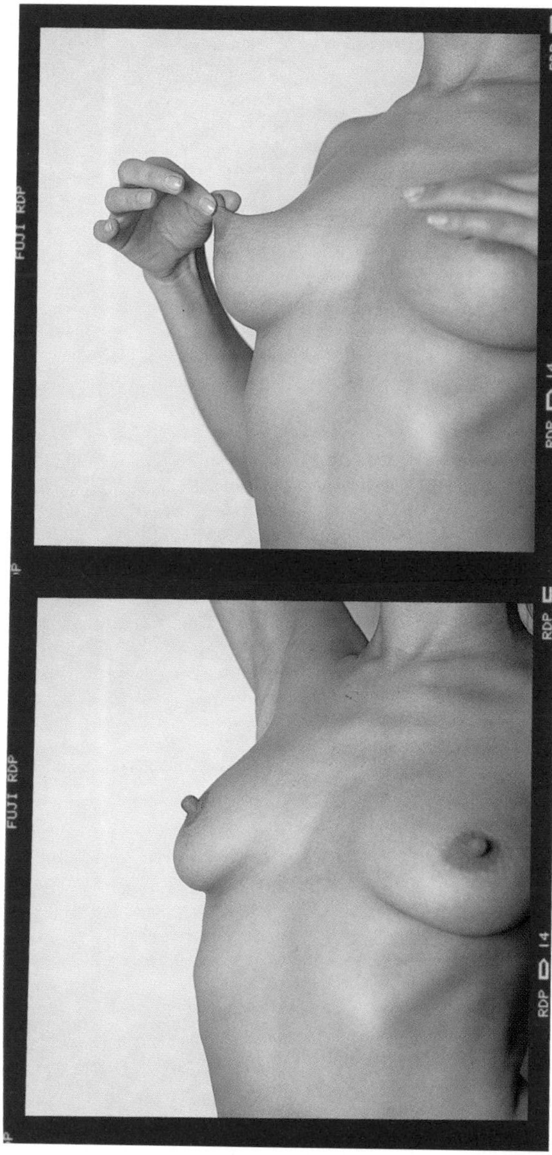

Breast shape and size

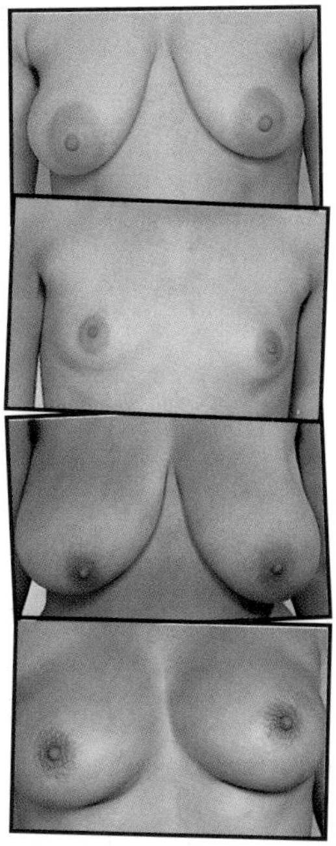

The initial growth of the breasts and their ultimate size are determined to some extent by genetic factors but primarily by hormone production: if a male is injected with the female hormone oestrogen he will develop breasts in the same way. It may be because of this hormonal factor that large breasts are sometimes seen as a symbol of fecundity. However, size is no indication of a woman's milk-producing capacity or her fertility. The variety in the size and shape of women's breasts is almost infinite, as is the range of people's notions of what size and shape is most attractive.

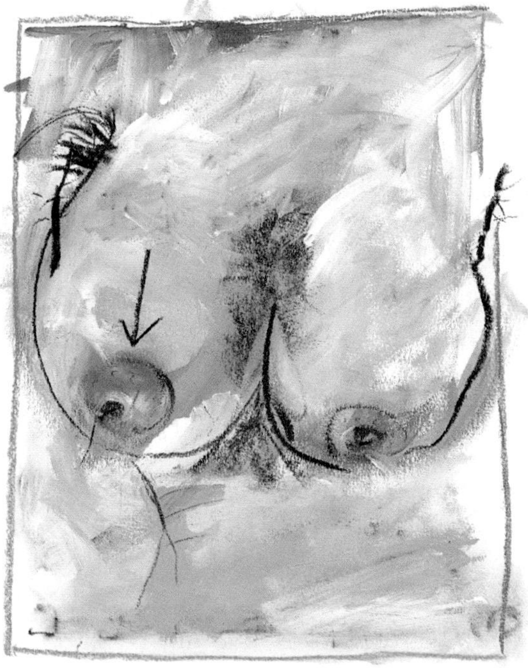

Slang terms
boobs, bosom, bust, cans, chabooms, chest, knockers, tits, Bristols, Manchesters, norks, zards, melons, brown eyes, headlights, trapfruits, hammocks, muffins, Vaticans, lungs, jugs, udders, wabs.

The breasts as erogenous zones

The 'sex flush' – together with the swelling of the areolae and the hardening of the nipples during sexual arousal – also draw attention to the breasts as powerful erogenous zones. This varies greatly from one woman to another. However, in research carried out by Masters and Johnson three of the 382 women questioned said that they could bring themselves to orgasm simply by manipulating their breasts, and others claimed to have come to orgasm during breast-feeding.

VAGINA

The vagina is the primary female sexual organ. The term derives from the Latin word meaning 'sheath', which serves as a male-oriented description of its function in sexual intercourse, 'sheathing' the penis. In reality the vagina's functions are considerably more complex than this description would suggest.

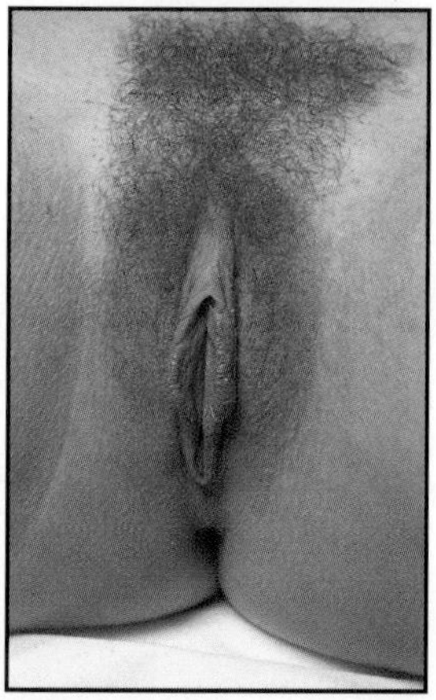

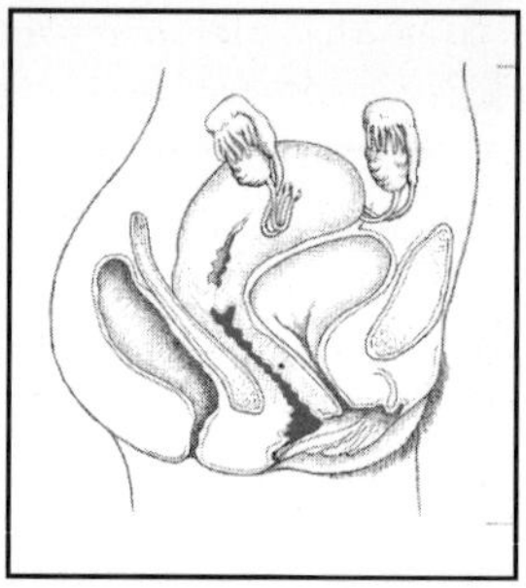

The vagina is the term for the passage which leads from the vulva to the cervix. It is marked in red on the cross-section diagram above. The top photograph shows the vaginal opening and lips.

Physiology of the vagina

The vagina is the passage which leads in from the vulva and vestibule (the outer parts of the female genitalia) to the cervix (the neck of the uterus). Apart from its role in sexual pleasure, the vagina has three main functions: to enable the male's sperm to enter the womb and fertilize an egg, and to enable both menstrual fluids and a developed foetus to leave.

It is a fibro-muscular structure, covered with a thin mucus membrane. The various layers of muscle – together with the numerous folds of skin by which they are covered – give the vagina great capacity for expansion and contraction. This means that most vaginas can accommodate any size of penis, as well as, potentially, a developed foetus.

See also:
penis
clitoris
growth and change
sexual intercourse
health and hygiene

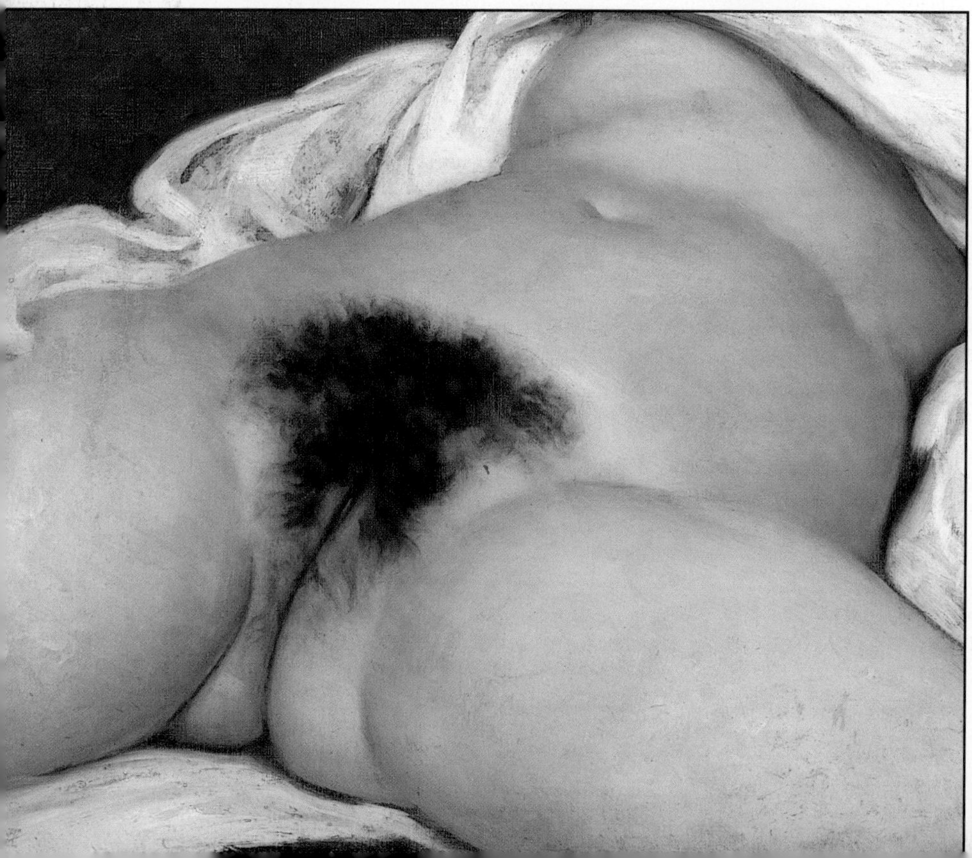

L'origine du monde (The Origin of the World) by Gustave Courbet (1866) is a celebration of female sexuality – emphasizing both sensuality and fecundity.

There are two main types of muscle in the vagina. The smooth muscle within the vaginal wall is not under voluntary control and will relax and stretch during sexual arousal and penile penetration without conscious effort. The muscle fibres surrounding the outer third of the vagina are under voluntary control, enabling the woman to 'grip' the penis by tensing the pelvic floor muscles. It is these muscles which may go into involuntary spasm in the condition known as vaginismus; they may also be damaged during childbirth.

Facts and fictions about the vagina

● It is widely believed that the size of both a man's penis and a woman's vagina is partly determined by race. There is, however, no conclusive medical evidence for this.

● It is often thought that smaller vaginas give greater pleasure to the partner in penetrative sex. While this may be true in some cases, it is a fact that in the latter stages of arousal all vaginas distend and balloon, reducing friction for both partners.

● In a virgin the vagina may be partially covered by a thin membrane known as the hymen. Traditionally taken as evidence of virginity, the hymen can in fact be broken quite easily, through bicycle- or horse-riding or gymnastics, or when using a tampon, as well as by first intercourse. When broken it may bleed a little, but this is rarely painful. In some women, the hymen is retained and may need surgical attention to allow penile penetration.

● In 1950 Dr Ernst Grafenburg wrote of 'an erotic zone ... on the anterior wall of the vagina'. The term G-spot was later coined, referring to the small area of tissue containing nerve endings situated inside the front of the vagina, behind the pubic bone. Its male equivalent is the prostate gland. Controversy about the nature of the female G-spot and indeed its very existence continues today. However, some research has concluded that in some women this area swells in the course of arousal and may even lead to the production of an 'ejaculate' of clear fluid at orgasm.

The vagina's self-care system

The vagina has a unique system which, if not interfered with in any way, ensures that it remains healthy and functions correctly.

One kind of fluid is constantly present. It is formed through the fermentation of the vagina's natural bacteria on its walls, creating a slightly acidic environment which maintains the vagina's health and natural bacterial balance.

Another fluid is produced during sexual arousal to provide lubrication and to aid the passage of the sperm into the cervix when the woman is at her most fertile. This was originally thought to come from the cervix or the Bartholin's glands on the inner side of the inner labia. It is in fact produced as droplets, like sweat, on the walls of the vaginal barrel, the quantity of which may vary according to the individual, her age, and her state of arousal.

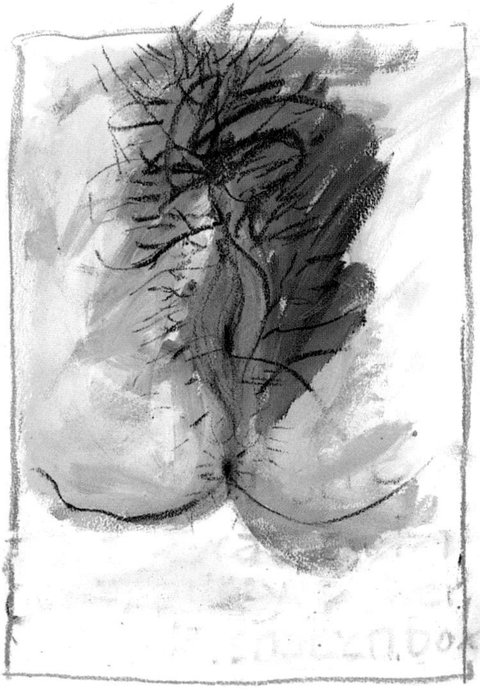

Slang terms

pee-hole, hole, coozy, pussy, twat, bearded clam, fanny, quim, cunt, slit, crack, box, doughnut, snatch, beard, beaver, badger, brownie, cherry pie, cooch, fern, fur-burger/pie/sandwich, gash, muff, poon tang, tail, nook, nooky, happy valley, trench, snapping turtle, Y, minge, money box, mousetrap, jelly roll, garden, hatch, promised land, rattle, snake canyon.

CLITORIS

The clitoris has long been recognized as the key to women's sexual pleasure: in fact the very word comes from the ancient Greek 'kleitoris', meaning 'key'. It is fundamental in two senses: firstly in that for most women direct or indirect stimulation of the clitoris is the most important part of sexual arousal and, for many, essential to reaching orgasm. Secondly, sexual arousal initiated in any part of the body can seem to the woman to be focused on the clitoris. It is unique in that its sole function seems to be as receptor and transmitter of sensual pleasure.

The word clitoris comes from the ancient Greek 'kleitoris', meaning 'key'.

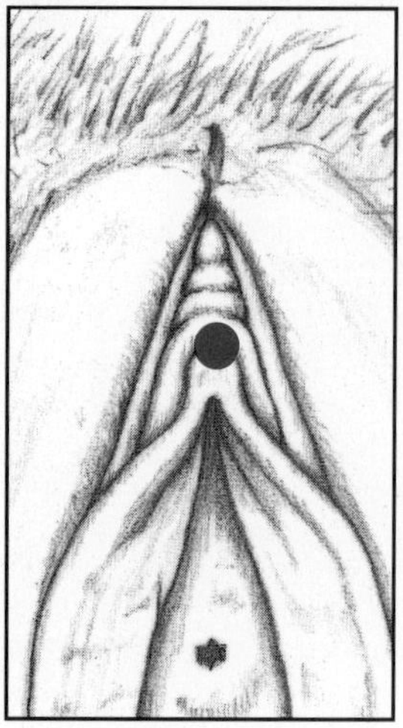

Location of the clitoris

The clitoris is situated about 2.5 to 3.5 cm above the vaginal opening, where the inner labia meet. The whole organ is generally about 2 to 3 cm long, although all but the head or glans, located at the tip of the shaft and only 0.3 to 1.3 cm in diameter, is hidden by a hood or prepuce formed by the inner labia. There is great variety in size and shape.

Self-exploration

Unlike the male sexual organs, those of the female are not immediately visible and consequently may be a little mysterious – or simply misunderstood. A healthy and fulfilling sex life depends on both partners knowing about their own and each other's sexual organs and how they look and feel.

This is particularly important with regard to the clitoris, probably the most mysterious of all the sexual organs – even now, it is not known exactly what happens to the clitoris at orgasm. However, knowing where it is and how to stimulate it can, in most women, be the key to sexual satisfaction.

The clitoris and sexual arousal

When a woman becomes aroused, the shaft of the clitoris thickens and may grow longer as it becomes engorged with blood. The glans also swells slightly, sometimes up to as much as

See also:
vagina
masturbation
sex positions
sexual intercourse

Female and male development
The clitoris is in fact the female equivalent of the penis. In the development of embryos of both sexes a small bud of tissue forms between the legs. This then develops into a penis in the male and a clitoris in the female. Other physiological equivalents include the nipples in both sexes, the ovaries and the testes, the labia majora and the scrotum, and the G-spot and the prostate.

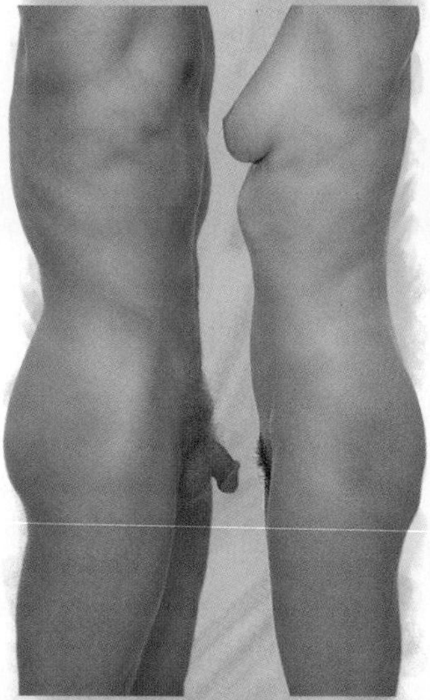

PARALLELS BETWEEN CLITORIS AND PENIS

- they develop from the same lump of tissue in the embryo
- the head of the clitoris and the penis is made up of sensory tissue
- the shaft contains erectile tissue
- they are surrounded by soft tissue
- the small head of the clitoris and the glans of the penis contain the same number of nerve endings
- their size and shape are no indication of their capacity to give or receive sensuous pleasure

The main difference between the clitoris and the penis is that the penis has other, non-sensual functions, such as carrying the urethra. The clitoris responds to sexual arousal much more gradually. While a man's erection is one of the first and most visible signs of arousal, the changes in the clitoris are slower and more subtle.

twice its normal size, making it more exposed and sensitive. However, during the plateau stage of sexual arousal, just before orgasm, the head or glans withdraws completely beneath its hood, making it impossible to know what happens to the clitoris during orgasm, even though pressure on the clitoral area continues to arouse the woman. After orgasm the glans quickly goes back to its usual position, normally within ten seconds, returning to its unstimulated size within five or ten minutes.

Clitoral and vaginal orgasms

The long-standing debate about the nature of the female orgasm has led to two main points of view.

Medically there is no difference between clitoral and vaginal orgasms. The main muscle involved in the muscular contractions associated with the female orgasm encircles the vagina and contains fibres which are also attached to the shaft of the clitoris. While it is known that the clitoris develops from the same tissue in the foetus as the penis in the male, the existence of a female G-spot like the male's prostate has not been conclusively proved.

The other point of view is based not on scientific evidence but on women's reports of their own experience. It is now widely accepted that a woman can have an orgasm without vaginal penetration and without a man. For most (but not all) women sexual arousal seems to be focused on the clitoris, and for many direct stimulation of the clitoris is necessary for them to achieve orgasm. However, the clitoris can be stimulated indirectly and women can reach orgasm through stimulation of the vagina, the breasts and other erogenous zones. Many women can come to orgasm just through fantasy.

For some women the clitoris is more important, for others it is the G-spot. An orgasm may seem to be focused on the clitoris, the G-spot or both. Some women are aware of the uterine contractions which occur at orgasm, some are not. A woman's ability to have an orgasm can even vary, as can the nature of the orgasm itself. Both can be affected by the menstrual cycle, by stress or by other factors.

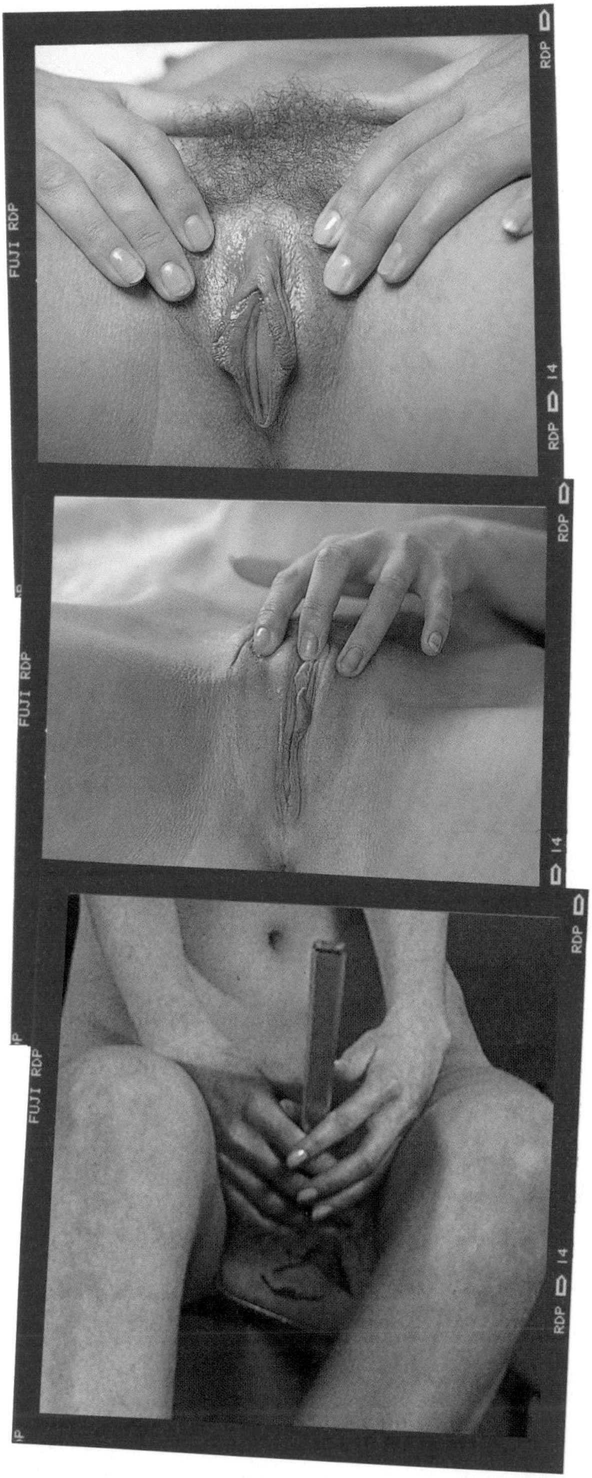

Self-exploration

For a woman to examine herself, she can squat down over a small mirror, or sit in front of one, with her legs apart (bottom). By opening the labia majora, the various parts of the vulva can be identified. The head of the clitoris can be seen when the labia minora are gently pulled apart (top); it is hard and can be felt by drawing a finger forwards from the vagina (centre).

MALE ANATOMY

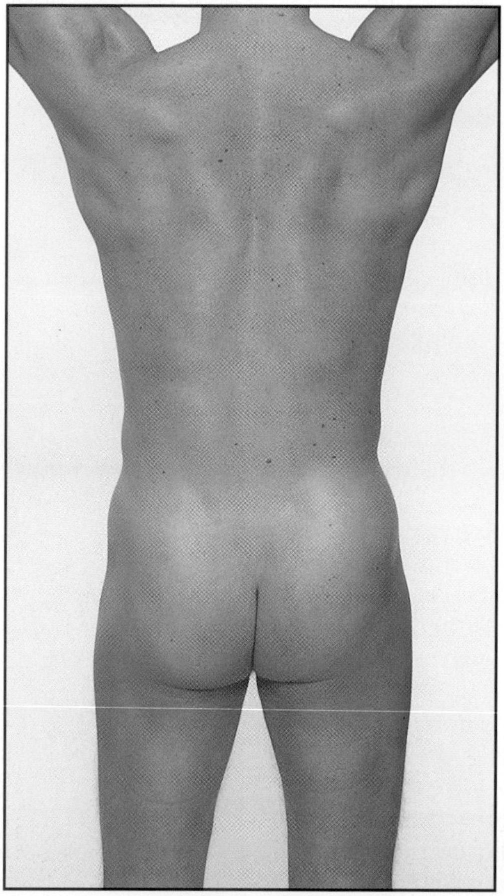

THE MALE BODY AND REPRODUCTIVE SYSTEM

❶ **The epididymis** the duct leading from each testis, in which the sperm are matured and stored until being passed into the vas deferens when needed. Each one is 5 to 7 metres long, tightly coiled and doubled back on itself.

❷ **The vas deferens** the duct which carries the sperm from the epididymis to the prostate gland.

❸ **The prostate gland** the organ in which the two vasa deferentia meet each other before joining the urethra. It produces secretions which form part of the seminal fluid and is also responsible for sealing off the exit from the bladder to prevent urine from being passed while the penis is erect. It is the site of the most common male cancer.

❹ **The urethra** the tube through which urine is passed out of the body from the bladder and semen is passed on ejaculation.

❺ **The Cowper's glands** join the urethra below the prostate. They produce a mucus substance whose purpose is to neutralize the acidity of any urine left in the urethra which could kill the sperm. This helps to lubricate the tip of the penis prior to ejaculation and forms part of the seminal fluid.

❻ **The perineum** the area of skin and underlying fibrous and muscle tissue between the scrotum and the anus. It includes a central ridge termed the median raphe.

❼ **The rectum** is the last part of the intestine, leading to the anus.

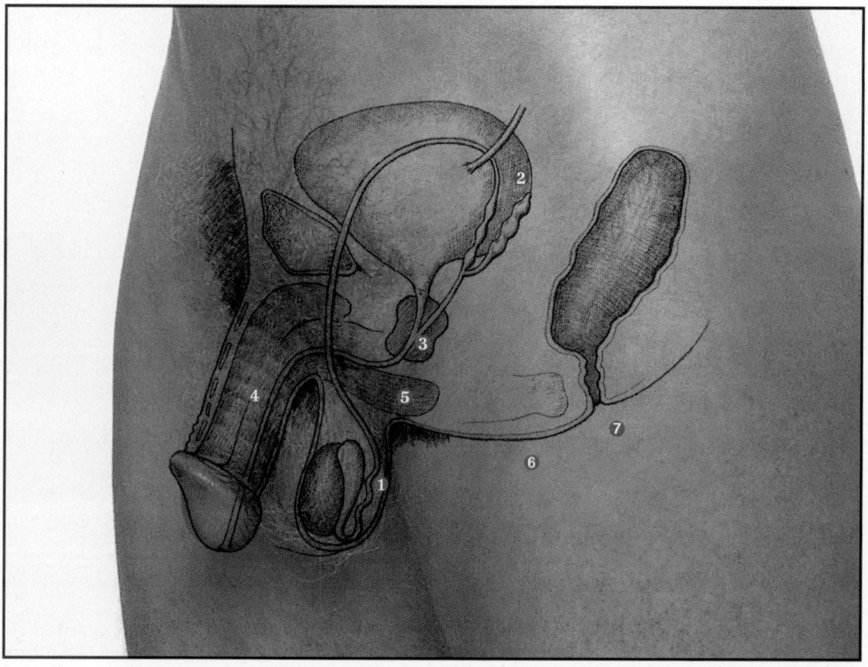

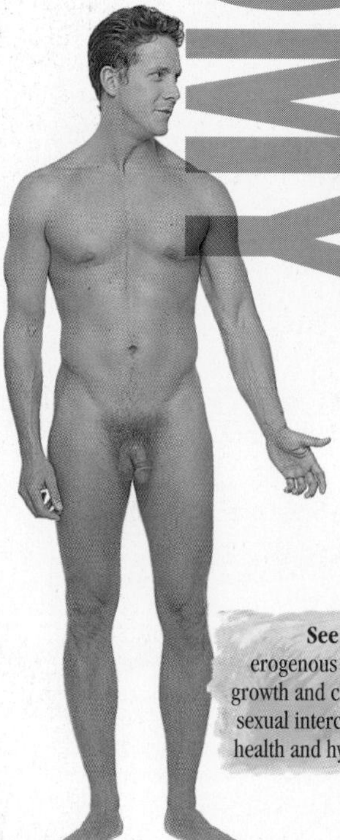

See also:
erogenous zones
growth and change
sexual intercourse
health and hygiene

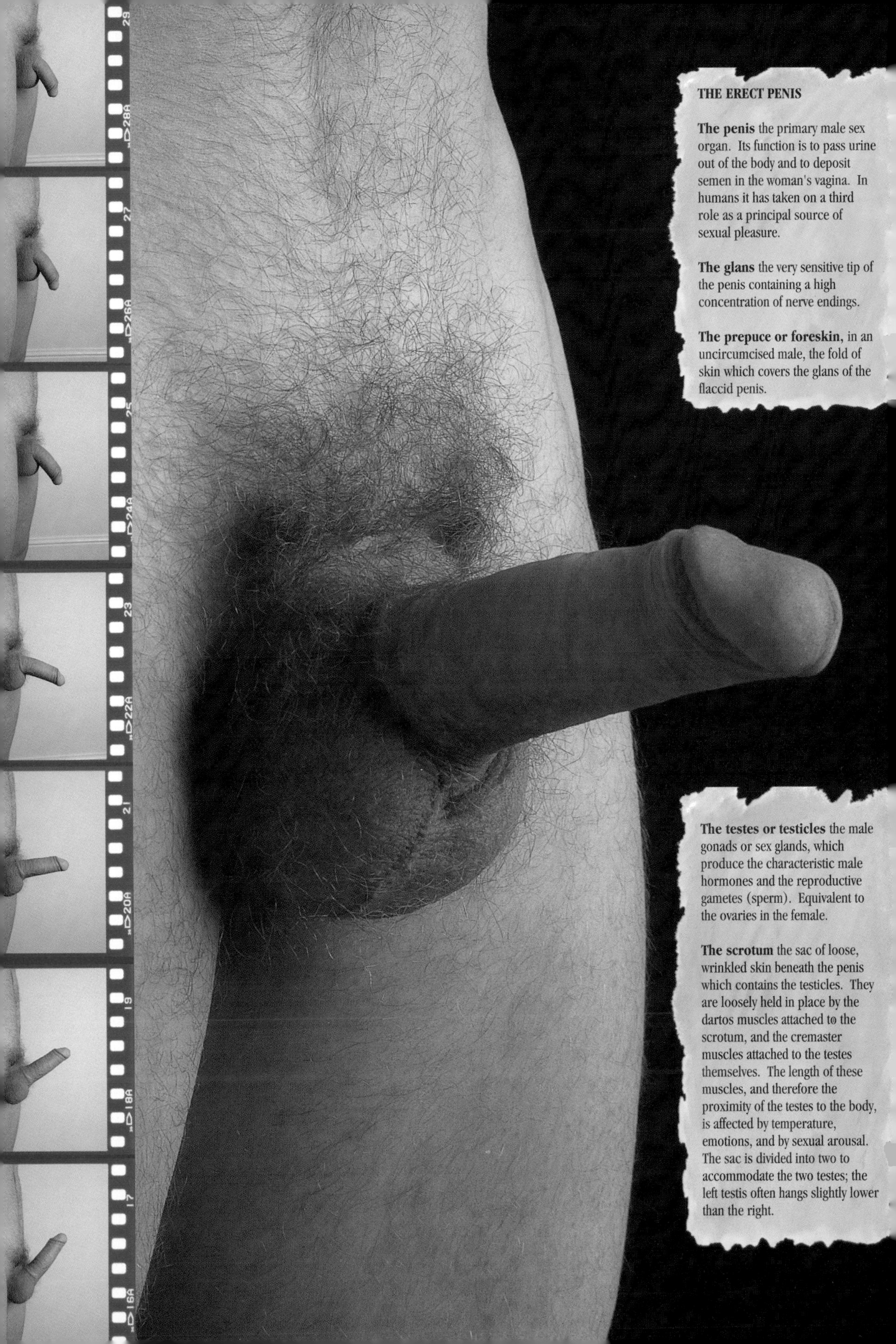

THE ERECT PENIS

The penis the primary male sex organ. Its function is to pass urine out of the body and to deposit semen in the woman's vagina. In humans it has taken on a third role as a principal source of sexual pleasure.

The glans the very sensitive tip of the penis containing a high concentration of nerve endings.

The prepuce or foreskin, in an uncircumcised male, the fold of skin which covers the glans of the flaccid penis.

The testes or testicles the male gonads or sex glands, which produce the characteristic male hormones and the reproductive gametes (sperm). Equivalent to the ovaries in the female.

The scrotum the sac of loose, wrinkled skin beneath the penis which contains the testicles. They are loosely held in place by the dartos muscles attached to the scrotum, and the cremaster muscles attached to the testes themselves. The length of these muscles, and therefore the proximity of the testes to the body, is affected by temperature, emotions, and by sexual arousal. The sac is divided into two to accommodate the two testes; the left testis often hangs slightly lower than the right.

PENIS

Throughout time and in almost all cultures the penis has been a powerful symbol – of male sexuality, of potency, of the force of life, and of virility. However, no other organ of the human body has been surrounded by as many myths and misconceptions as this, the primary male sex organ.

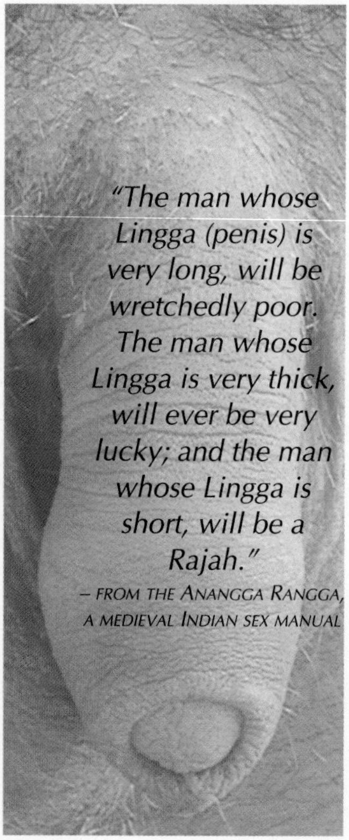

"The man whose Lingga (penis) is very long, will be wretchedly poor. The man whose Lingga is very thick, will ever be very lucky; and the man whose Lingga is short, will be a Rajah."

– FROM THE *ANANGGA RANGGA*, A MEDIEVAL INDIAN SEX MANUAL

Physiology of the penis

The penis is made up of erectile and muscular tissue, supplied with many sensory nerves. The erectile tissue lies in three columns, two on the back forming the corpora cavernosa, and one on the front forming the corpus spongiosum and extending to form the glans or head. This tissue is arranged in the form of a honeycomb. When the penis is flaccid the muscle fibres which form this honeycomb are contracted. During sexual arousal, the muscles relax to let more blood in. The many blood vessels and spaces in these structures become engorged with blood, causing the penis to become erect.

The urethra is the tube through which urine is passed out of the body from the bladder and semen is passed on ejaculation. It passes from the bladder, through the prostate gland, along the length of the penis through the corpus spongiosum, to its opening in the tip of the glans.

The penis is covered with loosely-attached, fatless skin, which folds back on itself at the tip to make up the prepuce or foreskin. This covers the glans of the flaccid penis in an uncircumcised male. Part or all of this section of skin may be removed in the traditional practice of circumcision. The prepuce is attached to the inner side of the glans by an extremely sensitive band of skin termed the frenulum. When the penis becomes erect, the prepuce is pulled back and the glans revealed.

See also:
vagina
clitoris
sexual intercourse
health and hygiene
sex aids
masturbation
oral sex
circumcision
testes

Man has proportionately the largest penis of all primates. As Dr Desmond Morris put it, "Men are apes with oversize penises."

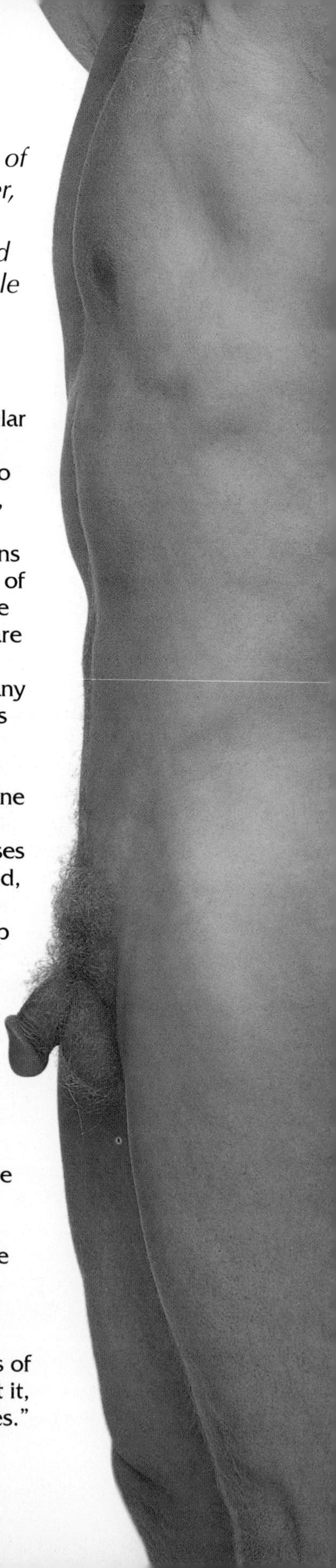

Penis size and sexual potency: some myths dispelled

One of the greatest myths about sex relates to penis size.

The focus on the penis may well be due to the fact that this organ is to such an extent the source of male sexual pleasure. Perhaps it is also for this reason that it has been widely assumed in many male-dominated societies that the penis is equally the primary source of sexual pleasure for the female. This leaves many men preoccupied with the size of their penis. Surveys suggest that almost all men – regardless of their sexual orientation – wish they had a larger penis. However, while some women may find a large penis attractive, others are concerned about being unable to accommodate it or about finding it painful. Generally, the girth of the penis is thought to be more important for sexual pleasure than the length.

A few basic facts:

- While there is some variety in flaccid penis size, the variation is somewhat diminished when the penis is erect. Smaller penises grow proportionally much more than larger ones, some even doubling in length.
- The vagina has great capacity for expansion enabling most women to accommodate almost any size of penis. A long penis may apply some pressure on the cervix. Some women find this painful but for others it is pleasurable; either way the depth of penetration may be controlled through particular positions for intercourse. Above all it is important for men to recognize that the most sensitive parts of the female genitalia are the clitoris and, in some women, the G-spot in the outermost section of the front wall of the vagina.
- Amongst homosexual men, surveys suggest that almost as many consider penis size to be completely unimportant as consider it important. It is largely a question of personal preference.
- Penis size is only related to fertility in that both are influenced by the male sex hormones produced in the testes. Ultimately, the variety in both size and shape is as great as in any other part of the body, and bears no relation to sexual potency or fertility.

The Examination of the Herald
Illustration by Aubrey Beardsley (1872–98) from *Lysistrata*.

"Most men fear that their sex organs are too small. A woman's reassurance seldom helps to allay these fears, but business success sometimes helps."
THEODORE I. BUBIN

Slang terms
cock, prick, dick, cong, prong, pecker, willie, Peter, pistol, Percy, tool, rocket, rod, joy stick, meat, machine gun, hot dog, pud, shaft, stick, sweet meat, wand, wanger, wee-wee, wiener, Johnny, John Thomas, organ, one-eyed trouser snake, bishop, skin flute, Hampton Wick, poker pole, canary, dingus, hammer, Mickey, member, one-eyed monster, putz, winkle, old man, plonker, nob.

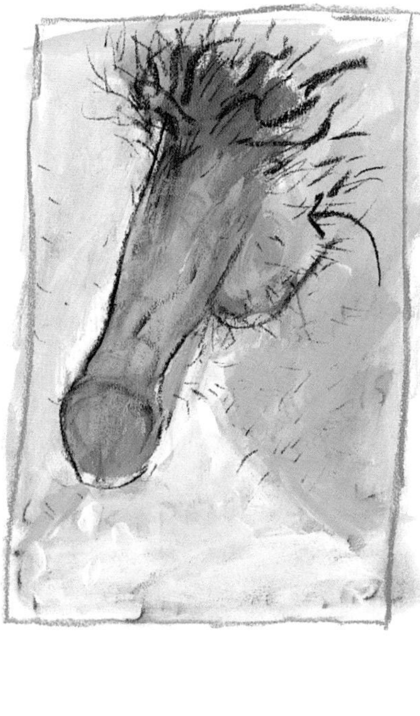

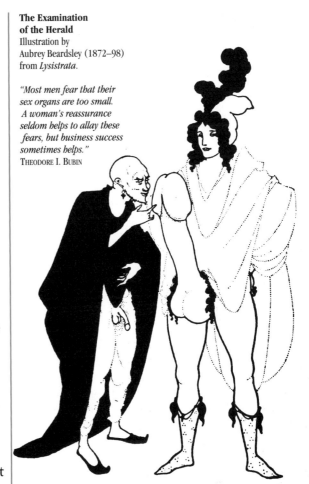

TESTES

While not as powerful a symbol as the phallus, the testes are often seen as the source of a man's 'masculinity'. In reality, they are just as important as the penis, if not more so.

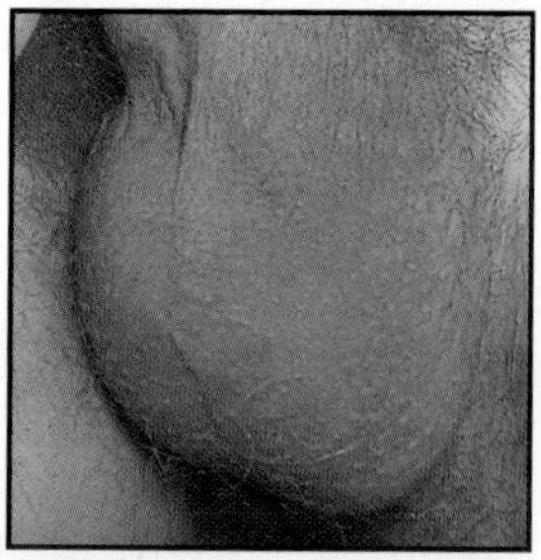

Slang terms
balls, bollocks, knackers, cobblers, marbles, bags, goolies, nuts, basket, lunch box, groceries, orchids, family jewels

Physiology of the testes

The testes or testicles are the male gonads or sex glands. They are equivalent to a woman's ovaries and develop from the same tissue in the embryo. They are responsible for producing male hormones as well as the male reproductive cells, sperm.

They are situated inside the scrotum, the sac of skin beneath the penis where they are loosely held in place by the dartos muscles attached to the scrotum, and the cremaster muscles attached to the testes themselves. To the touch, the testes are two firm, smooth, oval masses within the scrotal sac, which is divided into two to accommodate the two testes. They are protected by four layers of covering which correspond to the linings of the abdominal wall.

The sperm are produced in what are known as semniferous tubules. There may be as many as a thousand tubules in each testicle, very narrow and tightly coiled together and each over 60 cm long. These tubules produce sperm constantly, maturing

Self-examination is important for both men and women, for getting to know one's genitals and to detect any signs of infection.

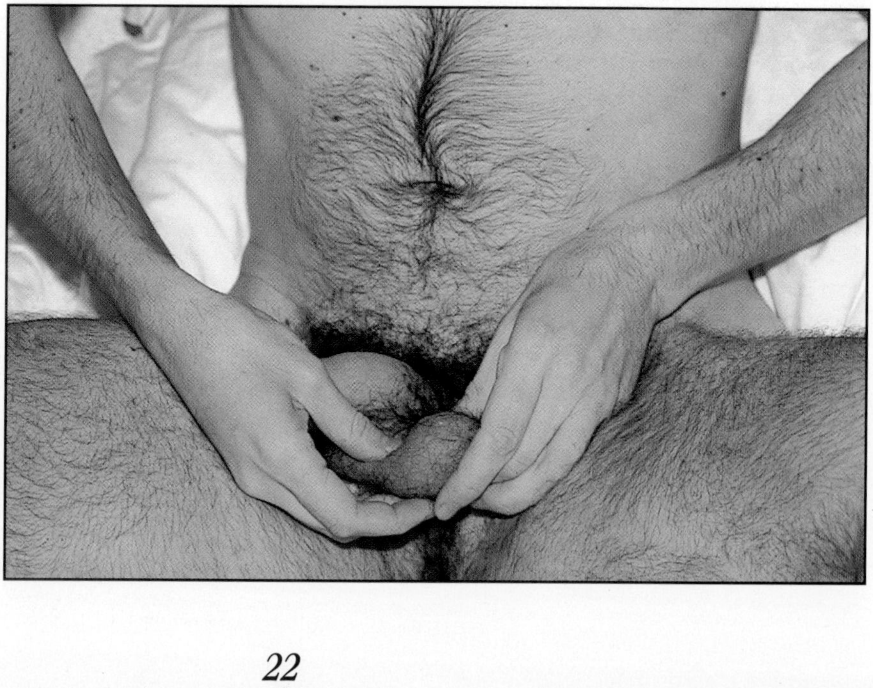

See also:
penis
sexual intercourse
sexual feelings – male
growth and change
oral sex
erogenous zones

and nourishing each one for some forty-five days in sertoli or nurse cells attached to the tubule's lining. They are then released into the epididymis, the duct where they are matured and stored until needed. Sperm are produced constantly, throughout the man's adult life. However, if ejaculation occurs more than once or twice a day it can take five to seven days to replenish the supplies which generally provide 200 to 400 million sperm for each ejaculation.

Sperm production and the position of the testes

The testes hang 'outside' the man's body because the sperm are produced at up to 8°C below normal body temperature. For this reason, it has been suggested that wearing tight trousers or underwear may reduce a man's sperm production, as tightly-fitting clothes hold the testes closer to the body than normal, and therefore at a slightly higher temperature.

Normally, the proximity of the testes to the body is controlled by the dartos and cremaster muscles, which relax and contract to keep the testes at the optimum temperature for sperm production. Therefore, when the man is cold, his testes are drawn closer to the body.

The height of the testes is also affected by the man's emotions and by sexual arousal. In the course of arousal the skin of the scrotum may thicken and darken with the increased blood flow to the genital area, and the testes are drawn tighter to the body, particularly just before orgasm. If pain is inflicted on the testes, or even with the threat of pain, the testes are again drawn closer to the body. The testes are extremely sensitive to pressure, which can produce excruciating pain.

FACT: Men's sperm counts are going down throughout the world.

FACT: One testis usually hangs lower than the other, and may be slightly larger. In right-handed men the right testis is generally higher; in left-handed men the left is higher.

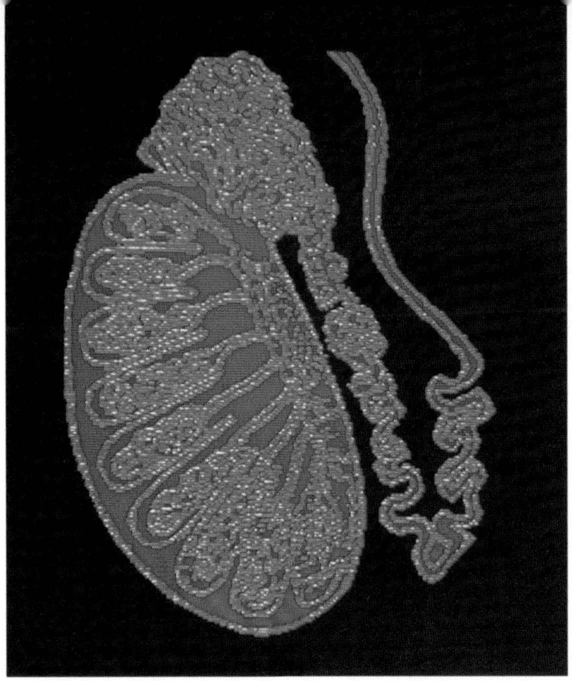

Colour-enhanced section through a testis, clearly showing the tightly coiled semniferous tubules in which the sperm are produced, and the epididymis into which they are released to mature and be stored until needed. Up to 200 to 400 million sperm are needed for each ejaculation.

The testes are emphasized in this advertisement, even though the penis is the more common symbol of masculinity. The testes have also been associated with virility in other ways, as in the phrase 'to have balls' meaning to have strength and bravado.

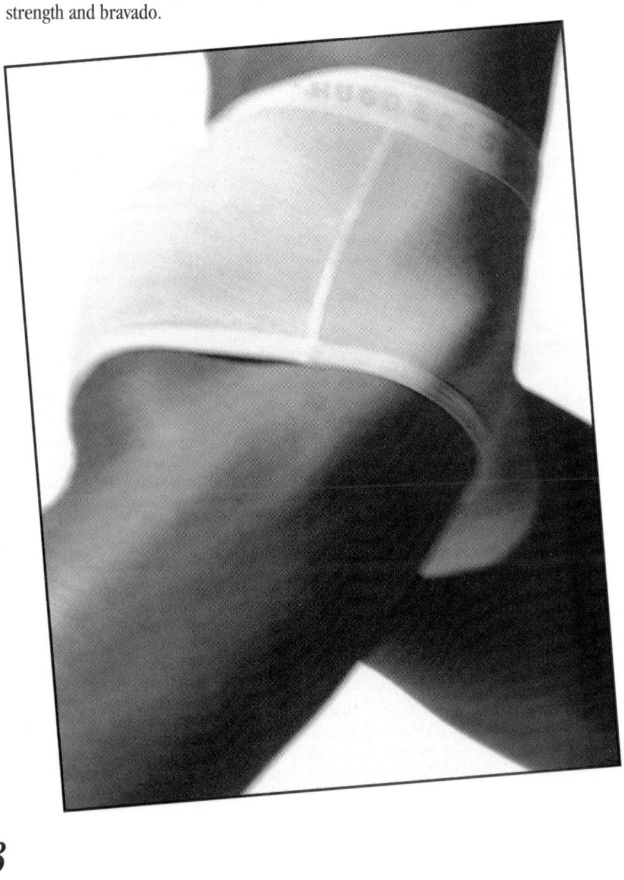

SEXUAL INTERCOURSE

Sexual responses begin in the brain as we react, consciously or unconsciously, to certain stimuli. These responses manifest themselves in a series of physical changes and sensations. The nature and intensity of the sensations experienced vary greatly from one person to another and may be affected by numerous independent, circumstantial factors.

Sexual intercourse is the broad term for genital play between two people; coitus is the specific term used for the penis-in-the-vagina act between a man and a woman. This section deals with male and female physical responses to sexual activity of all kinds, but with some specific reference to this basic sexual act.

The succession of changes may be broken down into four stages: arousal, plateau, orgasm and resolution.

FEMALE RESPONSE

AROUSAL

Blood flow to the pelvic area increases. The vagina dilates and its walls darken and start to 'sweat' a lubricating substance. The labia darken and swell: the labia majora may separate, with the labia minora protruding between them. The clitoris emerges from beneath its hood, or prepuce, as it lengthens and thickens. The uterus moves upwards and forwards so that the cervix protrudes less into the vault of the vagina. This movement lengthens the vagina, which also starts to distend to form a balloon shape at the upper end, near the cervix.

Physical responses to arousal occur in other parts of the body, as the nipples become erect and the areolae start to swell. Many women also experience a so-called 'sex flush', with a rash appearing on the skin of the abdomen, throat and breasts.

See also:
anatomy of sex
conception to childbirth
orgasm
sex positions
contraception
health and hygiene
sexual feelings

Excitement triggers the release of the hormone adrenaline into the bloodstream, causing a rise in blood pressure and pulse rate, muscle-tensing, dilation of the pupils, heavier breathing and some perspiration.

PLATEAU

The labia may continue to swell, and their colour continues to darken. Vaginal lubrication decreases, causing greater friction between the vaginal walls and the penis.
The entire outer part of the vagina – including the inner labia – swells to form what is termed the 'orgasmic platform'. This is the area from where the sensations of orgasm will spread. The upper end of the vagina continues to expand, and the uterus continues to tilt and be drawn up into the body. Just before orgasm, the clitoris withdraws beneath its hood.

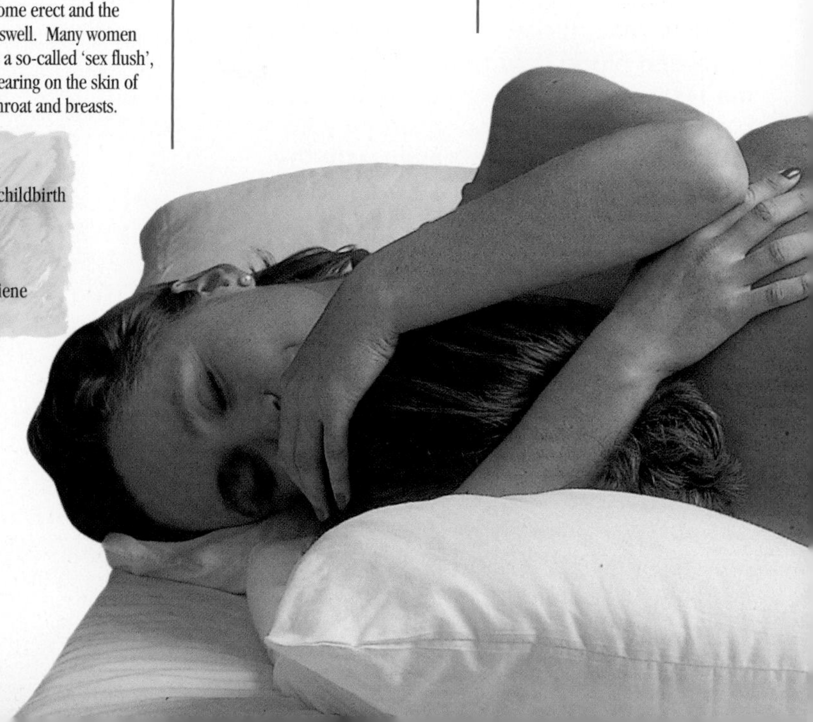

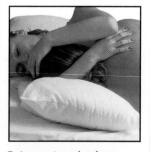

Sexual intercourse
When both partners are sufficiently aroused, the man's erect penis is inserted into the woman's vagina. Movement of the penis within the vagina leads to further arousal, which may culminate in orgasm. Many of the sexual responses seem, in some way, to be geared towards creating the ideal circumstances for fertilization to occur until finally, at ejaculation, the sperm is deposited as close as possible to the cervix. Its passage to the uterus may be further aided by female lubrication and by the uterine contractions of the female orgasm.

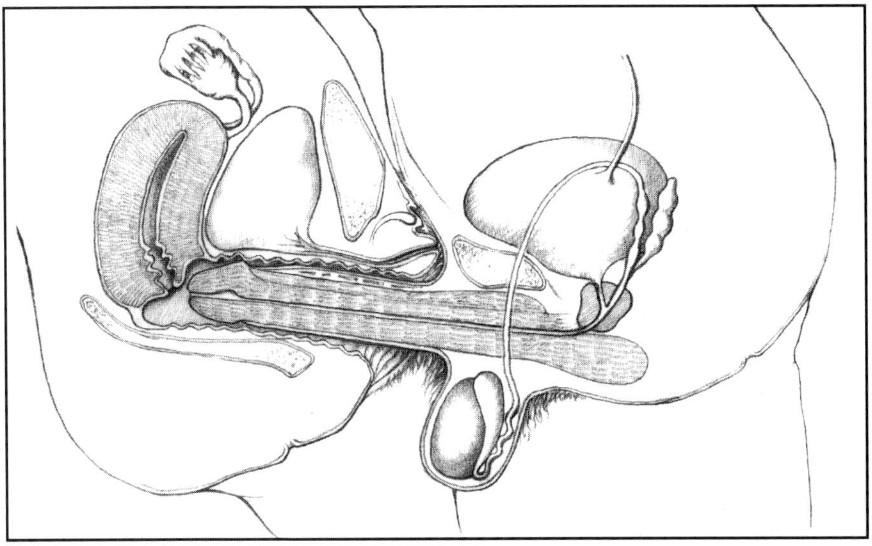

ORGASM
The orgasmic platform (see under 'Plateau') contracts rhythmically at intervals of 0.8 seconds (the same as in the man). There may be anywhere between three and fifteen of these muscle spasms, gradually becoming less frequent and intense. The muscles of the uterus also produce involuntary contractions. These contractions dip the cervix, raised in the course of arousal, back into the vagina. They also produce waves of intense pleasure throughout the body. At the same time, skin flushes may spread and deepen, and muscle spasm may occur in other parts of the body (such as the feet, hands, back and thighs). Blood pressure and pulse rate reach a peak.

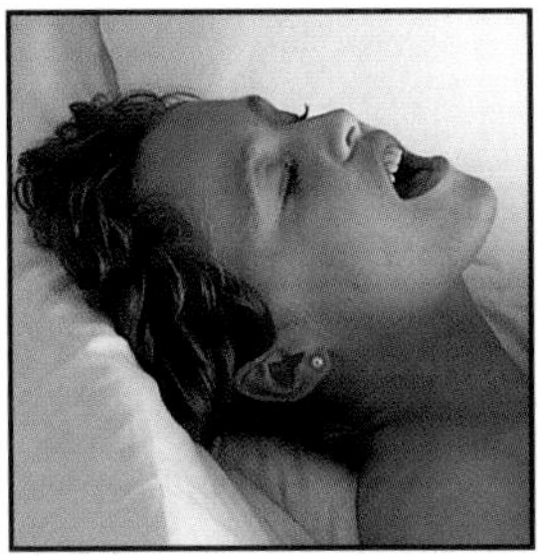

RESOLUTION
The sexual organs gradually return to their normal, unaroused state. Within five or ten seconds of the last vaginal contraction the clitoris returns to its normal position and the darker colour of the labia minora fades. It may take ten or fifteen minutes for the vagina to return to its usual size, shape and colour, and even longer for the swelling of the labia majora and the glans of the clitoris to subside.

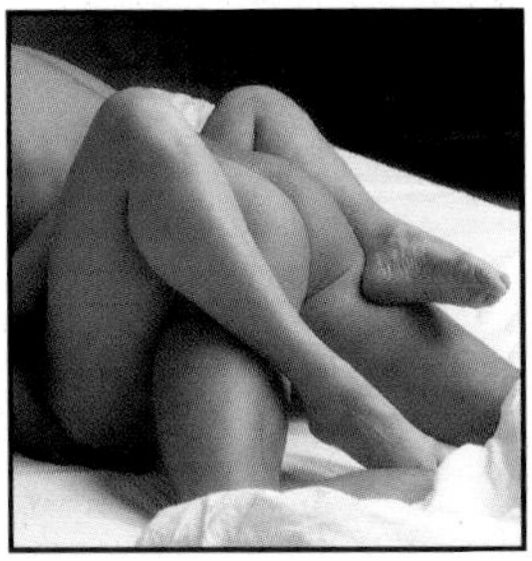

If orgasm has not been reached, the congestion in the blood vessels in the pelvic area may not have been released. This makes the resolution process much slower and may cause some slight pain, but this passes within a few hours.

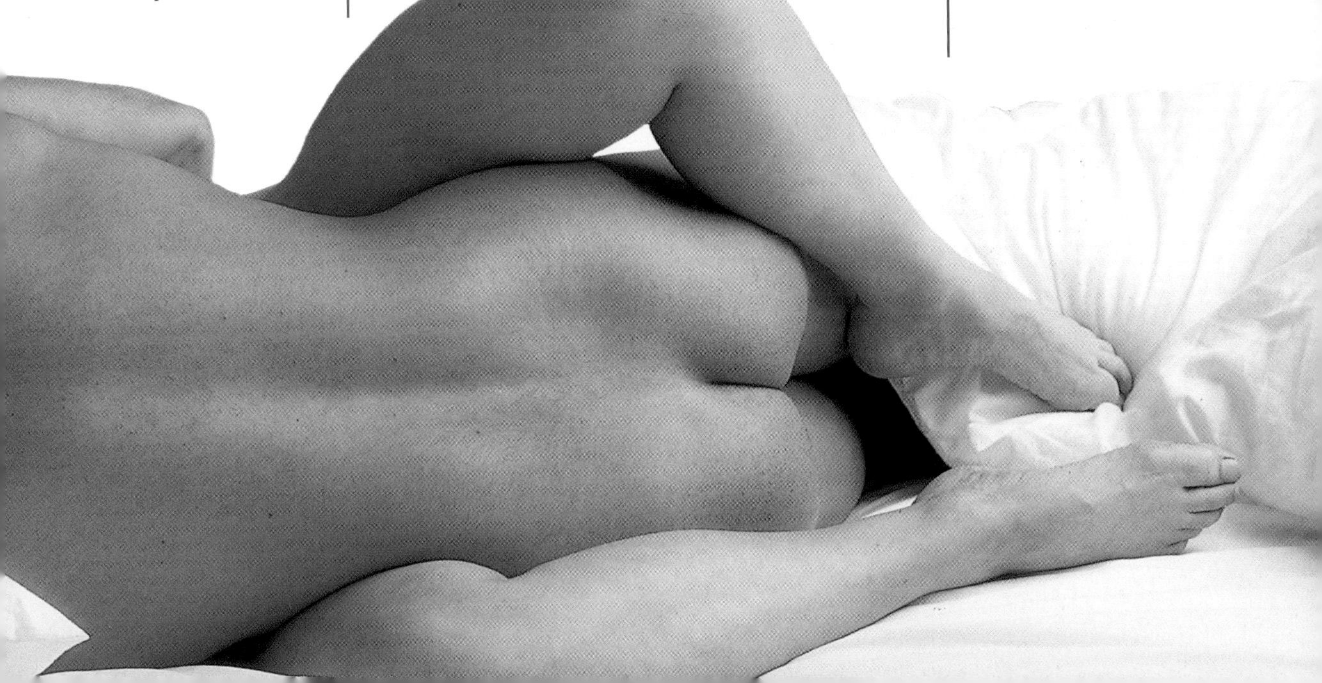

Patterns of arousal

In general, the process of becoming aroused and approaching orgasm follows distinct patterns for men and women. While the man can reach full physical arousal quite quickly before a marked plateau phase, for the woman the same process tends to be more gradual. However, while simultaneous orgasm is relatively rare, it can be achieved – particularly through getting to know one's own and one's partner's sexual needs and responses.

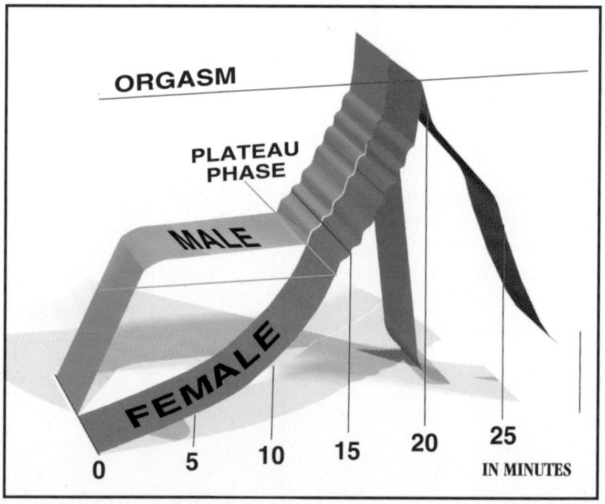

NB: TIMESCALES VARY WIDELY FOR DIFFERENT COUPLES. ALSO, SIMULTANEOUS ORGASM IS RELATIVELY RARE.

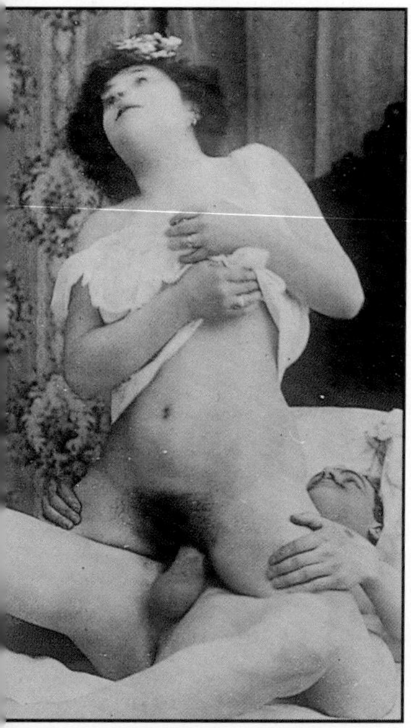

Sexual Ecstasy (and interesting position) shown in this 19th Century photograph

MALE RESPONSE

AROUSAL
The blood flow to the genital area increases, and the outflow of blood from the penis is reduced. The penis rapidly becomes engorged with blood, so that it stiffens, lengthens, and becomes erect. At the same time, the skin of the scrotum becomes thicker and firmer, and the testes are drawn visibly closer to the body. The increased blood flow darkens the skin in the whole genital area.

The skin may become flushed on other parts of the body (the so-called 'sex flush'), and the nipples

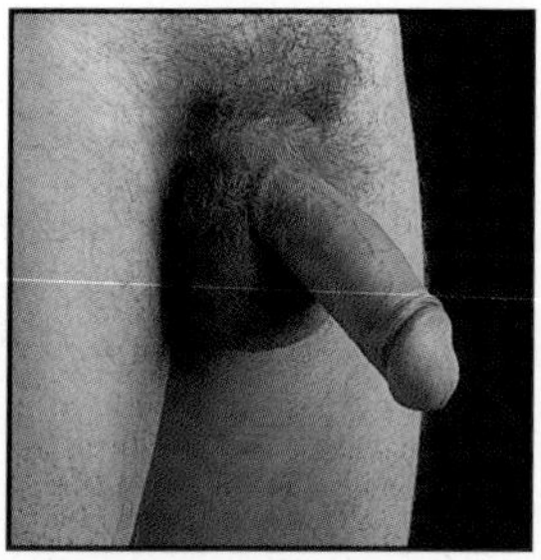

may become erect. Adrenaline makes the pulse rate and blood pressure rise, the muscles tense, and the pupils of the eyes dilate. Perspiration may increase and breathing become heavier.

PLATEAU
As the man starts to approach orgasm the glans of the penis becomes swollen and darker in colour. If the man is uncircumcised the foreskin is pulled right back, leaving the sensitive glans fully exposed. The testes are drawn even tighter to the body, and may slightly increase in size.

FACT: World distance record for ejaculated semen: 2.6 metres.

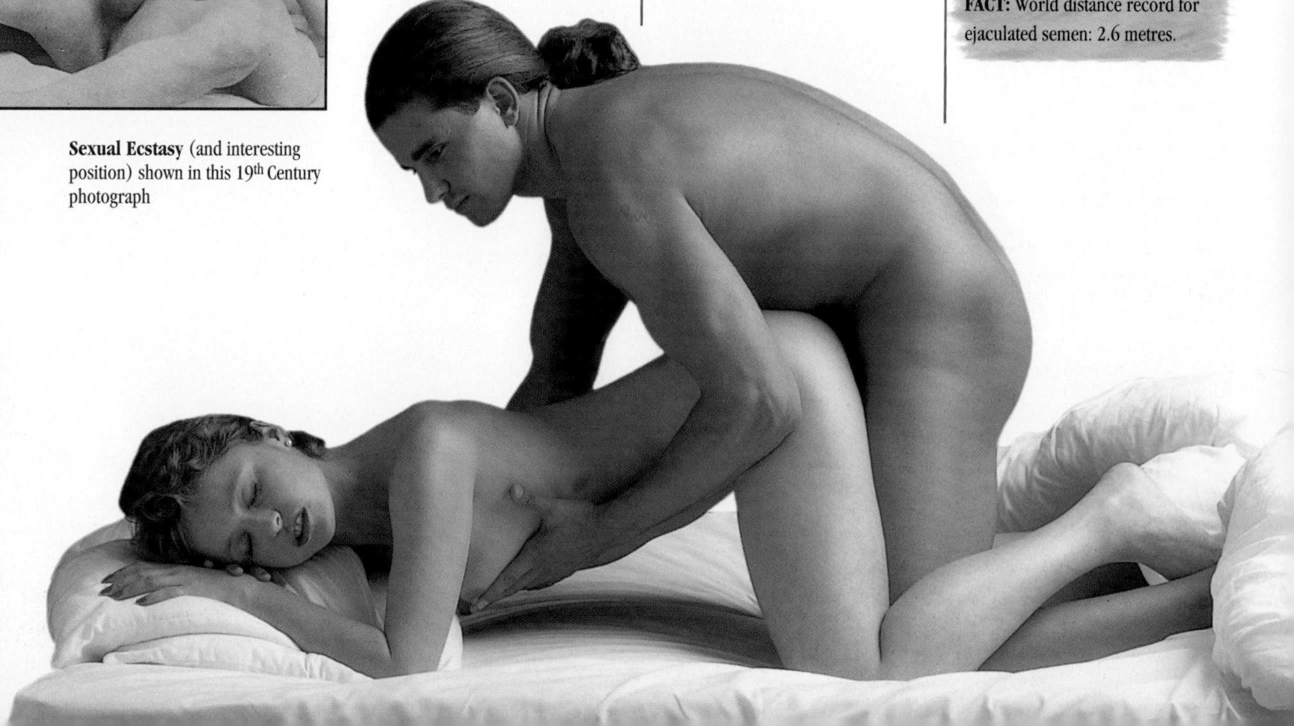

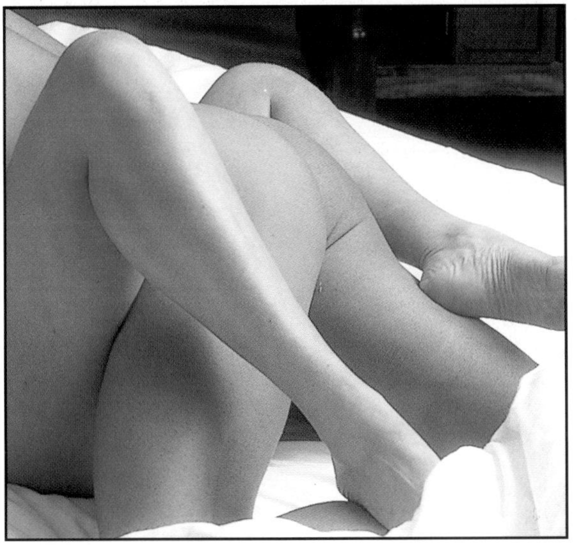

Differences between male and female response

The main difference between the male and female responses to intercourse is that some women are able to reach more than one orgasm during a single act of intercourse. Instead of passing from orgasm to resolution, the woman may repeatedly return to the plateau stage and reach orgasm several times. Unlike men, women tend to experience increasing pleasure with each orgasmic peak. Some also experience no refractory period, and can become aroused again and again almost immediately after each orgasm.

ORGASM

In men this has two stages. In the first stage the seminal fluid collects in the urethra, within the prostate. Involuntary muscle contractions are experienced in the pelvis, similar to the spasms that occur in female orgasm. This causes emission and is recognized as the period of ejaculatory inevitability, just two to four seconds before ejaculation, when the man is aware that orgasm is imminent and that there is nothing he can do to prevent it.

Finally ejaculation occurs. The muscles of the sex organs go into involuntary spasm, contracting rhythmically along the entire length of the urethra to expel the seminal fluid. The force of this may decrease with age, but in a young man the ejaculated semen can travel several feet and as fast as 30 mph. The muscles contract at the same rate as those of the vagina in the woman. They start at intervals of 0.8 seconds, and after three or four strong contractions rapidly reduce in force and frequency.

The greatest pleasure is felt with the first contractions, in which the largest volume of seminal fluid is ejaculated. Both gradually diminish with each contraction. The total volume of semen ejaculated is generally about 4 or 5 ml (half a teaspoonful). Ejaculation is usually accompanied by the intensely pleasurable sensations and release of tension of orgasm. Blood pressure, pulse and breathing rates reach a peak, skin flushes deepen, and muscle spasm may occur in many parts of the body as well as in the pelvic area. The man may perspire out of proportion with the physical effort exerted. It is possible to ejaculate without orgasm, and to have an orgasm without ejaculation.

RESOLUTION

After ejaculation the penis becomes flaccid again. This occurs more rapidly if the man removes his penis from the vagina immediately than if he remains in close proximity. The genitals return to their pre-arousal state, and any skin flushes fade. Breathing, pulse and blood pressure rapidly return to normal. Orgasm is followed by a refractory period, during which most men are unable to have another erection. The time varies from one man to another, and also depends on such factors as age and state of mind. If orgasm has not been reached, the congestion in the blood vessels in the pelvic area may not have been released. This makes the resolution process much slower and may cause some slight pain, although this passes within a few hours. Some men are able to maintain their erection after orgasm.

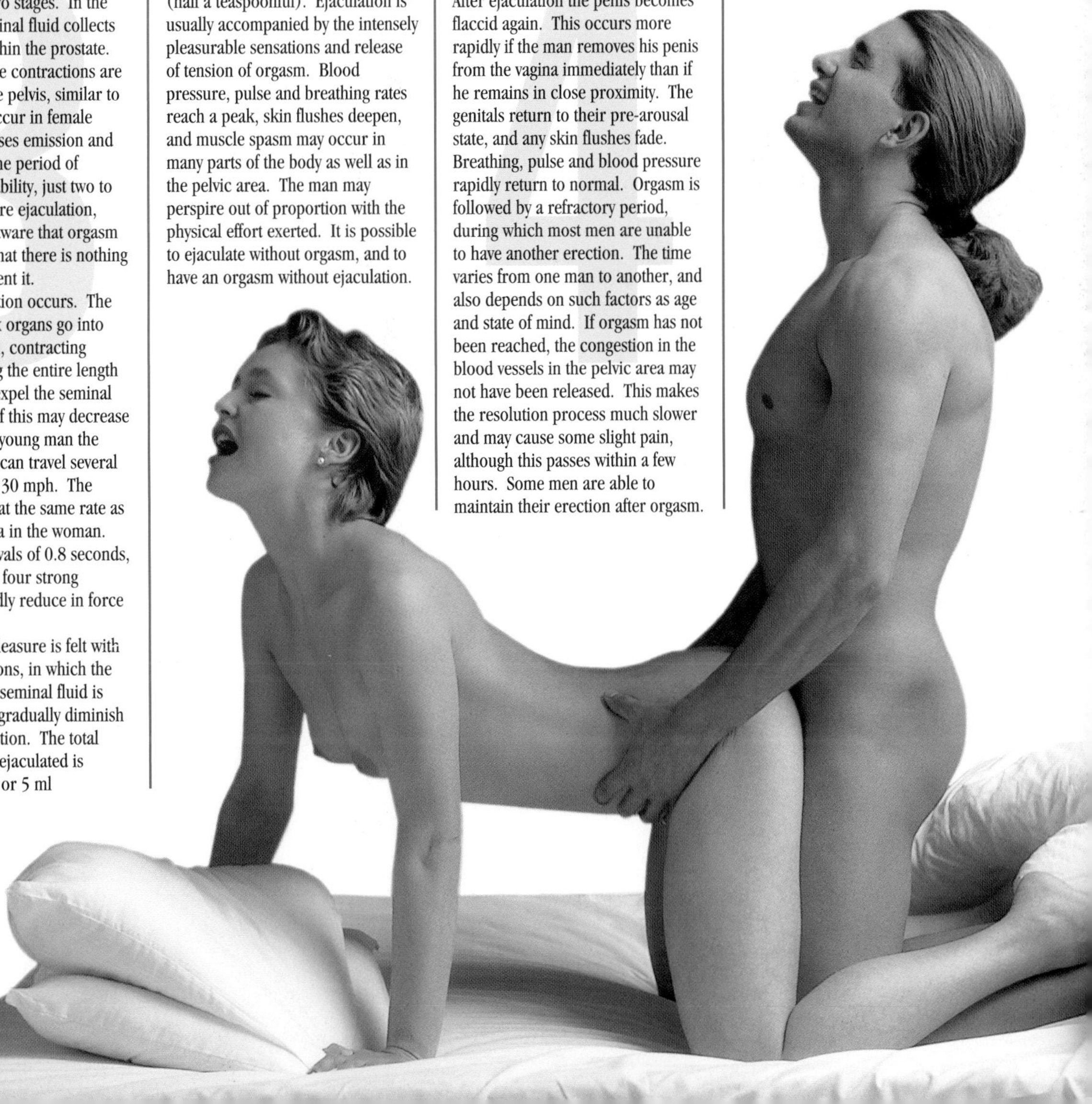

CONCEPTION TO CHILDBIRTH

Humans are unique in their enjoyment of the reproductive act. Indeed, where contraception is available and acceptable, the original purpose of sexual intercourse – to produce offspring – may seem secondary to the pleasure we derive from the act itself. It may even be that our enjoyment has evolved principally as a means of reinforcing the instinct for procreation in the human species.

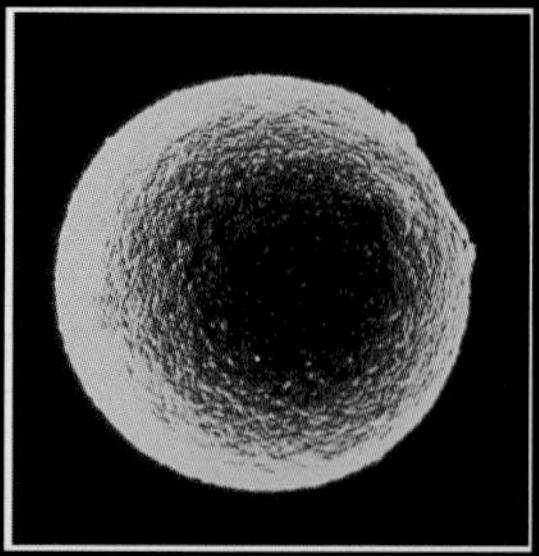

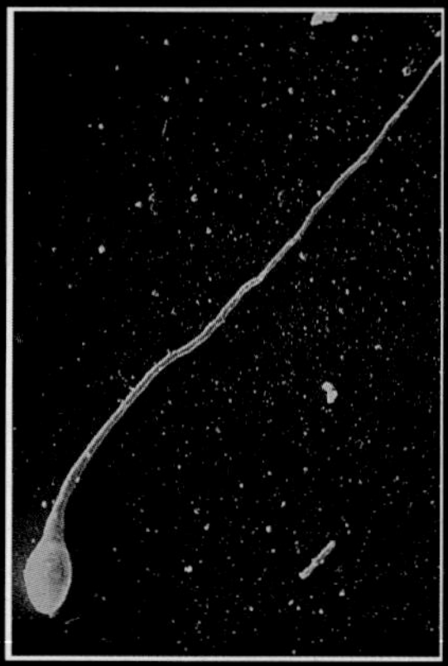

Human ovum (top)
Human sperm (bottom)

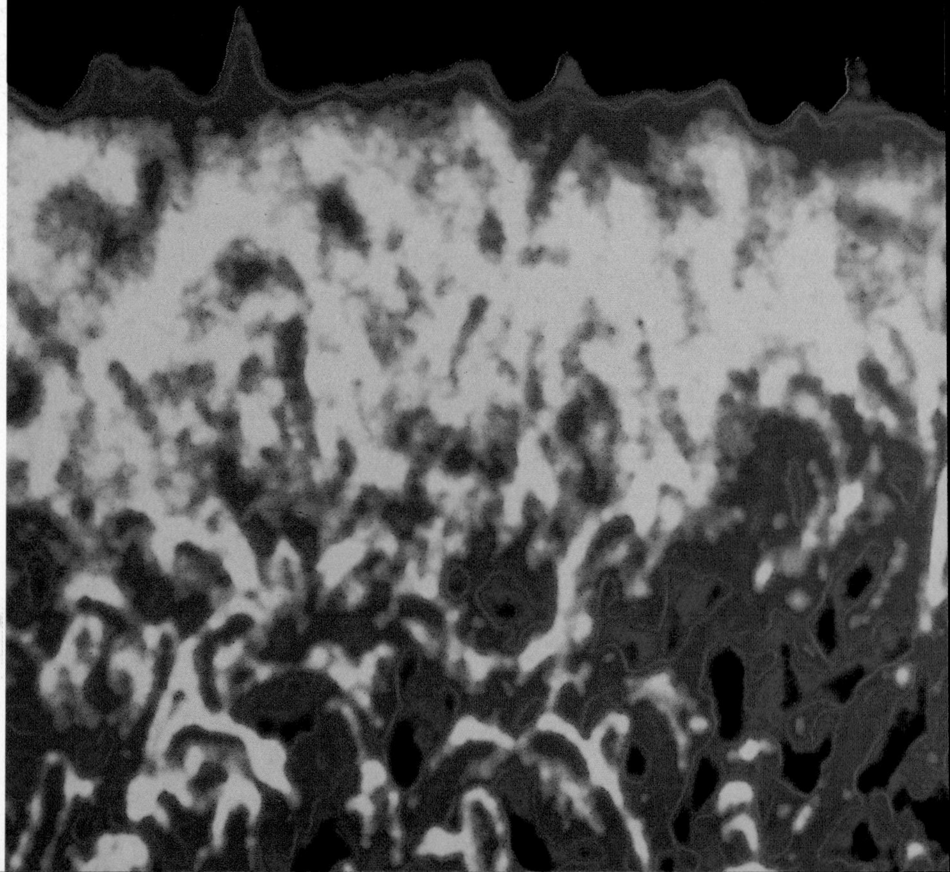

The moment of conception (main)

See also:
sexual intercourse
growth and change
contraception

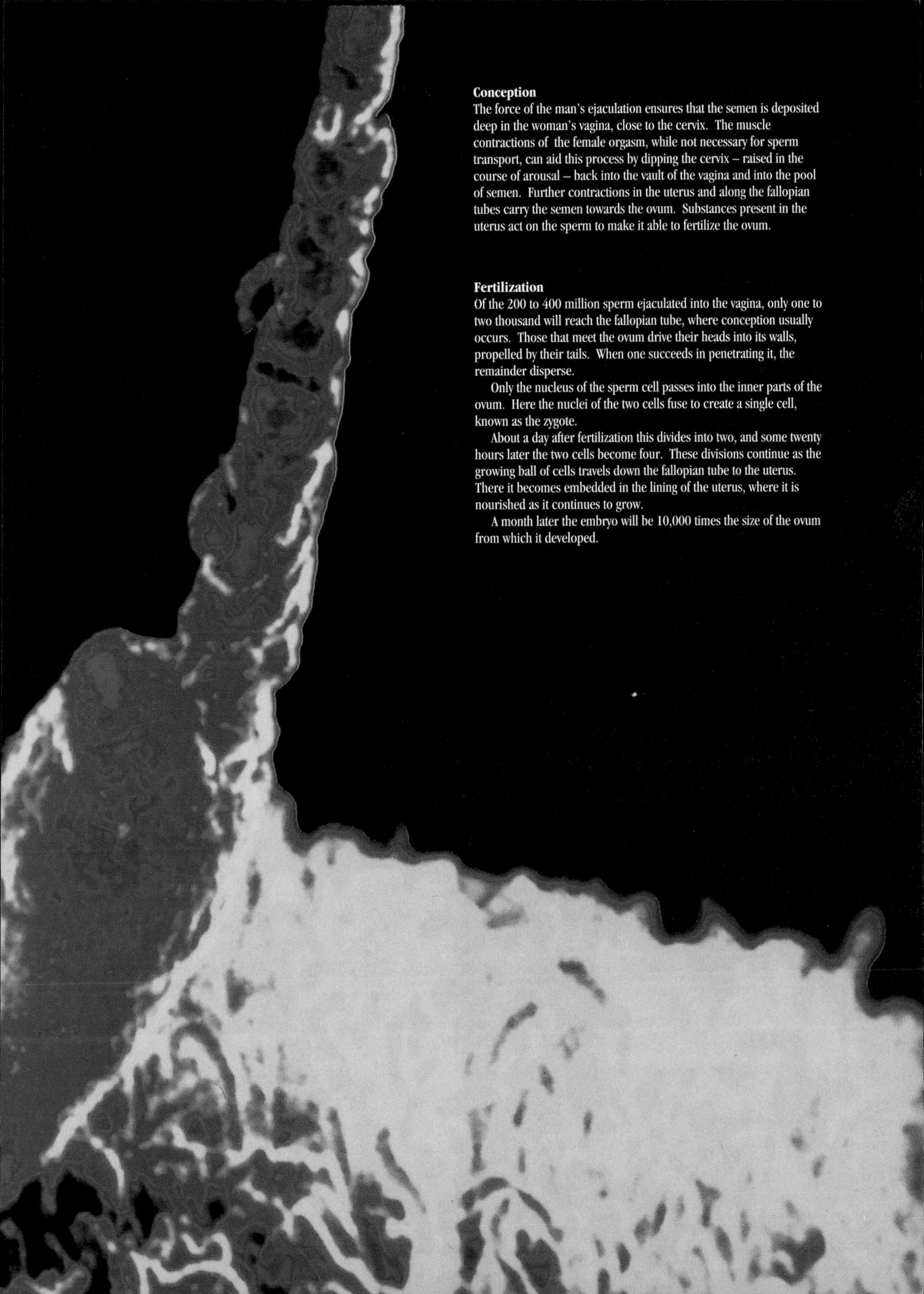

Conception

The force of the man's ejaculation ensures that the semen is deposited deep in the woman's vagina, close to the cervix. The muscle contractions of the female orgasm, while not necessary for sperm transport, can aid this process by dipping the cervix – raised in the course of arousal – back into the vault of the vagina and into the pool of semen. Further contractions in the uterus and along the fallopian tubes carry the semen towards the ovum. Substances present in the uterus act on the sperm to make it able to fertilize the ovum.

Fertilization

Of the 200 to 400 million sperm ejaculated into the vagina, only one to two thousand will reach the fallopian tube, where conception usually occurs. Those that meet the ovum drive their heads into its walls, propelled by their tails. When one succeeds in penetrating it, the remainder disperse.

Only the nucleus of the sperm cell passes into the inner parts of the ovum. Here the nuclei of the two cells fuse to create a single cell, known as the zygote.

About a day after fertilization this divides into two, and some twenty hours later the two cells become four. These divisions continue as the growing ball of cells travels down the fallopian tube to the uterus. There it becomes embedded in the lining of the uterus, where it is nourished as it continues to grow.

A month later the embryo will be 10,000 times the size of the ovum from which it developed.

Twins

There are two kinds of twin: fraternal (non-identical) and identical.

Fraternal twins are produced when two (or more) ova are released instead of one. Each of the ova can then be fertilized by separate sperm, to form two separate embryos which develop together in the uterus, each with its own placenta. The tendency to produce fraternal twins is thought to run in particular families.

Identical twins are rarer. They are produced when a single fertilized ovum divides into two separate, equal parts. These continue to divide and grow to form two embryos which share a single placenta.

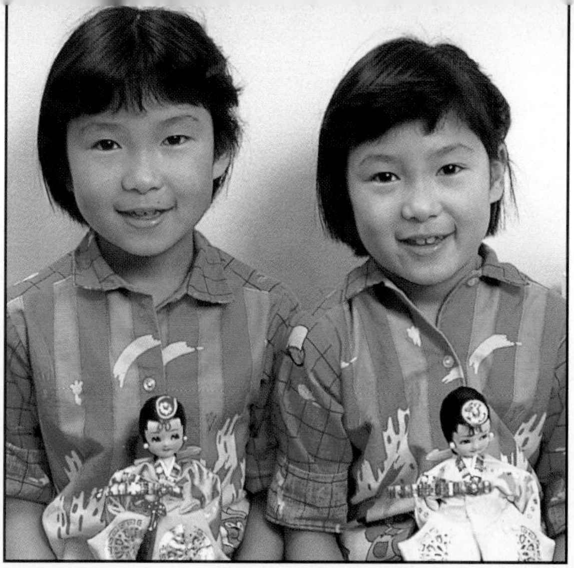

Twins from Asia

Gender and heredity

When the nuclei of the sperm and the ovum combine, so also does the genetic information contained by each one. In this way when an ovum is fertilized a new identity – a unique new set of genetic information – is created, with characteristics from both partners.

This genetic information also determines the sex of the child. Each ovum contains what is termed an X chromosome, while each sperm contains an X or a Y chromosome. An 'X' sperm produces a female embryo, and a 'Y' sperm produces a male.

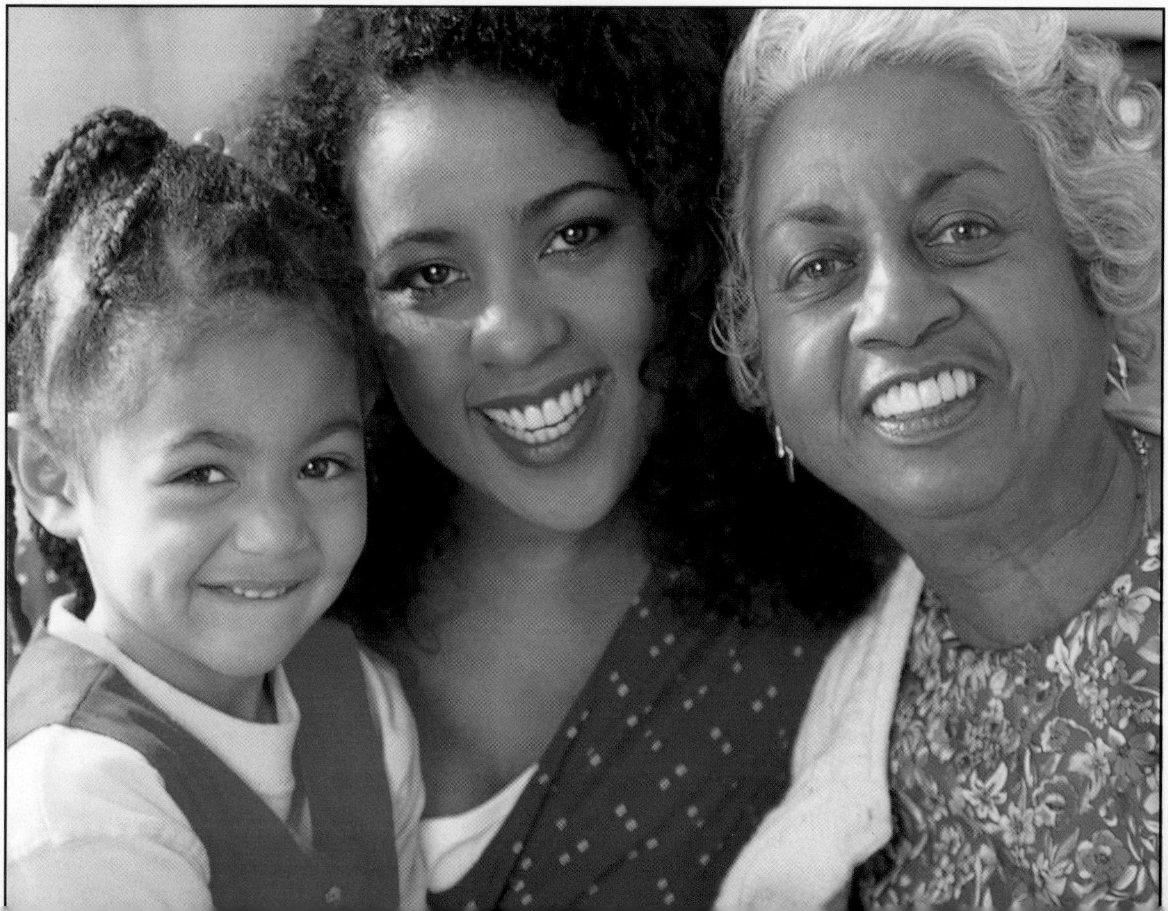

Three generations of one family
The extent to which genes determine our looks and personality remains a controversial issue.

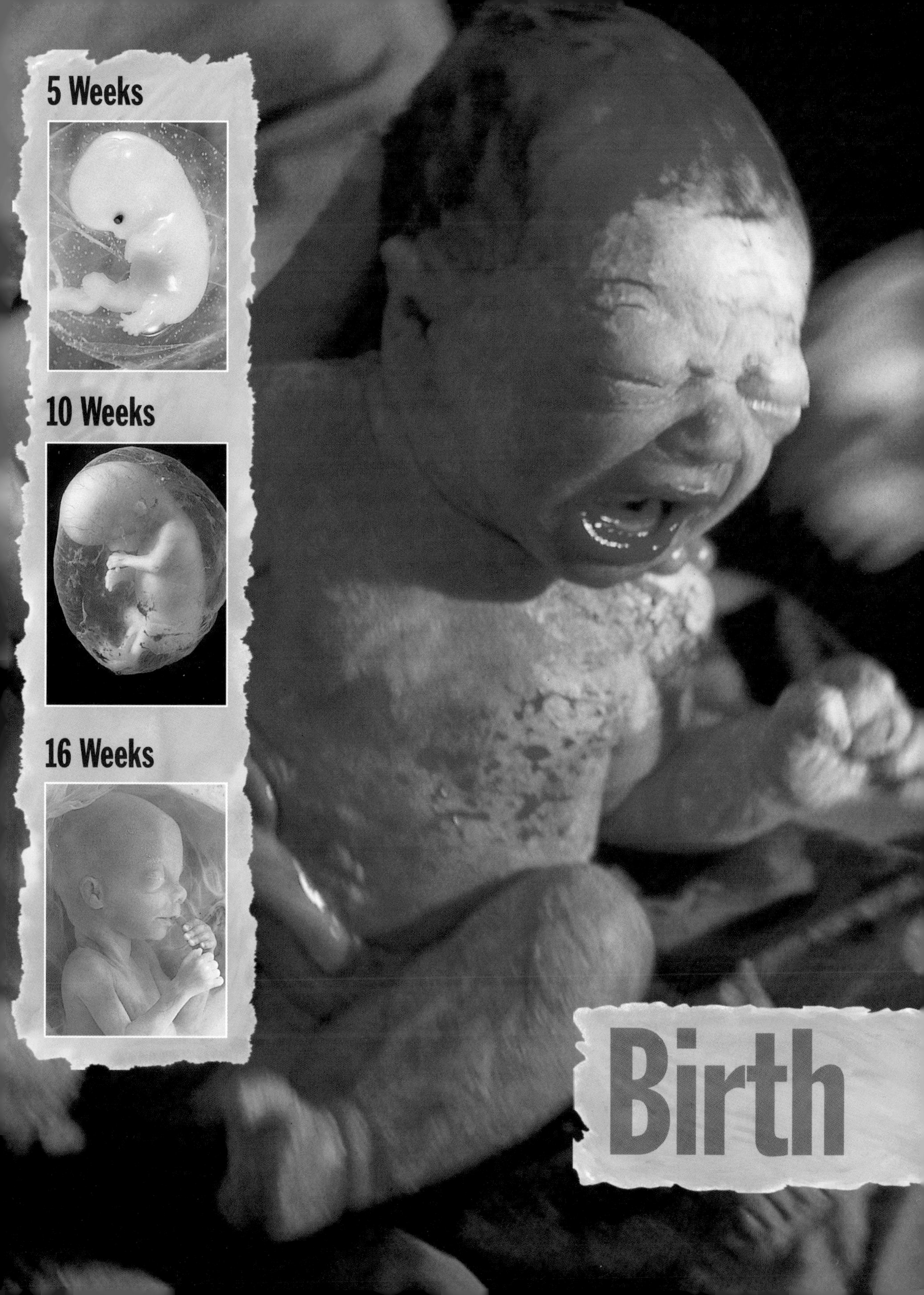
5 Weeks
10 Weeks
16 Weeks
Birth

GROWTH & CHANGE

The course of our sexual development is marked by a series of watersheds. These are the key points which mark the movement from one stage of development to another. Each of these entails a range of physical and psychological changes. The three watersheds are:

- *around the seventh week of pregnancy: the reproductive organs start to develop*
- *around the ages ten to sixteen: the reproductive organs become active*
- *later in life at the menopause: the reproductive system decreases its activity*

SEXUAL DIFFERENTIATION

At six weeks of pregnancy male and female embryos are still alike. However, just six weeks later the sex of the foetus is already quite apparent. Even though the gonads do not take their final shape and position until the thirty-fourth week of pregnancy, by the eleventh week the penis and the vulva are identifiable. At the same time, the female's fallopian tubes and the male's prostate are also beginning to form.

The changes initiated at this stage are caused by the production of the growth-stimulating hormone testosterone in the male and the growth-inhibiting hormone inhibin in the female. These and other sexual hormones are the key to our sexual identity. Ultimately this identity is determined by the pair of sex chromosomes created at fertilization, but its physical manifestations depend on the actions of the hormones. These are produced in the gonads at the stimulus of other hormonal messages originating in the brain, and bring about physical and emotional changes associated with sexual development throughout life.

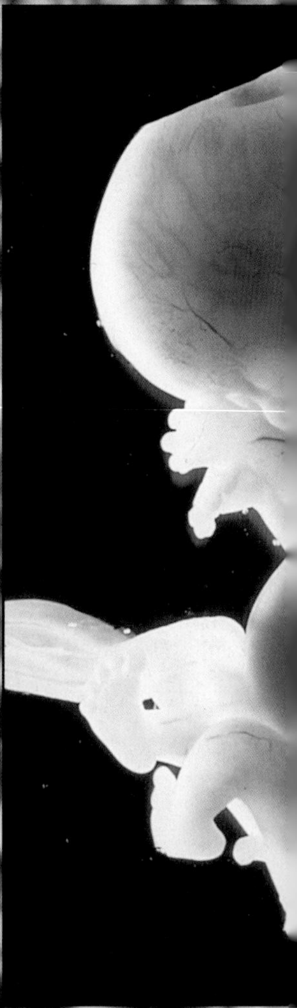

The foetus in the uterus, eleven weeks after conception.

See also:
sexual learning
anatomy of sex
masturbation
gender

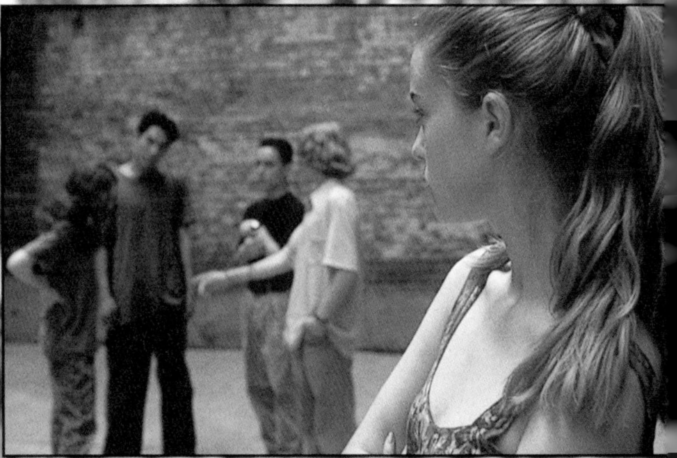

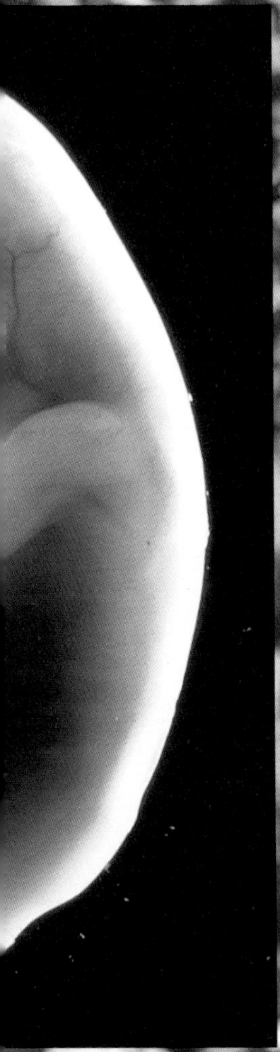

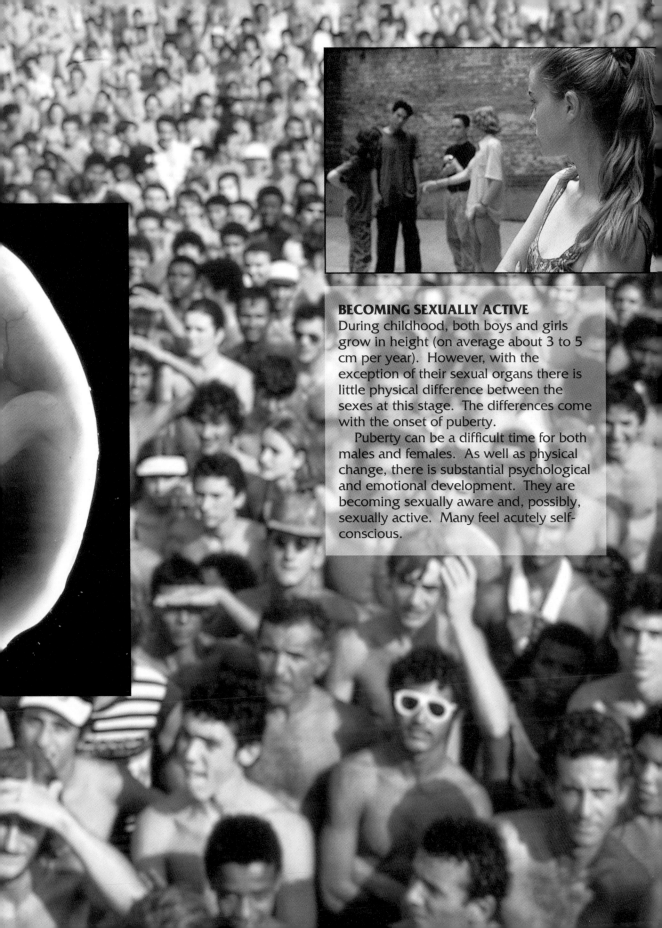

BECOMING SEXUALLY ACTIVE

During childhood, both boys and girls grow in height (on average about 3 to 5 cm per year). However, with the exception of their sexual organs there is little physical difference between the sexes at this stage. The differences come with the onset of puberty.

Puberty can be a difficult time for both males and females. As well as physical change, there is substantial psychological and emotional development. They are becoming sexually aware and, possibly, sexually active. Many feel acutely self-conscious.

GIRL TO WOMAN

In girls puberty generally occurs earlier than in boys, usually between the ages of nine and sixteen.

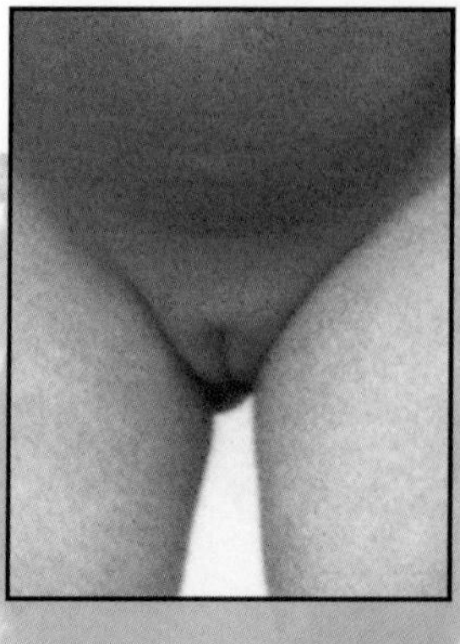

The maturing body
The differences in the bodies of four members of the same family demonstrate some of the changes that occur during puberty in women, as the pubic hair starts to grow and the vulva develops. The main changes in a woman's reproductive organs occur inside her body, in ovaries and uterus.

Frame

One of the first signs of puberty is the growth spurt, starting around the age of ten. Over the following four years many girls will come within a few centimetres of their full adult height, often growing as much as 10 cm within a single year. At the same time, the shape of the skeleton will be developing. In particular, the pelvis will widen to create the space where a growing baby can be accommodated. The different bones involved rarely grow all at the same rate, leaving many girls feeling 'gangly' or out of proportion for a few years.

Muscle and fat

Women's bodies naturally have a higher fat content than men's: generally twenty to twenty-five per cent as opposed to men's ten to twenty per cent. At the start of puberty, usually when the growth spurt begins, fat accumulates particularly on the breasts, upper arms, hips, buttocks and thighs. The result of this is that women tend to have softer and more rounded bodies than men, with a more curved and defined waist. However, this is by no means a universal truth. The shape of the adult body is determined by a number of factors, and in particular by heredity. Puberty is also the time when many women start to build greater body muscle. The proportions of bodily fat and muscle are strongly influenced by hormones and gender, but also by health, diet, exercise and heredity.

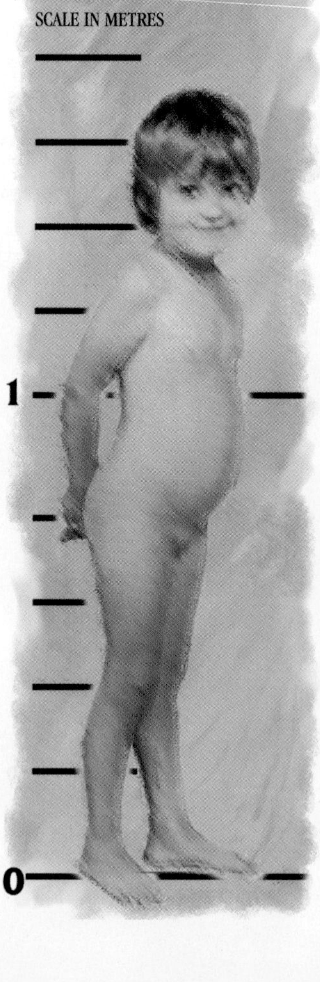

Skin

The change in hormonal activity also affects the skin. The sebaceous glands become more active, making the skin more oily and sometimes causing spots or acne on the face, chest and back. The activity of the sebaceous glands may also make the hair more greasy at this stage. At the same time the sweat glands develop, increasing individual body odour.

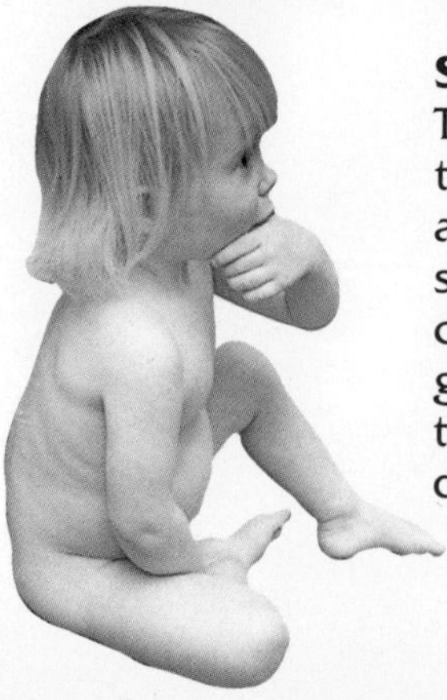

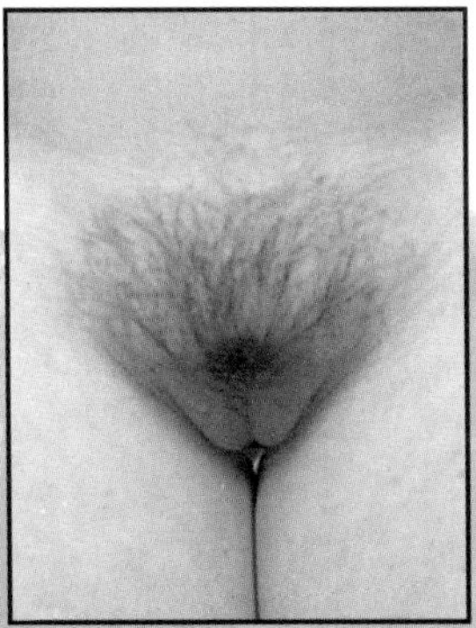

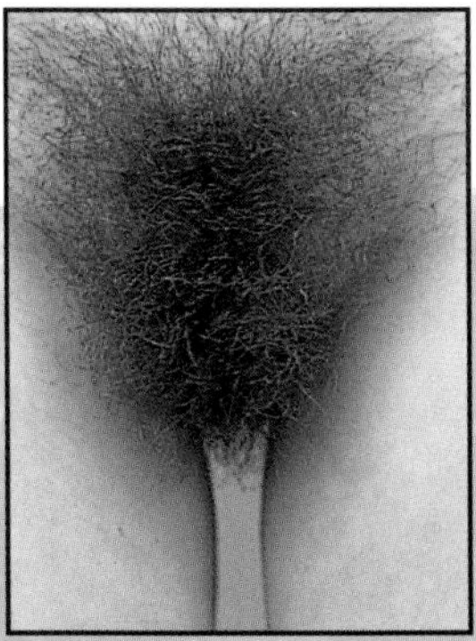

Body hair
Pubic hair, longer, darker and coarser than other body hair, grows first on the vulva before spreading over the mons pubis and towards the stomach and thighs in an inverted triangle. Pubic hair is not necessarily the same colour as the hair on the head. Further hair appears in the armpits, and the fine hair all over the body may also increase. The amount of body hair varies greatly from one woman to another and may be affected by hereditary factors.

Voice
As in men, women's voices tend to deepen during puberty, although to a much lesser degree.

Genitals
While the development of the genitals is much less noticeable than in boys, the same processes are in motion as the body prepares itself for sexual activity. Early in puberty girls will start to menstruate. The average age for first menstruation – known as the menarche – is 12.5 years, but this average appears to be gradually decreasing. The ovaries reach maturity and ovulation begins, usually one or two years after the first menstruation but often sooner. As the menstrual cycle becomes regular over the following two to three years vaginal discharge will also start to appear, keeping the vagina healthy. At the same time, the uterus grows to its full size, the vaginal wall thickens and the external genitals develop.

Breasts
The first sign of the development of the breasts is the swelling or 'budding' of the areolae. The nipple also enlarges, then the entire breast swells with the increased production of glands and fat. The size of the breasts depends on hormone levels and the amount of general body fat, as well as hereditary factors. It may vary throughout life with changing hormone levels, particularly in the course of the menstrual cycle. The breasts are often not of equal size or shape.

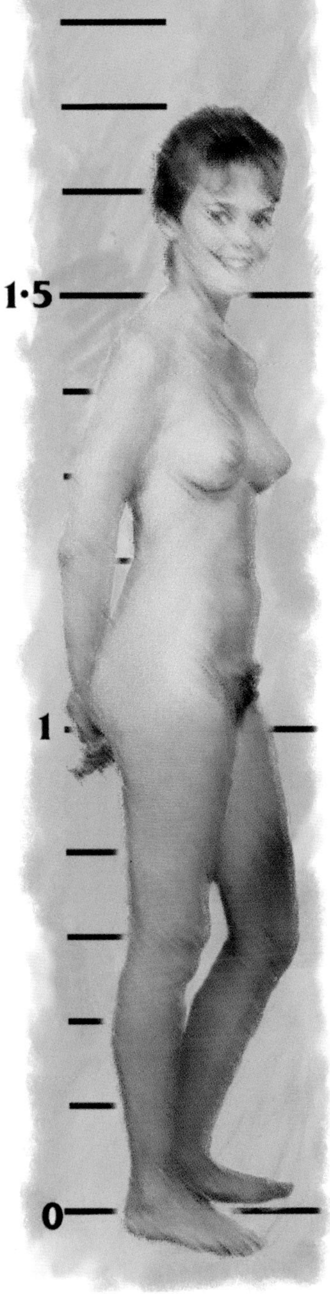

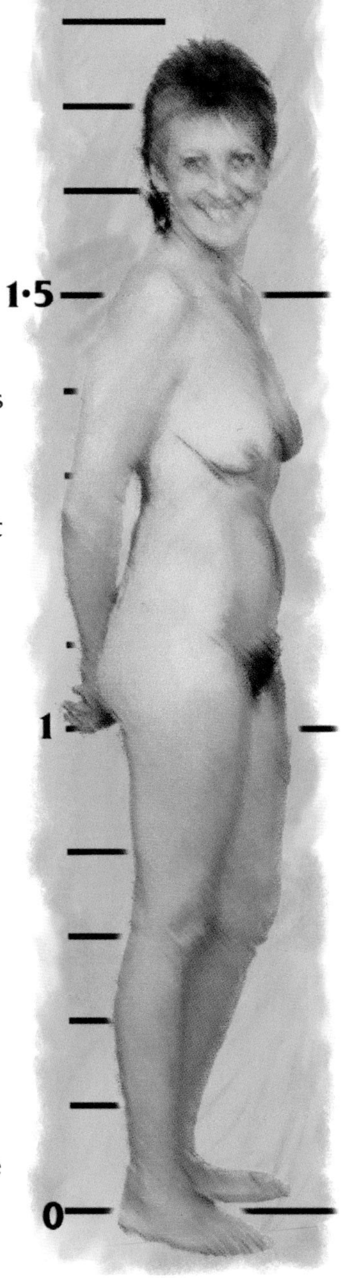

BOY TO MAN

In boys puberty occurs later than in girls, usually between the ages of eleven and seventeen.

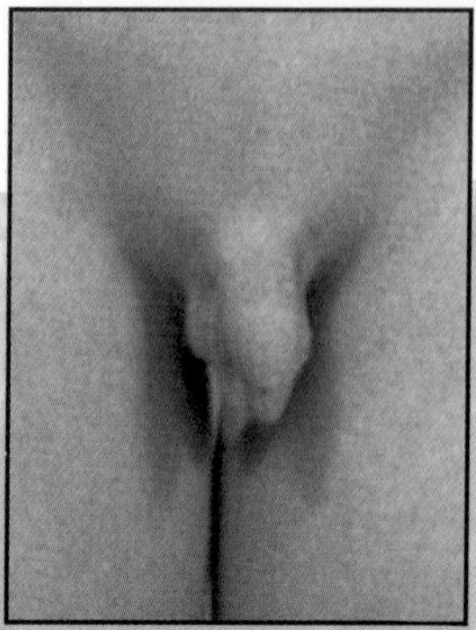

The maturing body
Four members of the same family show some of the visible differences to the genital area in the course of puberty as the pubic hair, the testes and the penis develop. These changes – and other less obvious ones – usually occur between the ages of eleven and seventeen.

Frame
The growth spurt associated with puberty begins around the age of thirteen in boys. They may grow up to 8 cm each year at this time, coming close to their full adult height by the age of eighteen. At the same time, just as women's hips widen, men's shoulders tend to broaden. The proportions of the different parts of the body to each other may vary at this time, as growth rates are rarely even and consistent. Many boys will feel uncoordinated or 'gangly', but this tends to pass as development progresses.

Muscle and fat
In general, men's bodies tend to be made up of less fat and more muscle than women's. Muscle often accounts for as much as forty per cent of an adult man's body weight, with only ten to twenty per cent fat. This is largely due to the actions of the male and female sexual hormones, whose effects are first noted during puberty. Indeed, artificial male hormones have often been used to aid muscle-building. A boy's physical strength may increase dramatically during the course of puberty. At the same time, some body fat may accumulate, particularly on the upper arms, chest and abdomen. Some boys may develop 'breasts' for a few months as the hormone levels readjust. While hormones play a significant part in determining the proportions of body fat and muscle, these are also dependent on general health, diet, exercise and heredity.

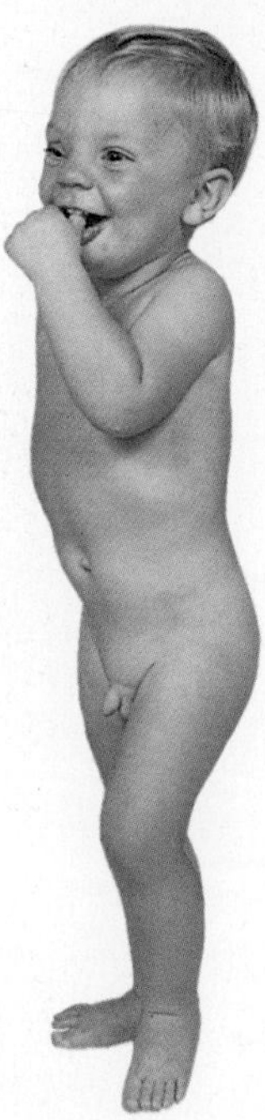

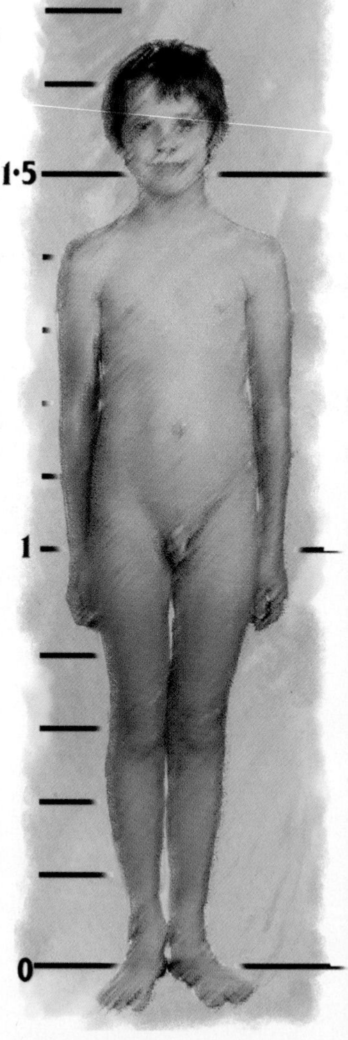

Skin
The hormonal changes of puberty also affect the skin and hair. The sebaceous glands become more active at this time, making both more greasy, and acne may appear on the face, chest and back. Body odour also increases as the sweat glands develop.

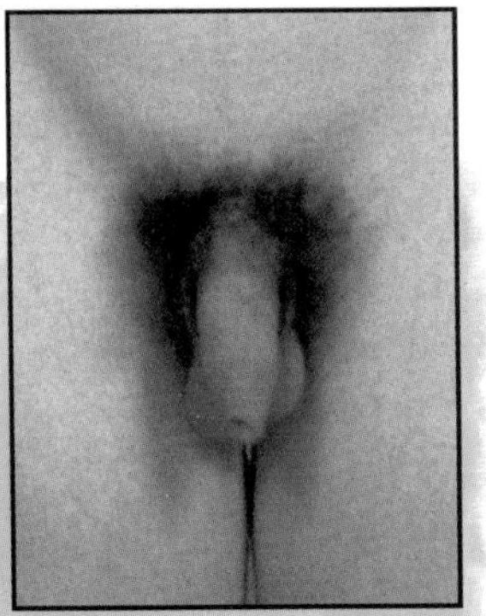

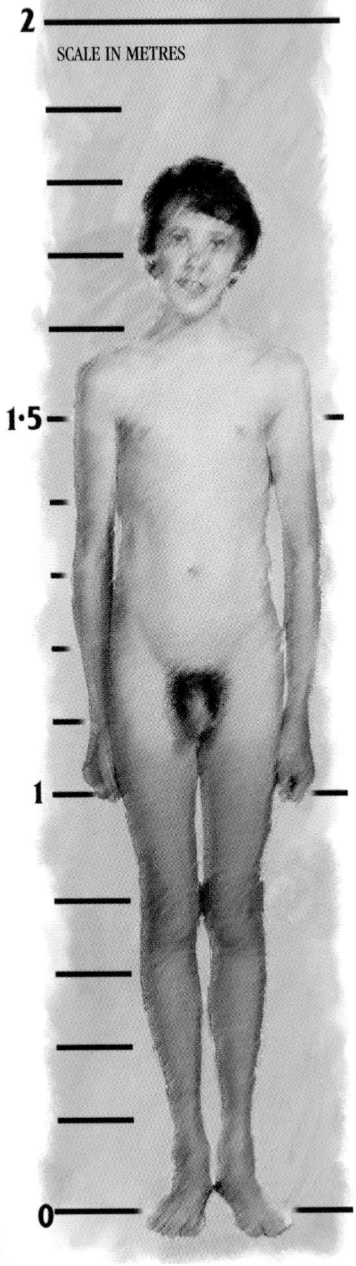

Body hair

The coarse pubic hair appears early in puberty at the base of the penis. From here it spreads to the scrotum and sometimes to the anus, and towards the stomach and thighs. It may be a different colour to the hair on the head, although it may turn grey with age. Hair also appears in the armpits, arms and legs, and sometimes on the chest, shoulders and back. Facial hair will also darken and thicken, and again may not be the same colour as the hair on the head. Body and facial hair tend to be much more abundant in men than in women. It is determined primarily by hereditary factors in terms of racial and family background, but is also influenced by any change in hormone levels.

Voice

In men puberty often causes the voice to change dramatically or 'break'. This is caused by changes in the larynx: namely the elongation and thickening of the vocal chords, together with the growth of the 'Adam's apple' from the thyroid cartilage. This can happen gradually or quite suddenly.

Genitals

These are probably the most noticeable changes in males. Around the age of ten or eleven the rate of growth of the external genitals increases dramatically. The testes grow in length and volume. The penis grows longer and wider, and its glans develops. The internal organs also develop and sperm and seminal fluid are produced (known as the spermarche). The penis can become erect and ejaculation can occur. Erections can occur from an early age, often without any sexual stimulus and at awkward moments. This tends to increase during puberty. Erections while asleep are common: if ejaculation occurs as well, it is known as a nocturnal emission or 'wet dream'.

FACT: Recent research has suggested that sperm counts in men are going down worldwide

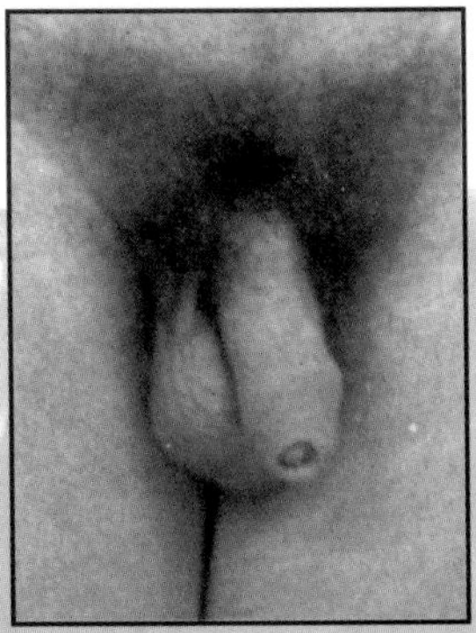

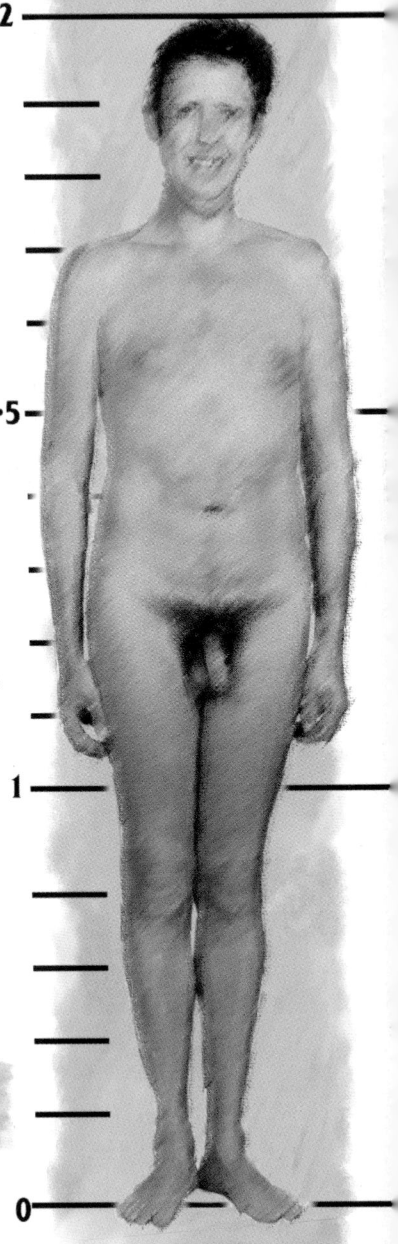

HORMONES

Hormones affect every aspect of our lives. Originating in involuntary chemical signals in the brain, they control many of our bodily processes, including the cycles related to reproduction. At the same time it is widely believed that it is in the cycles and variations of our hormones – and particularly the sex hormones – that lies the source of our emotions.

HORMONAL ACTION IN THE MATURE FEMALE

The menstrual cycle

The menstrual cycle is the method by which the female reproductive system is maintained. It is characterized by two hormones in particular, oestrogen in the first half of the cycle and progesterone in the second. If there are no problems, it ensures, along with hormones from the pituitary, that once each month a reproductive germ cell or ovum is released from an ovary, and that the uterus is ready to receive it if it is fertilized by its male equivalent, the sperm.

How the menstrual cycle works

Each ovary stores as many as half a million potential egg cells or ova. Each month the pituitary gland stimulates the growth of a follicle in one of the ovaries. In this follicle a single ovum is matured and oestrogen is produced. About halfway through the cycle the ovum is released, leaving an empty follicle, now called a corpus luteum, which starts to produce progesterone. This is the hormone which prepares the uterus lining for pregnancy. If the ovum is not fertilized, the levels of oestrogen and progesterone in the blood stream fall after about fourteen days, at which time menstruation – or the

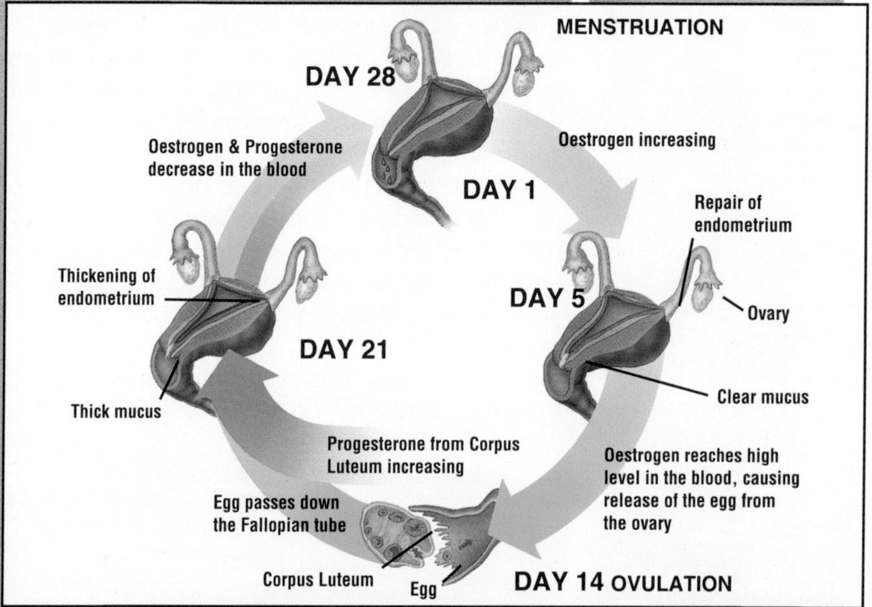

See also:
anatomy of sex
sexual feelings – male
sexual feelings – female
aphrodisiacs
sex drive
health and hygiene

menstrual period – will occur. The uterus lining is broken down and passed out of the body, ready for the cycle to begin again.

On average this cycle lasts twenty-eight days, although cycles between twenty-six and thirty-two days are quite common. If day one is the first day of menstruation, ovulation takes place around fourteen days before. Menstruation itself generally lasts for three to six days. About 30 ml to 150 ml of blood are lost each month.

There is nothing 'unclean' about menstrual bleeding or menstruating women, so long as basic personal hygiene is maintained. During menstruation some pain may be experienced. Known as dysmenorrhoea, this is a common occurrence which, if necessary, can be treated with pain killers or in extreme cases with hormonal preparations. There are various other disorders associated with menstruation, including amenorrhoea (stopped or missed periods), menorrhagia (heavy periods), and polymenorrhoea (over-frequent periods). These can often be treated.

Other effects of the female hormonal cycle

The menstrual cycle is marked by certain physical effects of the changing hormone levels. The oestrogen produced in the first half of the cycle tends to create feelings of well being. The hair and skin are in good condition. Vaginal discharge is minimal, becoming more profuse as ovulation approaches. The effects of progesterone in the second half of the cycle tend to be less positive. The breasts may become heavy and tender, spots may appear and hair may become greasier. Vaginal discharge becomes thicker and may have some odour. Many women suffer from water retention. Mood swings can also be a problem, with acute irritability, tearfulness and indecision, and in some cases severe depression and even violence. These symptoms are collectively referred to as the pre-menstrual syndrome (PMS). Once surrounded by superstition, PMS is now a medically recognized occurrence. It passes with the onset of menstruation, but if necessary can be medically treated.

*Crystals of **progesterone** in the female seen in a polarized light micrograph.*

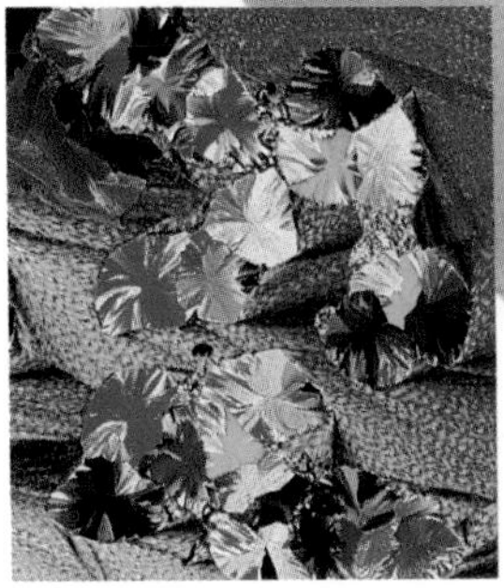

HORMONAL ACTION IN THE MATURE MALE

In men hormones do not follow a specific and regular cycle. Sperm are produced constantly and in vast quantities: there are on average 200 to 400 million sperm in each ejaculation. The male hormones sustain this production and maintain the whole male reproductive system.

How the male hormones work

The hormonal signals sent out by the pituitary gland act on the testes to aid and regulate the production of sperm and stimulate the production of testosterone. The sperm produced are matured and stored in the duct leading from each testis, the epididymis.

Other effects of the male hormones

Testosterone is one of several androgens, the steroids that stimulate the development of the male sexual organs and secondary sexual characteristics. It raises the rate at which proteins are produced, and lowers the rate at which they are broken down. The effects of this are increased muscle bulk and accelerated growth. Testosterone promotes aggression. It also sustains the male sex drive, although this can be self-perpetuating, as sexual activity – whether through intercourse or masturbation – is itself the best natural way of maintaining levels of testosterone.

*Crystals of **testosterone** in the male seen in a polarized light micrograph.*

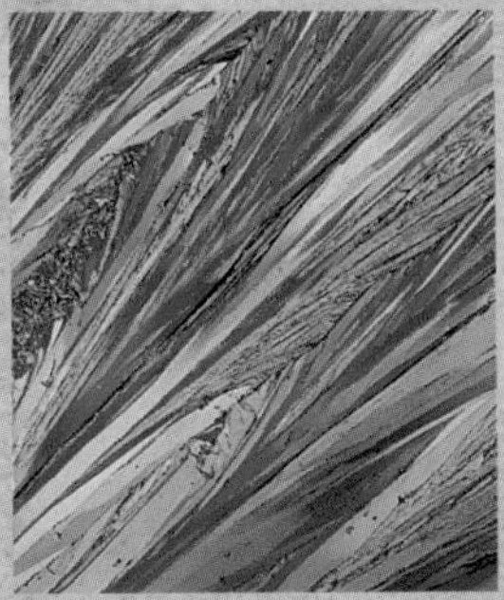

MENOPAUSE

This is the period in later life when the activity of the sexual organs declines.

Women and the menopause
The menopause is the term used to refer to the end of menstruation. It usually occurs between the ages of forty and fifty-six. Women whose periods started early tend to reach the menopause later, and vice versa. There is some evidence of heredity in the timing of both puberty and the menopause. The period of change tends to last one or two years as the system re-regulates itself – about as long as it takes for menstruation to become regular. It is at the menopause that the ovaries cease to be active. Ova are no longer released each month and the production of the sex hormones oestrogen and progesterone declines.

One of the first signs of the menopause is irregularity in the menstrual cycle, before menstruation ceases completely. All of the sex organs are affected: the uterus and ovaries shrink, the vaginal walls grow thinner, and the vulva may partially atrophy. Physical responses to sex tend to be slower and sometimes less intense, but not necessarily any less pleasurable. The 'plateau' stage of arousal may last longer. Orgasms tend to be less intense, but any decline in sex drive is usually gradual. Generally those who enjoy sex earlier in life will continue to do so for as long as their general health permits.

Different women's experiences of the menopause vary greatly. For some it is very straightforward and even a relief. However, for others it can be quite traumatic, and there are certain short-term symptoms caused by the change in hormone levels which can be disagreeable. These include hot flushes, night sweats, palpitations, headaches, fatigue, insomnia, irritability, mood swings and depression. More importantly, lack of oestrogen can lead to some of the major health problems affecting women in later life, such as heart disease and the brittle-bone disease osteoporosis. Treatment, including hormone replacement therapy (HRT), may be recommended.

See also:
sex drive
sexual feelings

The menopause usually occurs between the ages of forty and fifty-six in women and more gradually after the age of forty in men. It need not mean the end of an active and satisfying sex life.

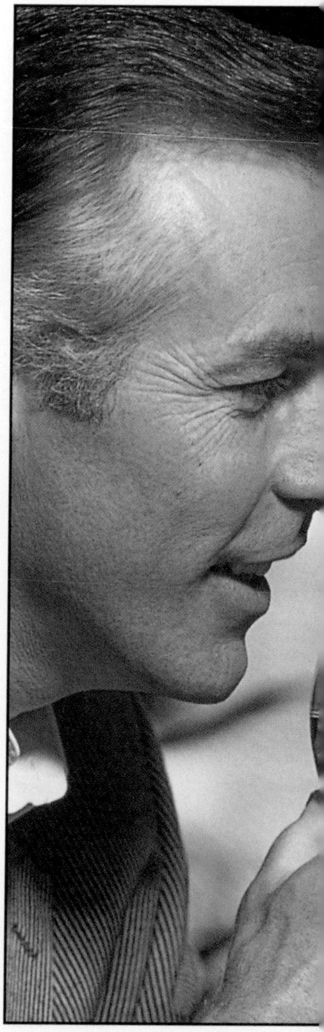

HRT replaces the hormones which the ovaries are no longer producing. It can eradicate the short-term symptoms of the menopause, and reduce the risk of heart disease and osteoporosis by up to fifty per cent. However, HRT may not be suitable for some women, while others may prefer natural methods of easing menopausal symptoms. These include dietary supplements and various alternative therapies, such as reflexology, acupuncture, aromatherapy and homeopathy. More and more treatments are becoming recognized, as more is learnt about how to ensure that women can continue to enjoy good health through and after the menopause.

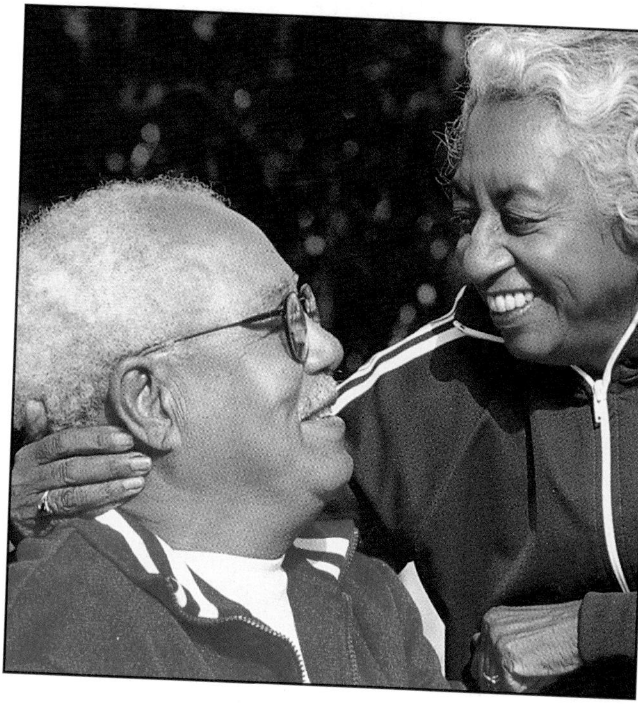

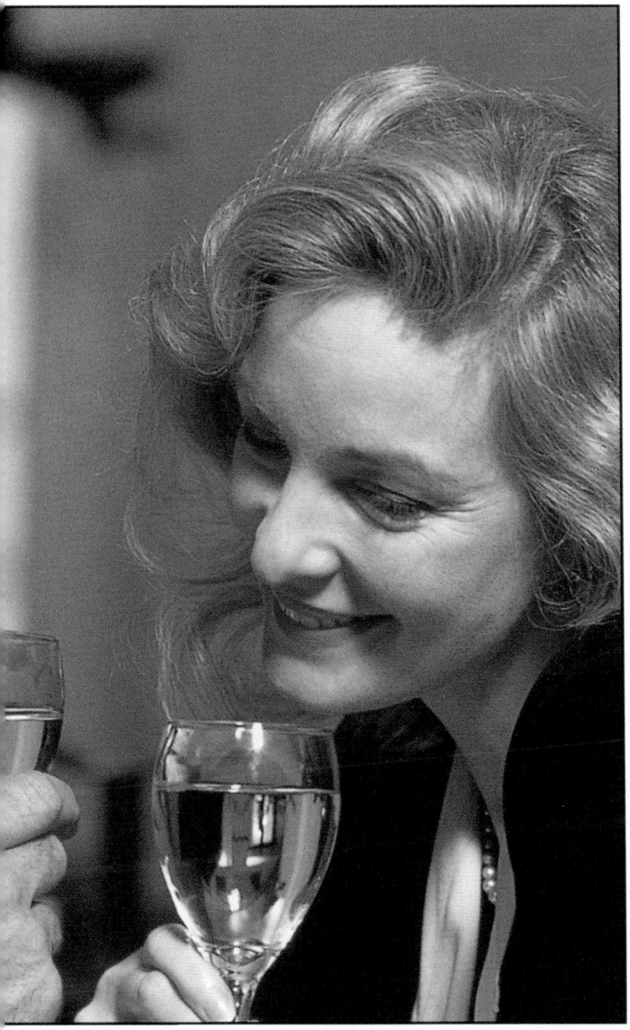

Men and the climacteric or 'male' menopause

The climacteric in men is less well-recognized than that which occurs in women. This may be because it tends to be less dramatic.

On the whole, the production of testosterone decreases very gradually from the age of about forty. By sixty this may have produced noticeable changes. The testes may shrink and become less firm, and the scrotal sac may grow looser and more wrinkled. Physical responses to sex may be slower and less strong. It may be more difficult to obtain an erection as the blood vessels in the pubic area harden and slow down the blood flow. However, many men can maintain an erection for longer than in earlier life and the 'plateau' stage of arousal tends to last much longer, even though orgasm is often more short-lived.

Along with testosterone, sperm production tends to decrease with age. However, in many men both continue to be produced well into old age, with the result that they may remain both sexually active and fertile.

CONTRACEPTION

Ever since the connection between sexual intercourse and conception was first recognized, people have been looking for ways to prevent pregnancy.

Four thousand years ago Egyptian women were using pessaries of honey and animal dung, while Arabian women mixed pomegranate pulp with alum and rock salt. The Greeks used a concoction of cedar oil, frankincense and olive oil, and even experimented with intrauterine devices. In China and Japan disks of oiled paper were used as rudimentary cervical caps. It is said that the idea of the intrauterine device developed from the Arabic custom of placing a stone in the uterus of a female camel to keep it sterile, although how the method first came to be used in humans is not known.

From tortoiseshell to 'teasers' – condoms have developed greatly from their origins. They are now available in an almost infinite variety of shapes, sizes, colours and flavours, and seem likely to remain one of the most popular forms of contraception.

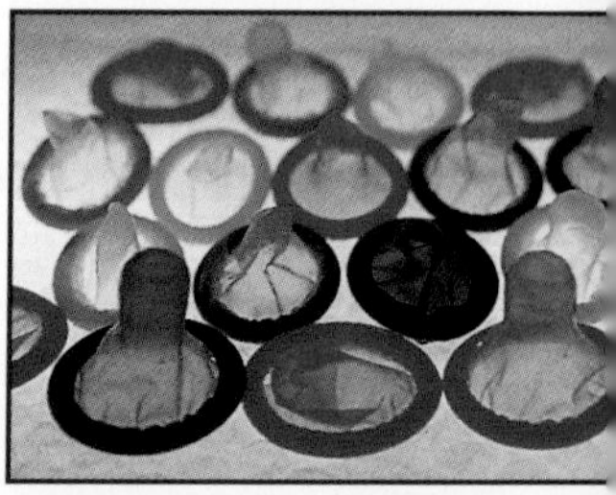

The base of the condom should be held on withdrawal to avoid spilling semen.

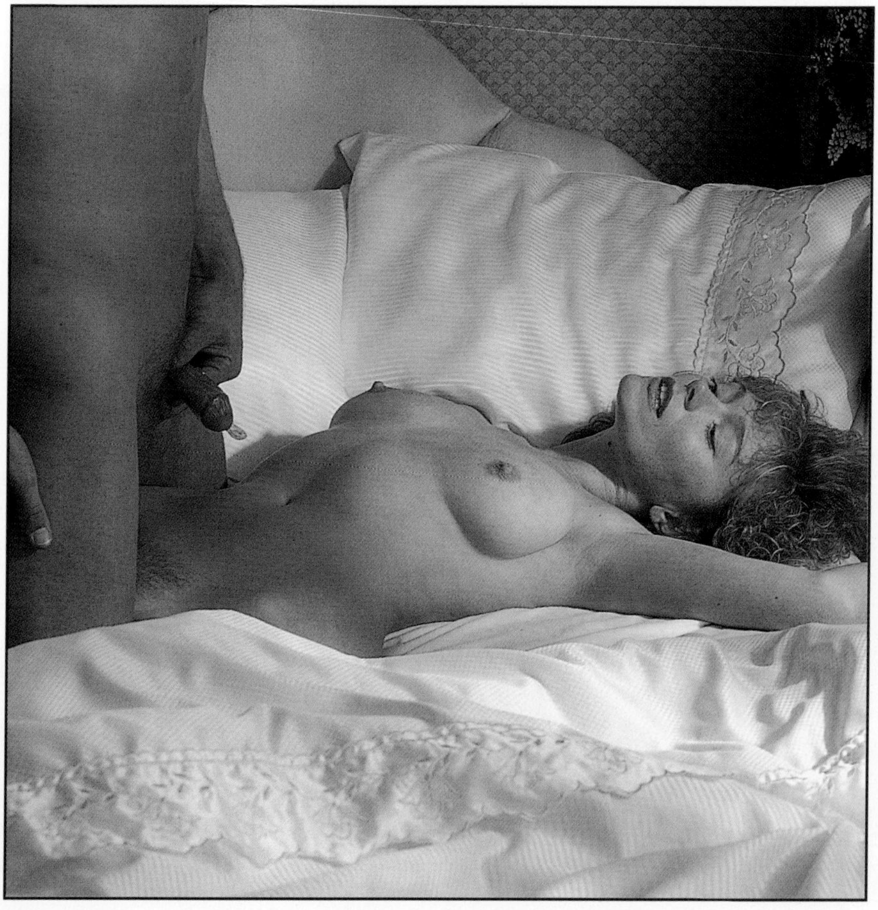

See also:
conception to childbirth
safer sex
making love
sex and religion

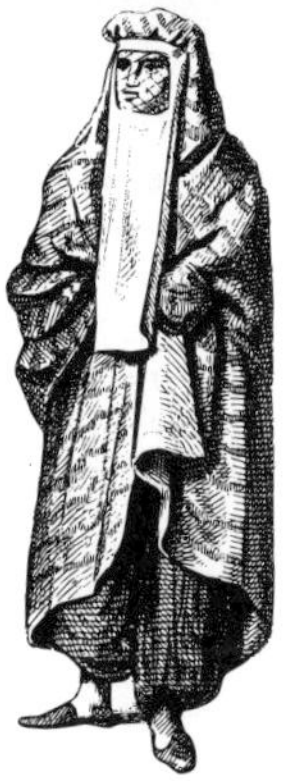

At one time in Persia it was recommended that the woman should jump backwards nine times then sit on her toes stroking her navel! In Japan, men wore sheaths made from tortoiseshell, horn or leather.

However, it was in the sixteenth century that the Italian Gabriel Fallopius developed a sheath made from chemically treated linen, although this was initially developed to prevent venereal infections. This rudimentary version of the condom was later replaced with animal intestines, and eventually with latex rubber.

The condom and the diaphragm have been used widely since the end of the nineteenth century. Since then both the variety and the reliability of methods of contraception have increased dramatically. Intrauterine devices (IUDs) were used at the beginning of this century, but with frequent damage to the wall of the uterus. Consequently it was not until the 1960s that a more modern and safer form of the IUD was produced – which achieved instant popularity. It was at this time that the first hormonal oral contraceptives were produced, as a result of research carried out in the mid and late fifties.

Many of the contraceptives available today are highly sophisticated, and continue to be developed further, providing us with a constantly growing range of choices. The social acceptability of their use has also increased. The key to successful use of contraceptives lies in the combination of having the motivation to prevent pregnancy, knowing how to use the chosen method correctly, and being sufficiently happy with that choice to use it consistently.

Contraceptives function by preventing the production of sperm or egg, or preventing them from meeting, or preventing them from surviving. Methods may be divided broadly into four main types: natural, mechanical and hormonal methods, and sterilization.

The range of methods of contraception continues to grow, under the influence of developments in scientific research and public demand. In many countries, a great variety is available, enabling most people to find a method appropriate to their own personal needs and preferences.

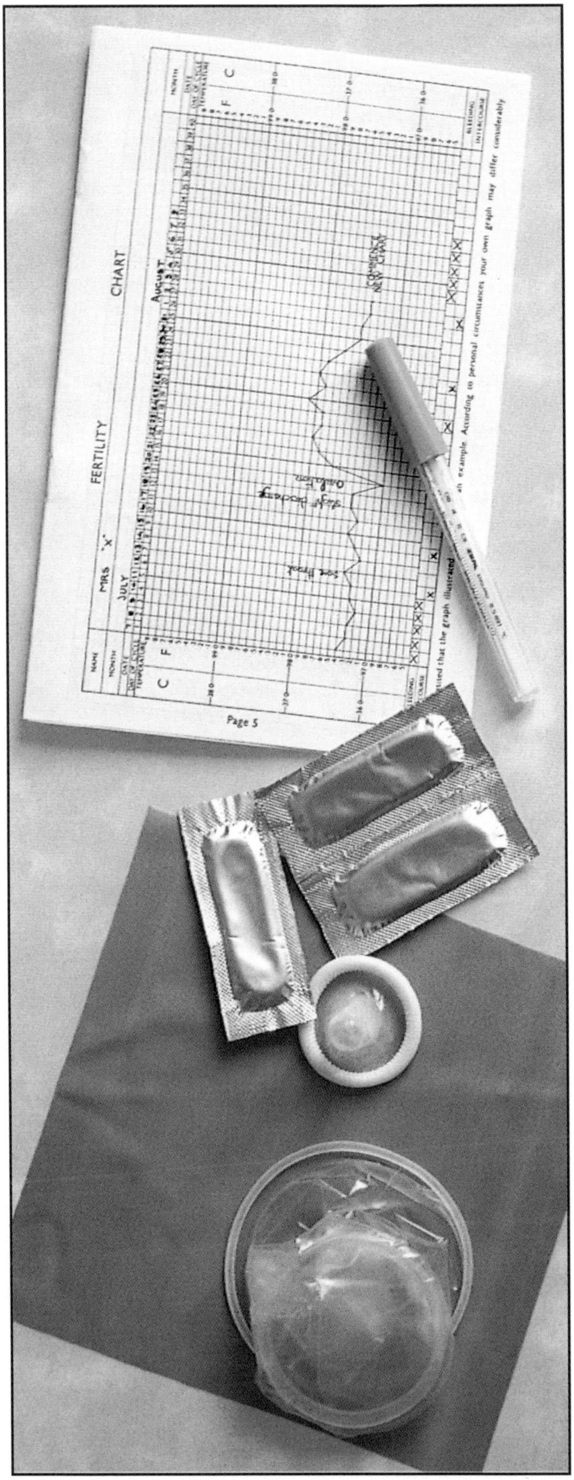

NATURAL METHODS

Natural methods of contraception do not involve any hormonal or mechanical intervention. Success or failure depends on using the technique correctly, and even then these methods may not be too reliable. The assistance of a teacher fully trained in natural family-planning methods is advisable.

Rhythm methods
These are based on the woman's natural body cycles, determining when ovulation is likely to occur, so that the couple can avoid intercourse when conception is most probable. It is the only form of contraception acceptable to some religions. The lifetime of the sperm is estimated at up to five or six days and that of the egg at just one or two, so the 'safe period' is taken from six days before ovulation to two days afterwards. There are three different ways of calculating the time of ovulation which are described here only briefly.

The obvious advantage of these methods is that they are entirely natural. They also give a woman a greater awareness of her own body, and enable her to know when she is most fertile should she wish to become pregnant. They are, however, far from reliable, especially for women who have irregular periods. Their effectiveness varies from two to twenty per cent failure, meaning that in every hundred women using the rhythm method, between two and twenty will become pregnant during the course of a year. The calendar method remains the least reliable.

For greater safety, all three methods should be combined and, if possible, should be explained in more detail by a trained natural-methods teacher. None of them provide protection against sexually transmitted diseases.

The calendar method
This is so unreliable that it is generally only recommended as a cross-check against other methods. A record must be kept of the length of the woman's menstrual cycle for at least six months, counted from the first day of her period to the day before the next period starts.

The first day of the fertile time is calculated by subtracting nineteen from the number of days of the shortest cycle (i.e. fourteen days after ovulation plus five days to allow for sperm survival); the probable last fertile day is given by subtracting ten from the longest cycle (i.e. fourteen days after ovulation minus four days to allow for ovum survival).

The cycle may change – and if it does, then the calculations must be altered accordingly.

The temperature method
This involves taking the woman's temperature early in the morning (before getting out of bed and before having anything to eat or drink) and recording it daily. The temperature rises by about 0.2–0.4°C for three days immediately after ovulation. However, body temperature may be affected by various other factors, making this a potentially unreliable guide on its own. With a record taken over some months, however, the 'safe period' may be estimated.

The cervical-mucus method
This involves observing the regular changes in uterine mucus. This increases in quantity and becomes more slippery and clear at the time of ovulation, so that the sperm can travel through it more easily. Intercourse is not safe until the discharge has become cloudy, sticky and thick once more.

Ovulation tests, which are not unlike pregnancy tests, have now been developed to indicate when ovulation has occurred.

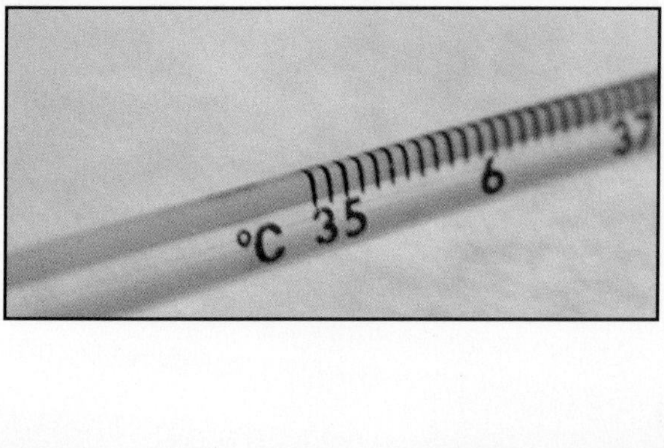

Withdrawal
In this method, also known as coitus interruptus, the man withdraws his penis from the vagina before ejaculation. While it has the advantages of other natural methods and is popular worldwide, it is probably the least reliable of all methods. It requires a degree of control which is not always possible and can result in extreme frustration for both partners. It is also very risky, as it is essential that not even a drop of sperm should be deposited in or near the vagina. Even the fluid that lubricates the penis in the earlier stages of arousal may contain sperm, so withdrawal prior to ejaculation may still be too late. It is estimated that each year as many as a quarter of the women regularly using this method become pregnant.

Non-penetrative sex
This is a way of enjoying sexual activity while avoiding conception. It may involve kissing, stroking, mutual masturbation and other activities, excluding full intercourse. Worldwide, anal sex is often used as a contraception method.

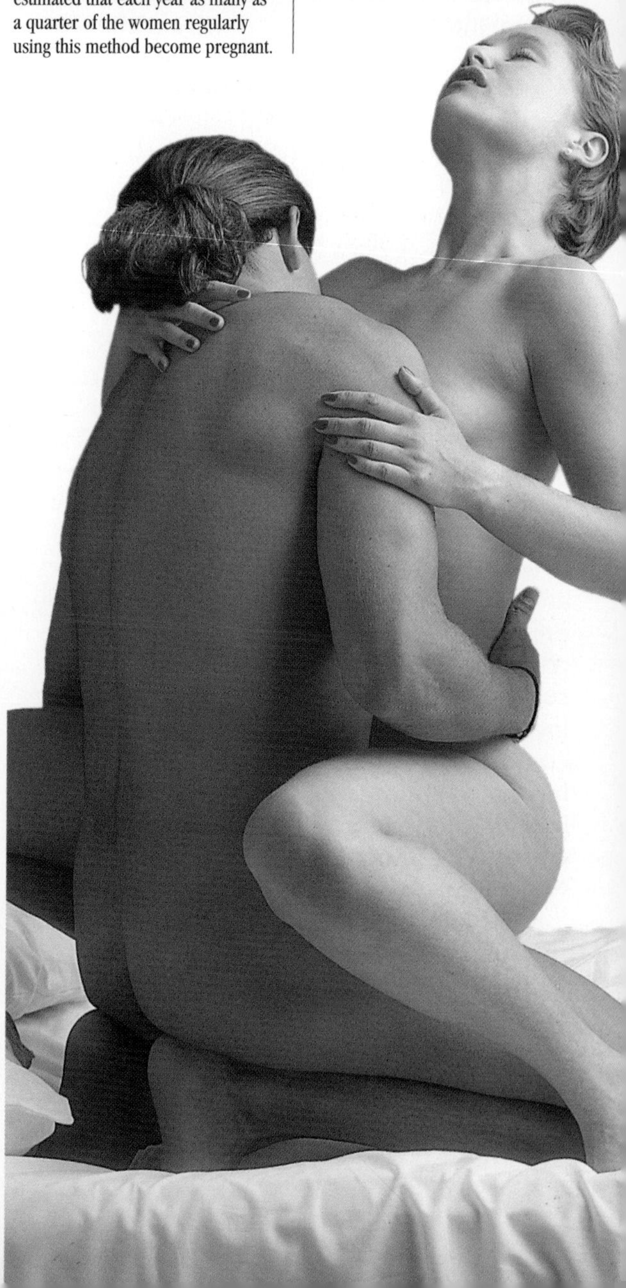

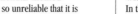

MECHANICAL METHODS

These are designed to allow full vaginal intercourse to take place without necessarily leading to pregnancy. They function in a variety of different ways and may be used in conjunction with one another or with other methods.

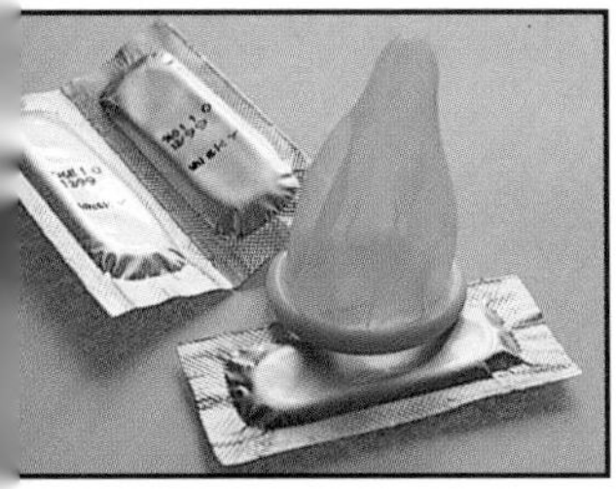

The condom
The male condom or sheath is the most common of the 'barrier' methods: that is, those which prevent the sperm from meeting the egg. It is also the only widely used male contraceptive. It is made of thin latex rubber, and functions by catching and retaining ejaculated semen. It must be rolled on to the erect penis before any contact with the vagina. This may be done either by the man or his partner, who may make it a part of foreplay. The air should be squeezed out of the end or the teat, if there is one, then the condom should be rolled gently over the tip of the penis leaving the teat (or the last half inch, if there is no teat) free to catch the ejaculate. The condom should not be pulled or tweaked, as this can damage it.

On withdrawal from the vagina, the condom should be held carefully in place at the base of the penis while it is still partially erect to prevent any sperm from escaping.

For extra security and lubrication condoms may be used with spermicides; spermicidally treated condoms are also available. For lubrication, only a spermicide or a water-based jelly should be used, as other substances (such as petroleum jelly) may damage the condom or irritate the vagina.

A new condom must be used each time intercourse takes place.

The male condom is one of the most popular and widely available forms of contraception. Available in a variety of shapes, colours, textures and flavours, its popularity has increased considerably in recent years as it provides a high level of protection against sexually transmitted diseases, including HIV infection.

The most common complaint is of reduced sensitivity, although this can be a benefit for those men who are prone to premature ejaculation. Another complaint is that the putting on of the condom can interrupt the growing excitement of sexual arousal, although this may be incorporated into foreplay. Occasionally allergic reactions to the rubber may occur; hypoallergenic condoms are now available.

Reliability is high: of a hundred women whose partners use the condom as the sole method of contraception, only two to four will become pregnant in the course of a year if it is used consistently and correctly. With less careful use, up to fifteen women in a hundred will become pregnant.

The female condom

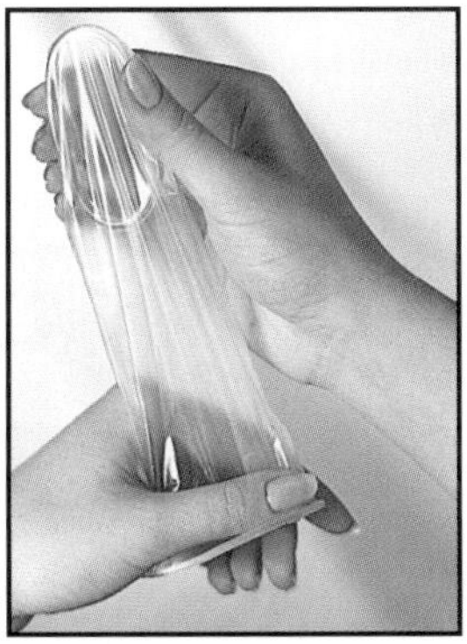

The female condom, which has been reintroduced recently, provides an additional barrier method for women. It consists of a tube of thin polyurethane plastic, closed at one end, with a flexible ring at each end to make it easier to insert and to hold it in place. The inner ring fits inside the vagina just behind the pubic bone, like the diaphragm. The outer ring lies flat against the vulva.

The female condom functions in the same way as the male equivalent. It is inserted before intercourse in order to catch and retain the ejaculated sperm, and provides a similar degree of security. However, it is expensive and care must be taken that the penis enters the condom and does not pass between the condom and the vaginal wall.

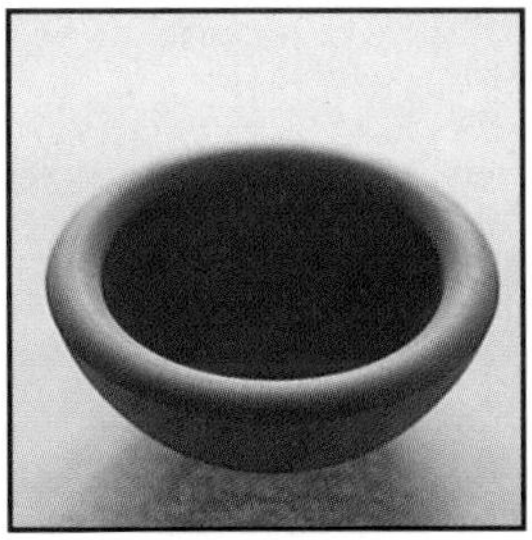

The diaphragm and the cap
These are also barrier methods, preventing the sperm from reaching the uterus. They both consist of a circular dome of thin rubber placed in the vagina. The diaphragm fits behind the pubic bone and blocks the entrance to the cervix. It is kept in shape by a pliable metal or firm rubber rim. The cap is smaller and covers just the cervix; it is held in place by suction.

Both are available from doctors and need to be fitted correctly. They should be checked by a family-planning nurse or doctor every six months, as the vagina can change shape, especially with weight loss or gain. They may be inserted any time before intercourse. However, the spermicide used with them must be topped up if intercourse occurs more than three hours after insertion, or if intercourse is repeated.

Both caps and diaphragms must be left in place for at least six hours after intercourse, but should be removed before more than thirty hours have elapsed. With careful use, the diaphragm and cap have a failure rate of only four to eight per cent, which rises to ten or fifteen per cent with less careful use.

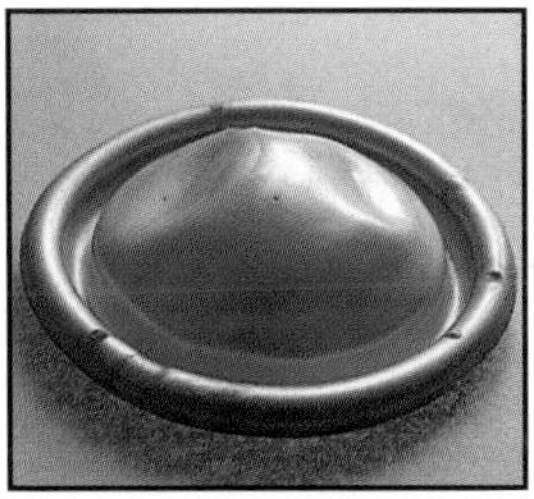

Intrauterine devices (IUDs)
The term 'intrauterine device' refers to devices that are inserted (by a trained health professional) into the woman's uterus. They function largely by preventing the sperm from fertilizing the ovum. Made of plastic and thin copper wire, they have one or two fine threads attached to the plastic frame that extend through the opening at the cervix, where they can be felt by the woman's fingers. They are also known as coils, 'T's or loops, although these terms are no longer strictly accurate.

IUDs can also be used as a form of emergency contraception, since they make the uterus hostile to the implantation of an embryo.

IUDs have to be inserted by a trained health professional, but provide immediate protection and can be left in place for between five and eight years, depending on the type of device used. They must also be removed by a health professional.

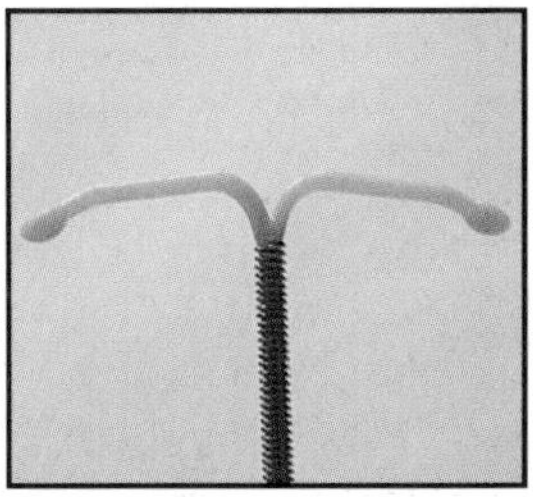

Their advantages lie in the fact that they do not require thought or preparation before lovemaking and do not involve the use of any hormones. However, there are possible problems. IUDs may cause pelvic inflammatory disease (salpingitis). This is more common among young users, particularly with changes of partner. If pregnancy does occur, ectopic pregnancy (where the embryo settles and starts to grow outside the womb, usually in a fallopian tube) and miscarriage are more likely. In some women, they may cause longer, heavier or more painful periods. IUDs provide no protection against sexually transmitted diseases.

However, IUDs remain almost as reliable as the pill, with less than one per cent of users becoming pregnant each year.

The intrauterine system (IUS)
The IUS, marketed under the brand name Mirena, is an IUD with a hormonal implant. It can be left in place for three years. This system is becoming increasingly popular, as in tests it has been shown to reduce blood loss, menstrual pain and the likelihood of some genital infections, as well as being highly effective as a contraceptive.

Spermicidal sponge
This is used in a similar way to the cap and the diaphragm in that it is placed in the vagina behind the pubic bone. It functions by both blocking and killing the sperm ejaculated into the vagina. However, it is less reliable than other methods and is consequently rarely used.

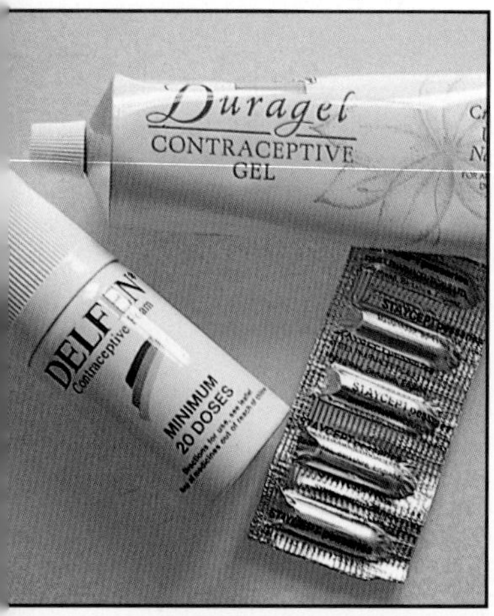

Spermicides
These are chemicals that kill the sperm inside the vagina. Available as creams, jellies, foams or pessaries, they are applied or inserted into the vagina before intercourse. On their own spermicides are not considered a reliable form of contraception, and are generally used in conjunction with another method – in particular with diaphragms, caps and condoms – for extra security.

HORMONAL METHODS

These involve the use of synthetic hormones similar to those produced naturally by the body during pregnancy. Taken either by pill, injection or implant, they have been one of the most popular female contraceptives since the 1960s. Research has also been carried out on hormonal contraceptives for use by men, but as yet none are available.

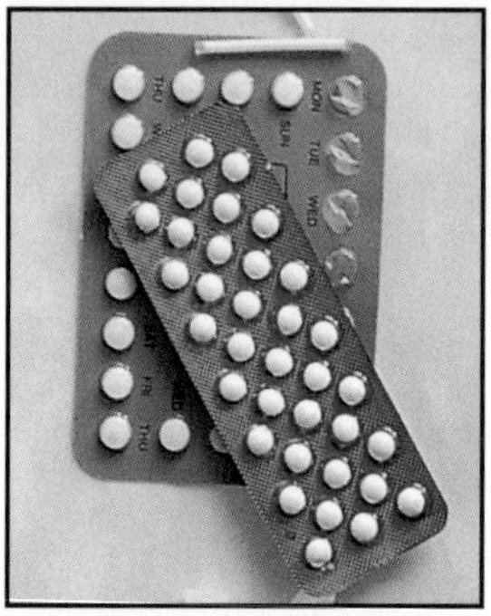

The combined pill
This contains both oestrogen and progestogen. Progestogen thickens the cervical mucus, making it less easy for the sperm to get through to meet the egg. It also makes the lining of the womb thinner, making it less likely to receive a fertilized egg. Oestrogen alters the body's hormonal cycle to stop the ovaries from releasing an egg each month. The exact amount of oestrogen and progestogen used depends upon the type and brand of pill.

Use of the pill is based on a standard twenty-eight day cycle. Hormonally active pills are taken for the first twenty-one days, followed by a seven day break to allow for the bleeding that takes the place of normal menstruation. The most common type of combined pill is monophasic, each of the twenty-one pills in the packet containing the same amount of hormone. There are also bi- and tri-phasic pills, which vary the amount of each hormone taken over the twenty-one days to follow the body's natural cycle more closely.

Finally there is the 'everyday pill', each packet of which includes seven inactive pills. It is therefore particularly useful for women who have difficulty in remembering to take their pill, as there is no seven-day break.

Whatever the type or brand, the combined pill is taken at approximately the same time every day.

The advantages of the combined pill are considerable. Firstly, it provides constant protection, with no mechanical devices and no interruption of intercourse. As well as this, many women find that it reduces bleeding, period pain and premenstrual tension. More significantly, it offers substantial protection against cancer of the ovaries and the womb. It can help prevent some pelvic infections and reduce the risk of fibroids, ovarian cysts and non-cancerous breast disease. The pill can be used by most women, up to the age of the menopause if they remain healthy (with regular blood pressure and smear tests) and do not smoke.

However, the pill is not suitable for some women, such as those who are very overweight or have any personal or family history of heart or blood-pressure problems or blood clots. Some research has suggested that use of the pill may slightly increase the risk of some kinds of cancer, but this is still very uncertain. Many of the potential ill effects of the pill have been linked with smoking. Generally speaking, the worst side effects experienced are headaches, weight gain or loss, reduced interest in sex, mood changes, and bleeding between periods. If these occur they will usually disappear within the first few months, or may be eliminated by a change of pill. The pill does not offer any protection against sexually transmitted diseases.

If taken regularly by suitable users, the pill is the most effective reversible method of contraception, with a failure rate of less than one per cent. Apart from failing to take it, the only things that can reduce the pill's reliability are vomiting within three hours of taking it, severe diarrhoea, and the effects of certain medicines.

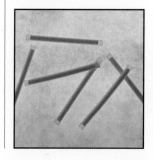

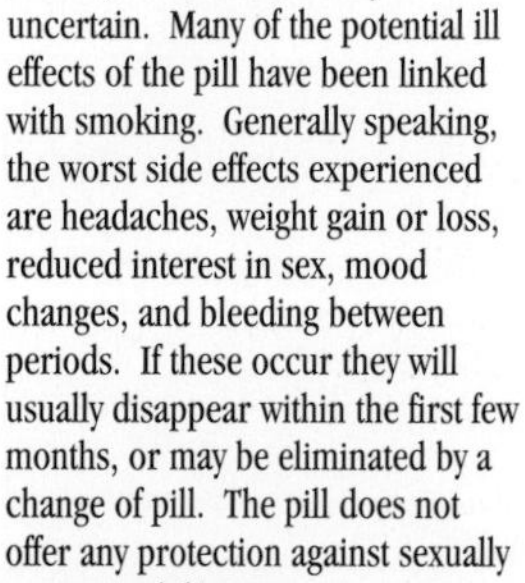

The progestogen-only pill
This is also known as the 'mini pill'. It contains no oestrogen, functioning simply by thickening the cervical mucus and making the womb lining thinner, although it can affect ovulation in some women (see under 'The combined pill'). Otherwise it is similar to the combined pill, but with less likelihood of side effects and only a marginally higher probability of irregularity in the menstrual cycle. It must, however, be taken at exactly the same time every day. It is useful for older women who smoke and should therefore not take the combined pill. The progestogen-only pill can also be used by breast-feeding mothers with no risk to the baby.

When it is used carefully, the progestogen-only pill has a failure rate of only one per cent, though this rises to four per cent with less careful use.

Injections and implants
Contraceptive injections give protection for either eight or twelve weeks. Implants, on the other hand, can provide protection for up to five years. They are small, soft tubes placed under the skin of the upper arm which gradually release a hormone into the bloodstream. Like the mini pill, they use just progestogen, which thickens the cervical mucus and, in the injection method, stops ovulation. They are only available from doctors specially trained in their use.

As well as the advantages of the progestogen-only pill, they have the great bonus of being effective for the full period, with no need to remember to take a pill at a specific time every day, or even to think about contraception. The main disadvantage of the contraceptive injection lies in the fact that it cannot be removed, so any unwanted side effects will continue throughout the eight or twelve week period, whereas an implant can be removed at any time.

Both injections and implants are extremely reliable, with less than one woman in a hundred becoming pregnant in a year. The statistics on implants suggest that about two women will become pregnant over the course of five years.

STERILIZATION

Sterilization of the male or female is a simple and relatively minor operation, which is highly effective. Failure rates stand at about one in five hundred for women, and for men one in a thousand, or less, during the first year after the operation, dropping to one in three thousand later.

Reversal of sterilization is possible, but requires a more major operation; the success rates stand at about seventy per cent for women, and between ten and ninety per cent for men. These figures vary according to the type of operation carried out and, for men, according to how long ago it was performed.

Sterilization should still be seen as a permanent step.

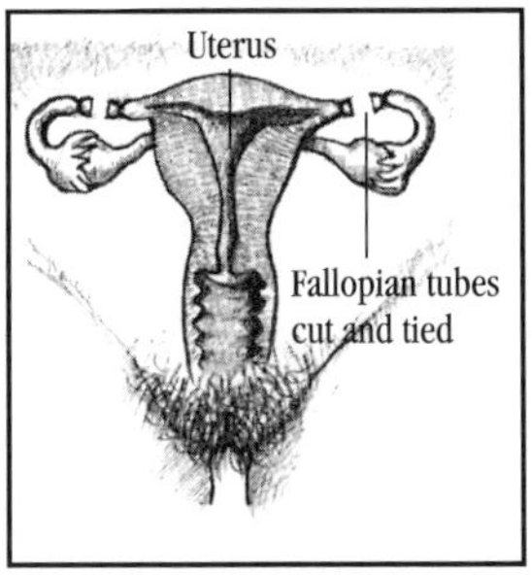

Female sterilization
This involves blocking or cutting and tying the fallopian tubes, in which the sperm and ovum meet. As in male sterilization, the body's natural cycles are unaffected: an egg is still produced every month, even though it cannot be fertilized. Enjoyment of intercourse is also unaffected.

The operation is usually carried out under general anaesthetic as a day case. Afterwards there may be some slight bleeding or pain for one to two weeks, and a couple of weeks' rest may be required. After this time periods continue as normal. Female sterilization is effective at once, although some women are advised to use another method of contraception until their next period.

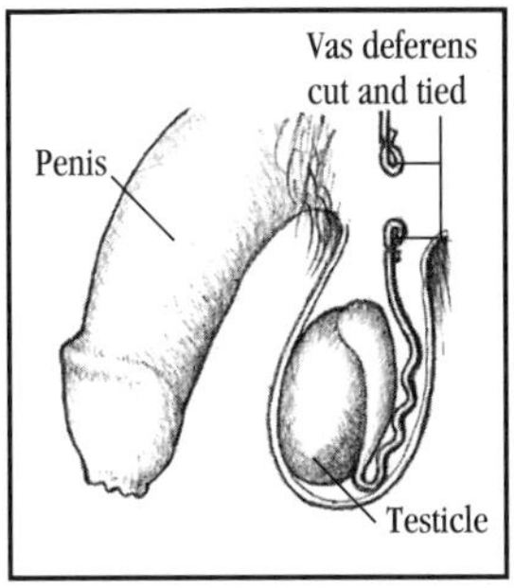

Male sterilization (vasectomy)
This involves blocking or cutting and tying both of the tubes (the vasa deferentia) which carry the sperm from the testicles to where they are mixed to form the semen. Hormones and sex drive are unaffected, as are the man's orgasm and ejaculation. The sole difference is that there are no sperm in the semen, and this is only detectable under a microscope.

The operation is performed under local anaesthetic and takes about ten minutes. The most common problem following the operation is bruising, swelling and pain, but usually this is slight and lasts no more than a week.

Vasectomy is completely reliable as a form of contraception after two clear semen tests, two to four months after the operation, to ensure that any sperm left in the tubes leading to the penis have gone. Failure of the operation stands at about one in every thousand within a few months of the operation, but this is usually shown by sperm tests. The chances of failure occurring some time later are estimated at between one in three thousand and one in seven thousand. Some men report a drop in sex drive, though others – safe from any likelihood of fertilization – report an increase. These variations are almost certainly psychological, not physiological.

EMERGENCY CONTRACEPTION

In many countries emergency contraception is available for women who have had sex without contraception and do not want to become pregnant, or for women who suspect their method of contraception may have failed. It is essential to seek advice quickly.

Emergency pills
Even though this method is also known as the 'morning after' pill, it may be taken up to seventy-two hours after having unprotected intercourse. It contains the same hormones as the combined pill but in larger quantities, functioning either by stopping an egg from being released or by preventing a fertilized egg from implanting in the womb. Two doses are taken twelve hours apart. There may be some nausea, and the emergency pill is not suitable for all women. It is ninety-five per cent effective in preventing pregnancy.

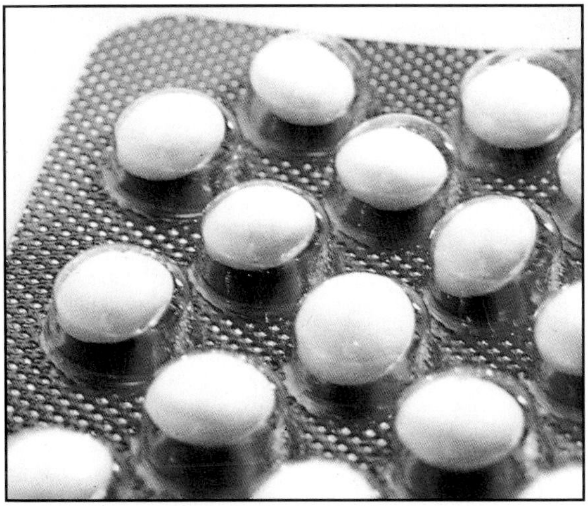

IUDs as emergency contraception
IUDs (see under 'Mechanical methods') can also be used for emergency contraception, but must be fitted within five days of having unprotected intercourse.

Check-ups are usually made three to four weeks after using emergency contraception.

HEALTH & HYGIENE

Part of enjoying a healthy sex life is looking after your sexual and reproductive system. Sexual health is a responsibility: it affects both partners.

Natural, pleasant bodily odour can be a fundamental source of attractiveness. Obsession with cleanliness has severely reduced the impact of personal odour as one of the most powerful sexual signals. However, it has also increased awareness of the importance of personal hygiene and helped eliminate offensive stale smells.

In fact, many parts of the body are looked after by the body's own processes. Nonetheless, minor problems can often be avoided by taking certain steps to maintain a basic level of hygiene, such as washing the genital area and anus once a day and wearing clean underwear. Strong soaps should be avoided, as they may cause irritation in this sensitive area. Urinating soon after intercourse can also help prevent infections in the urethra.

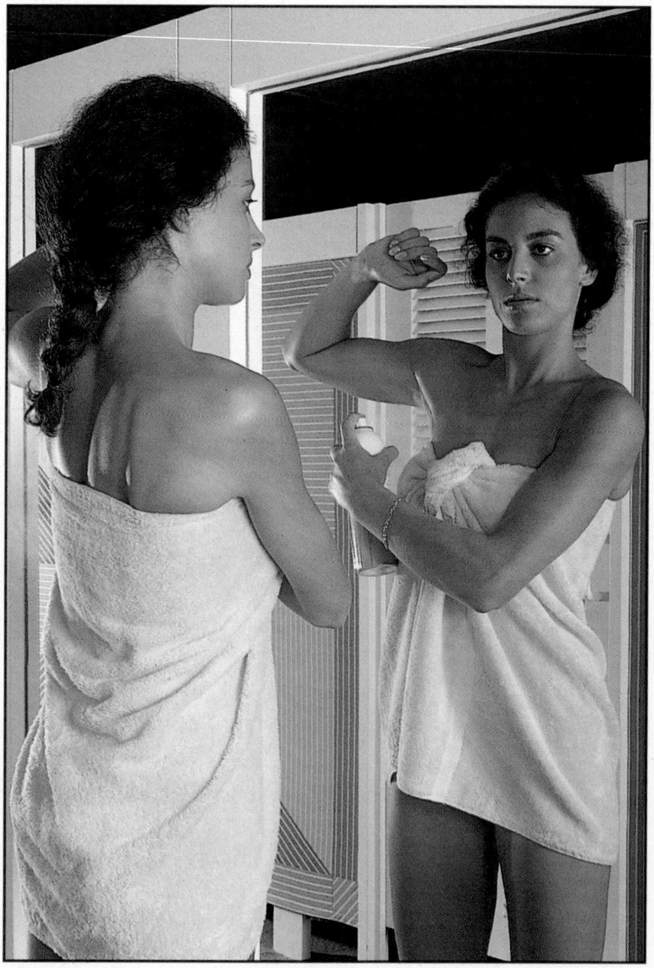

FACT: A recent survey suggested that while women tend to wash their hands more frequently than men, men are more likely to do so before having sex.

Body odour
The Western obsession with cleanliness has severely reduced the impact of personal odour as one of the most powerful sexual signals. However, it has also increased awareness of the importance of personal hygiene and helped eliminate offensive stale smells.

See also:
penis
vagina
HIV and AIDS
safer sex

Hygiene for women
Some vaginal discharge is normal and necessary for maintaining a healthy environment in the vaginal and vulval area. However, its delicate balance may be upset by use of strong soaps, or too much soap, and by vaginal deodorants or perfumes.

Some slight 'yeasty' odour is normal and healthy. However, any changes which do not coincide with the usual menstrual pattern may be a sign of infection.

After using the toilet, women should always wipe themselves from front to back (from vagina to anus), to prevent bacteria from the anus entering the vagina and possibly causing infection.

Hygiene for men
Males of all ages should wash the penis at least once a day. Particular attention should be paid to the area just below the head of the penis, where a glandular secretion known as smegma can accumulate. If the man is uncircumcised, he should draw back the foreskin while washing. Penile discharge is not normal and should be investigated.

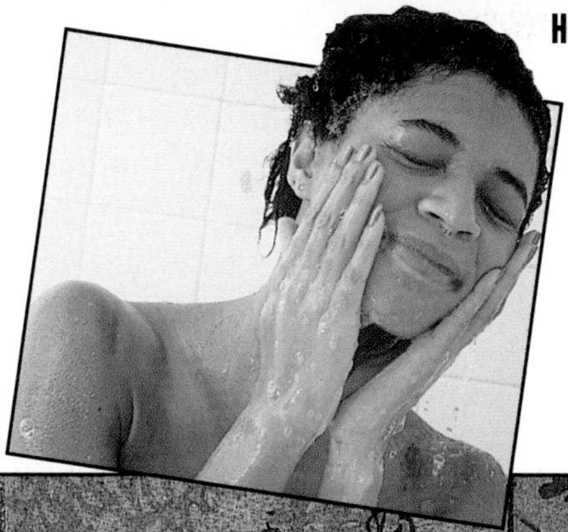

This Japanese woodcut from the nineteenth century by Kunimori II shows a man's penis being cleaned by his female companion. Animals groom each other – and this can be part of human relationships as well.

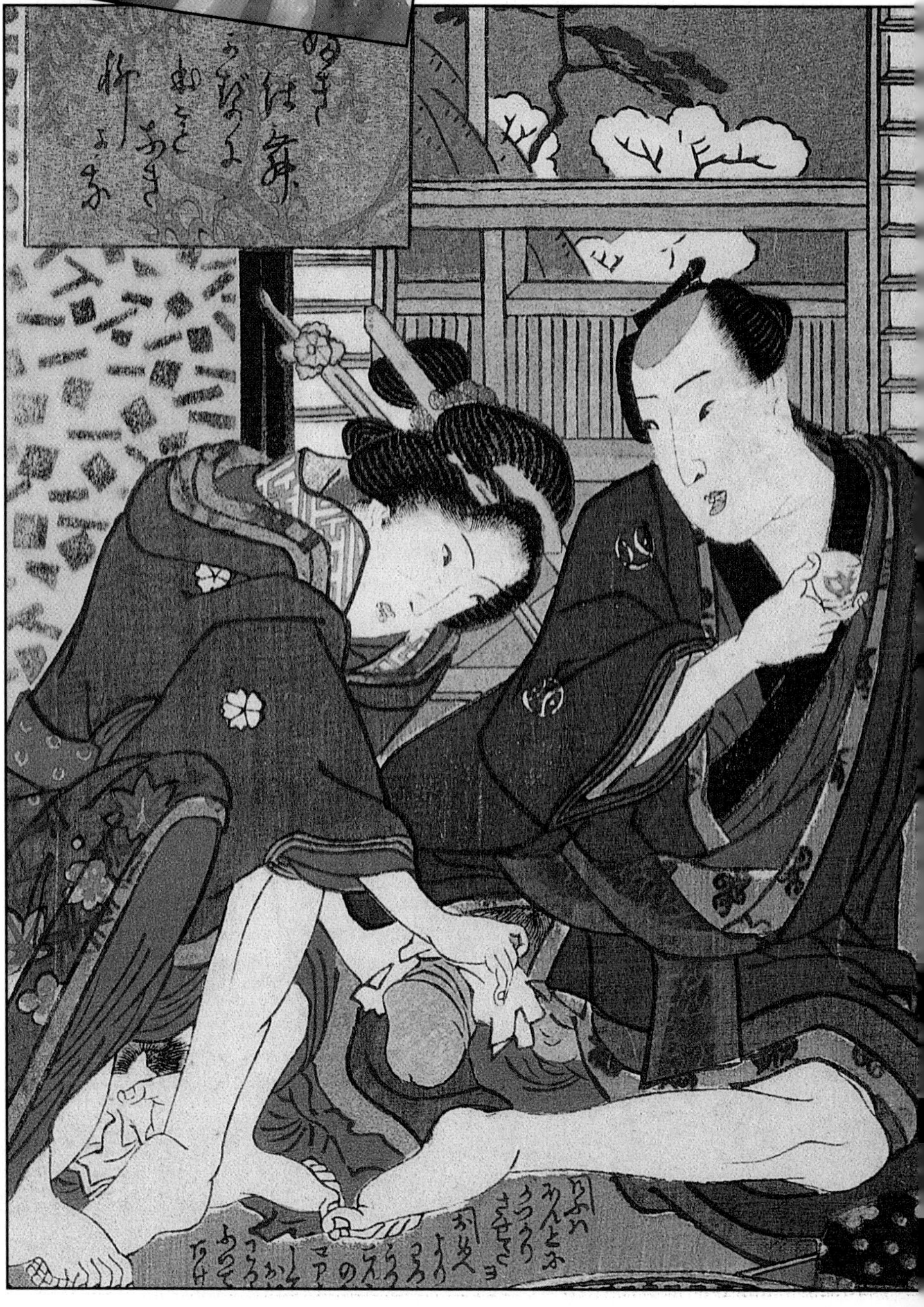

CIRCUMCISION

Male and female circumcision have been traditional in some cultures since ancient times, and are still performed today. Female circumcision is an emotive and much debated issue.

Uncircumcised penises

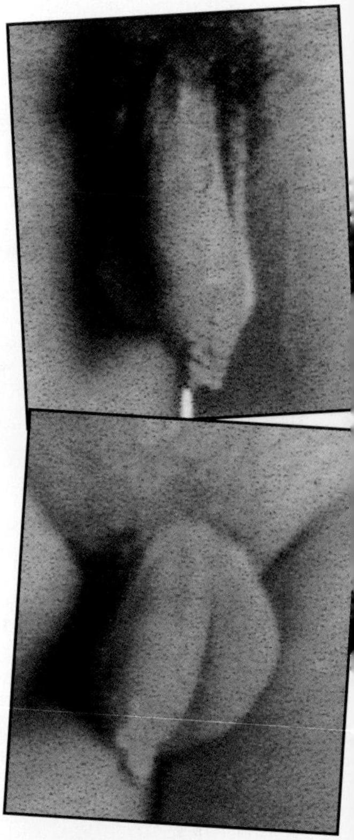

Male circumcision

Male circumcision is both one of the oldest surgical operations (it was already well established in Egypt by 4000 BC) and the most widespread. It is currently estimated that about half of the world's male population is circumcised.

There are several varieties of male circumcision, but the most common consists of the removal of the whole of the foreskin. This is a religious practice amongst Jews and Muslims, and is also customary in many parts of Africa, the Middle East and Australia. The operation may be carried out on babies or small children as a religious birth rite, or on adolescents to mark the passage into manhood. By the twentieth century it had become widespread in societies in which it had no traditional basis, in particular Britain and the United States.

Circumcised penises

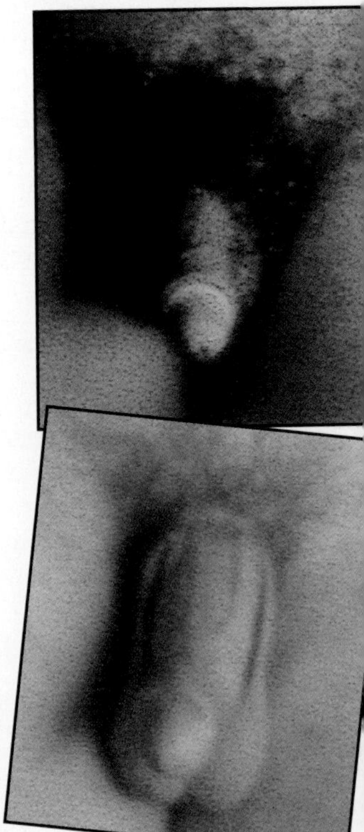

Now the main argument in favour of circumcision is hygiene, as removal of the foreskin eliminates any potential problems with the accumulation of the glandular secretion known as smegma. Circumcision has also been linked with the prevention of various kinds of cancer, as occurrences of both cervical cancer in women and penile cancer in men are significantly less frequent in societies where male circumcision is practised.

In physical terms, the operation is almost always unnecessary. In adults it is intensely painful and there is a risk of complications, such as infections and withering of the penis. However, the use of anaesthetic and hygienic medical procedure reduces these dangers, so that this ancient custom can be carried out more safely.

See also:
penis
vagina
sexual attraction

FACT: There is no clinical evidence to suggest that circumcision affects sexual capacity in any way.

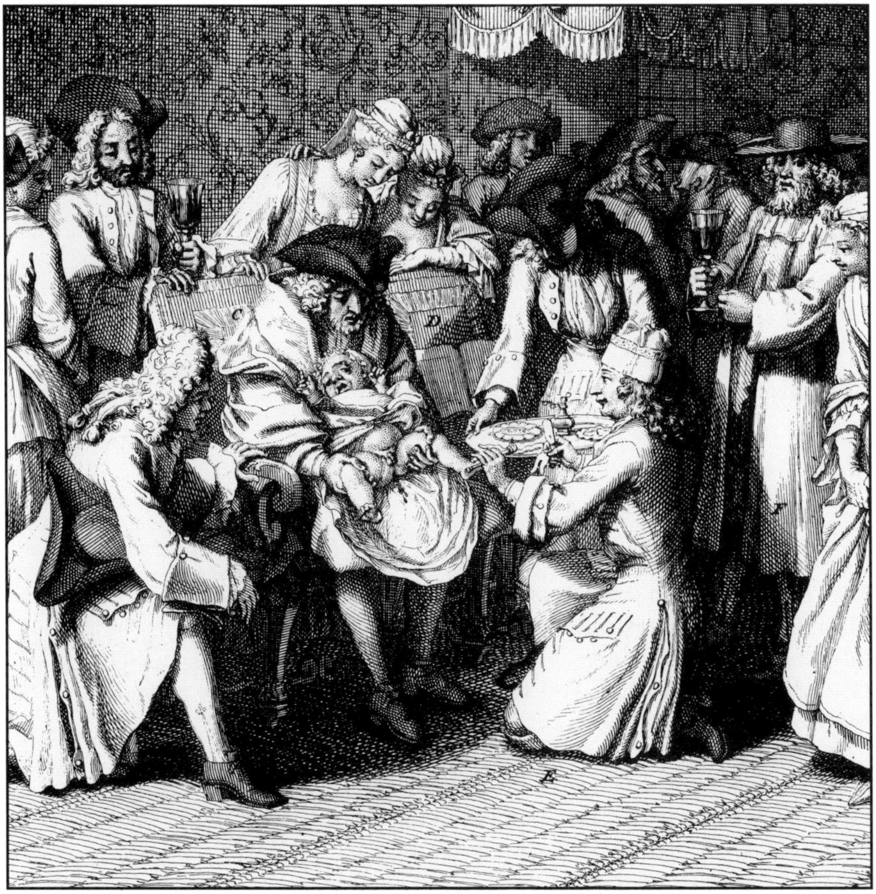

A Portuguese Jewish circumcision ceremony, depicted in an eighteenth century engraving. The child's father is standing at the back on the left, with a glass of wine in his hand, while his mother is not permitted to attend the ceremony.

FACT: There is enormous variety in the nature of circumcision practices and in their origins. For example, the Hottentots of southern Africa are said to have cut off one of the testicles before marriage as this was believed to prevent the conception of twins, which was deemed extremely unlucky. Meanwhile some Australian societies practise subincision of the penis, cutting along the length of the underside of the penis as deep as the urethra. It is thought that the intention may be to imitate the wider, two-headed penis of the kangaroo, whose sexual prowess is admired.

Female circumcision

Female circumcision is less frequent than male, but it is the subject of considerably more controversy. It is estimated that it has been carried out on 90 to 100 million women alive today.

The most common forms of female circumcision are clitoridectomy and infibulation. Clitoridectomy involves the removal of the clitoris and sometimes other parts of the vulva. Infibulation is the sewing together of the labia majora, leaving only a very small hole for urination and menstruation; it usually involves the removal of parts or all of the clitoris and labia minora. Female circumcision is carried out in children or young women before puberty and marriage. Clitoridectomy is quite common throughout Africa and in some Islamic groups. Infibulation is most common in eastern Africa. Both are also becoming increasingly common among immigrant populations in Britain and the USA.

A circumcised girl from Somalia, where female circumcision is still widely practised.

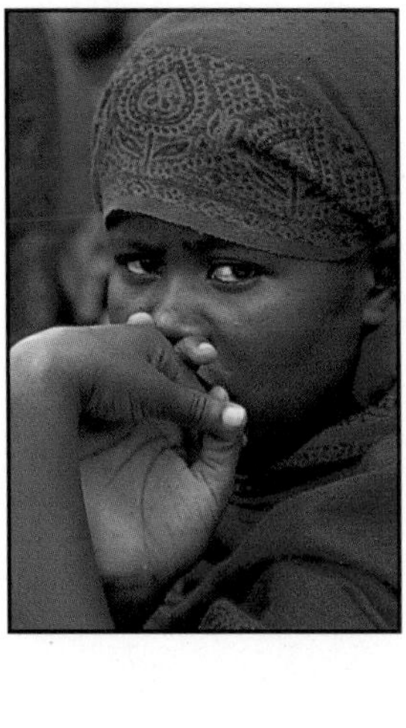

The origins almost certainly lie in a specific intention to reduce or eliminate women's sexual pleasure, as the operation holds no benefit for the woman at all outside social convention. The number of deaths resulting from complications or infections remains high. It is surrounded by controversy, as on the one hand it is seen as a brutal and dangerous practice inflicted on women by a male-oriented society, but on the other it is also an ancient and deeply-rooted tradition.

SAFER SEX

'Safer sex' is the term used for the various ways of adapting sexual activity to reduce the risk of sexually transmitted infections. These may range from minor infections such as thrush, to HIV, the virus which can lead to AIDS. The point of safer sex is to minimize these risks while making sexual activity as enjoyable and varied as ever – and perhaps even more so.

Basically, safer sex means sexual activity in which body fluids are not mixed. The forms which it can take are almost endless.

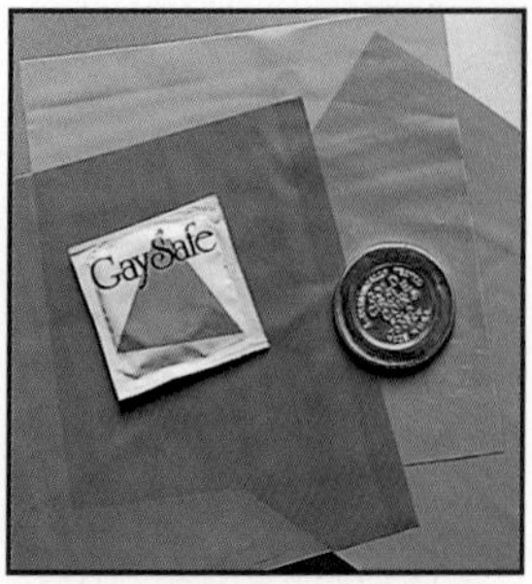

Special condoms for anal sex and dental dams for oral sex, to be used as part of safer sex practices.

Spermicides and microbicides
Spermicides are chemicals which kill sperm. In tests they have also been shown to be capable of killing HIV and various kinds of bacteria. However, as yet they are not sufficiently effective on their own, and are best used in conjunction with other methods such as condoms.

Research is also being carried out on chemicals which function not as contraceptives but just as microbicides: that is, chemicals which kill infection-carrying microbes or bacteria. Effective viracides are also being sought.

Condoms

The most common modes of transmission of STDs and AIDS are vaginal and anal intercourse. If used carefully, the condom is one of the most reliable and widely available methods of making these activities safer. Condoms should be used with a water-based lubricant, particularly for anal intercourse. Oil-based substances such as Vaseline, body lotion or massage oil should be avoided, as they weaken the latex of the condom, often causing it to split. Many brands of condom are bought pre-lubricated with spermicides, which can themselves kill some infections.

Extra-strong condoms should be used for anal intercourse. The female condom can also be used for both vaginal and anal intercourse. Made of polyurethane instead of latex, it is less vulnerable to damage from oil-based lubricants.

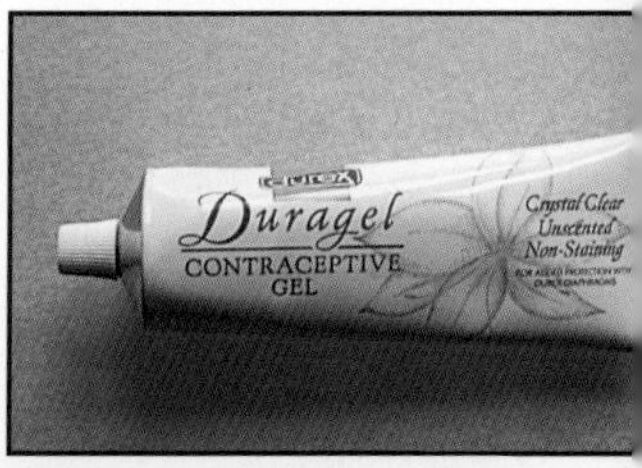

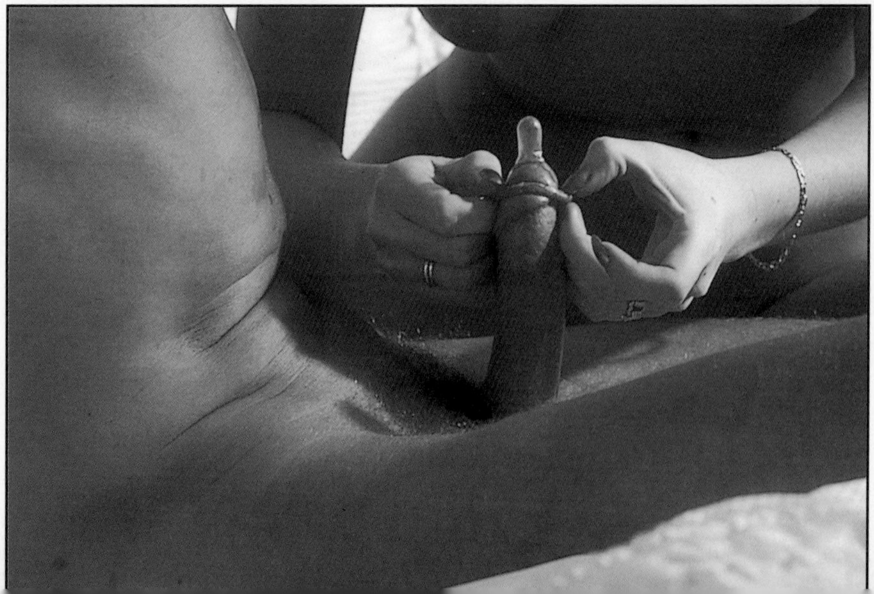

See also:
sexual practices
contraception

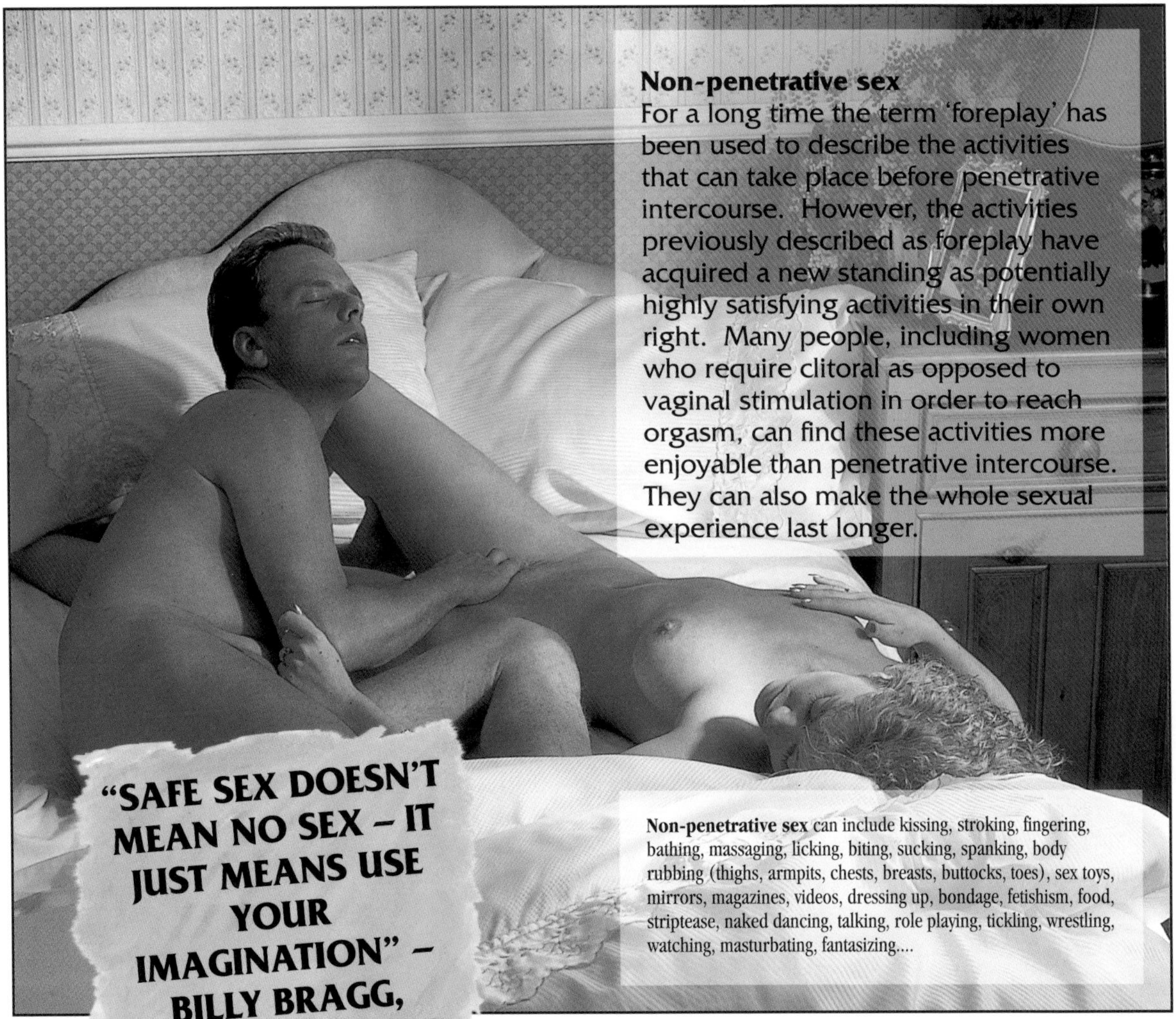

Non-penetrative sex

For a long time the term 'foreplay' has been used to describe the activities that can take place before penetrative intercourse. However, the activities previously described as foreplay have acquired a new standing as potentially highly satisfying activities in their own right. Many people, including women who require clitoral as opposed to vaginal stimulation in order to reach orgasm, can find these activities more enjoyable than penetrative intercourse. They can also make the whole sexual experience last longer.

Non-penetrative sex can include kissing, stroking, fingering, bathing, massaging, licking, biting, sucking, spanking, body rubbing (thighs, armpits, chests, breasts, buttocks, toes), sex toys, mirrors, magazines, videos, dressing up, bondage, fetishism, food, striptease, naked dancing, talking, role playing, tickling, wrestling, watching, masturbating, fantasizing....

"SAFE SEX DOESN'T MEAN NO SEX – IT JUST MEANS USE YOUR IMAGINATION" – BILLY BRAGG, 'SEXUALITY' TOUR.

Oral sex

Oral sex does involve some risk of transmission of certain infections and diseases to the person performing the oral sex. However, it is considerably less than the risk associated with unprotected penetrative sex and can be all but eliminated by using condoms or dental dams. A dental dam is a square of latex that is placed over the vulva or anus; a condom cut down one side can be used in the same way. Flavoured dams and condoms are available

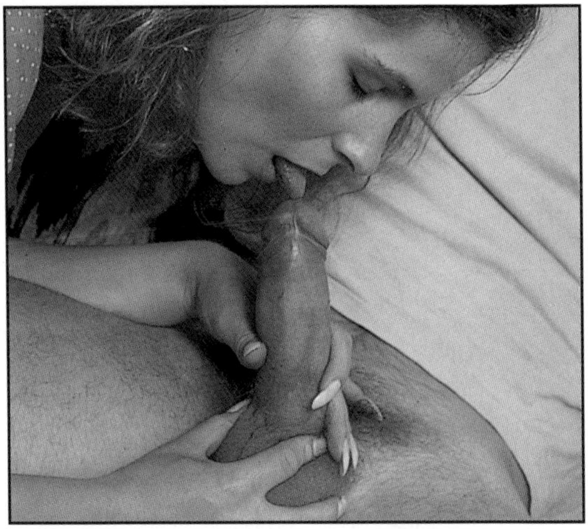

DISORDERS

INFECTIONS & DISEASES OF THE SEXUAL AND REPRODUCTIVE ORGANS

References to sexually transmitted diseases (STDs) appear in the early writings of most cultures. They can be found both in the Bible and in early Hindu mythology. Two of the oldest are syphilis and gonorrhoea, which have been widespread for centuries. Their origins are unknown. They have been referred to as 'the French pox', 'Indian measles', 'the Italian disease', and 'the Portuguese illness', each country keen to blame another and thereby absolve itself from responsibility. Historically they have been spread by voyages of discovery and military campaigns in particular.

Control and elimination

Two major breakthroughs were the discovery of the microscope, which facilitated diagnosis, and penicillin, which provided the first safe, reliable cure. Before these advances diagnosis had been haphazard and treatment had been localized, unreliable or simply dangerous. The mass production of penicillin after the Second World War and the increasing availability and use of condoms brought new hope for the control – if not the elimination – of the gravest sexually transmitted infections and diseases. With the scare induced by HIV/AIDS, the incidence of STDs dropped for a few years. However, recently their spread has increased once more.

NOTICE

EFFECTIVE TREATMENT
MEDICAL HELP SHOULD BE SOUGHT IF AN INFECTION OR DISORDER OF THE SEXUAL OR REPRODUCTIVE ORGANS IS SUSPECTED. TREATMENT IS EFFECTIVE IN MOST CASES IF INITIATED IN THE EARLY STAGES OF INFECTION.

Pubic lice (pediculosis pubis) clinging to pubic hair.

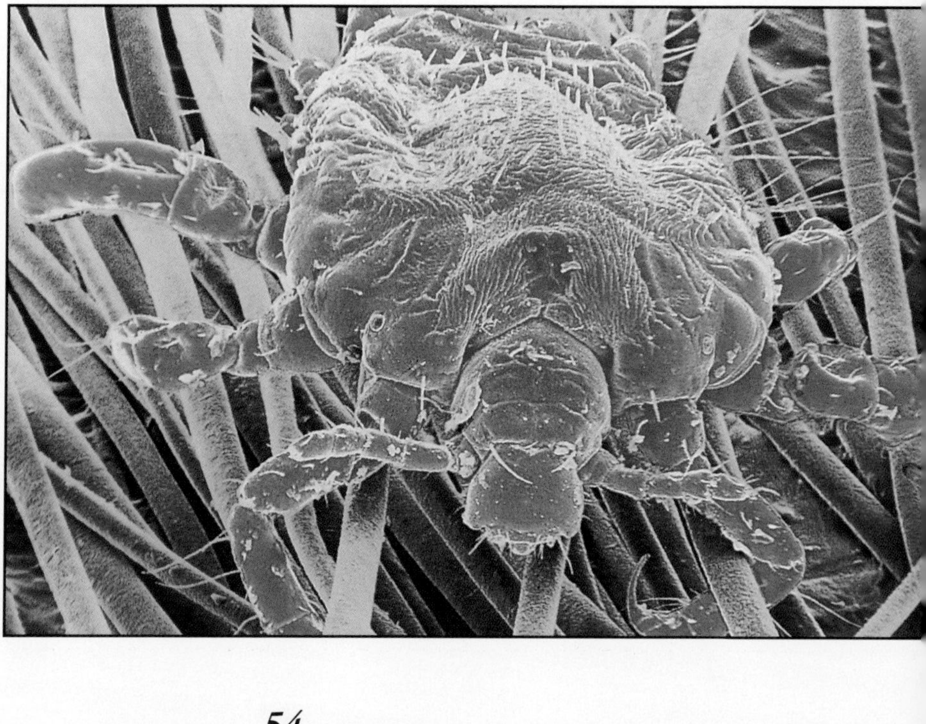

See also:
HIV and AIDS
safer sex

INFECTIONS/DISORDERS CAUSED BY SEXUAL CONTACT AND NON-SEXUAL MEANS

NON-SPECIFIC GENITAL INFECTIONS

These cover a large group of infections which are some of the most common disorders of the sexual and reproductive organs.

They include:

cystitis (inflammation of the bladder)

vaginitis (inflammation of the vagina)

salpingitis (inflammation of a fallopian tube)

urethritis (inflammation of the urethra)

balanitis (inflammation of the glans penis)

posthitis (inflammation of the foreskin)

proctitis (inflammation of the rectum)

Causes: various bacterial and non-bacterial germs, allergies or friction. They may also occur as symptoms of other infections or diseases.

Symptoms: any unusual discharge, irritation or discomfort in the genital area may indicate an infection.

Treatment: there are various options available for most non-specific infections, often including antibiotics.

PUBIC LICE
(pediculosis pubis)

Cause: pubic lice are wingless parasites. They infest the hair in the pubic area and occasionally on other parts of the body. They feed on blood by biting into the skin. Eggs are laid and attached to the root of the hairs, hatching a week later. They are passed from one person to another through close bodily contact and occasionally from infested clothes, towels or bedding.

Symptoms: the bites may cause acute irritation, but there are often no symptoms at all.

Treatment: DDT emulsion or powder. Shaving is not necessary, although it does provide a rapid cure.

THRUSH

Cause: a fungus called candida albicans, a type of yeast which exists normally and harmlessly in the skin, mouth and gut. Under certain conditions it can multiply and cause discomfort in genital areas and sometimes in the mouth in both men and women. Factors that can lead to infection with thrush include:

- wearing tight trousers or nylon underwear
- using perfumed soaps or genital deodorants
- taking certain antibiotics
- diabetes
- pregnancy
- ill health
- sexual contact with someone who is infected with thrush

Symptoms in women may include:

- irritation and soreness around the vagina, vulva or anus
- thick, white, yeasty vaginal discharge
- swollen vulva
- pain on urinating or having sexual intercourse

Symptoms in men may include:

- irritation or soreness on the tip of the penis or under the foreskin
- thick, white discharge under the foreskin
- difficulty in pulling back the foreskin

Treatment: fungicidal cream applied to affected areas in men and women, or fungicidal vaginal pessaries in women.

BACTERIAL VAGINOSIS
(also known as Gardnerella)

Cause: multiplication of bacteria which occur naturally in the vagina, as in thrush. This bacteria seems to affect women only.

Symptoms: watery, grey vaginal discharge with 'fishy' odour, especially after sexual intercourse.

Treatment: a short course of antibiotics.

INFECTIONS/DISORDERS CAUSED BY SEXUAL CONTACT AND NON-SEXUAL MEANS

SCABIES (the 'itch')

Cause: a parasitic mite. The disease is spread by close physical contact and poor hygiene, including infested clothes, towels and bedding. The mites survive by burrowing into the outer layers of the skin, most commonly on the hairy parts of the body, although they can also affect the hands, particularly the web of the fingers. They can also spread to other parts of the body. The female also lays eggs in these burrows.

Symptoms: the burrows appear as fine black or white lines surrounded by inflamed skin and with a blister at one end. The saliva and droppings produced by the mites cause acute irritation.

Treatment: application of a lotion such as benzyl benzoate or malathion all over the body from the neck down. The treatment may have to be repeated several times.

GENITAL HERPES

Cause: the herpes simplex virus, which affects the genital and anal areas and occasionally the mouth. It is passed through genital or oral-genital contact. People are particularly infectious when they have the characteristic genital blisters or oral cold sores, and intercourse should be avoided at this time; however it is also possible, although more rare, for the virus to be passed on when there are no symptoms. It can be passed from the genital area to the mouth and from the mouth to the genital area.

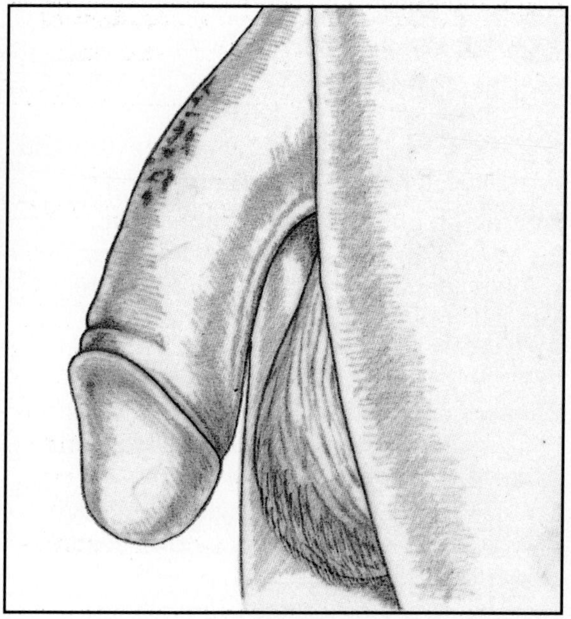

Symptoms may include:

- in the genital or anal area small, painful blisters form then burst to leave red ulcers. These usually heal within one to two weeks.
- stinging, tingling or itching in the genital or anal area
- (particularly in women) pain or burning sensation when passing urine
- cold sores on the mouth
- general flu-type symptoms such as headache, backache, fever or swollen glands

These symptoms tend to occur within a week of infection. Relapses are common, but the first outbreaks are usually the worst.

Treatment: no cure for herpes has yet been found. However, there are various remedies which can ease the symptoms and help to ward off attacks.

HEPATITIS B

Cause: a virus present in the blood and other bodily fluids of an infected person, causing inflammation of the liver. It is passed on by sexual contact and contact with other body fluids, including blood, saliva and urine.

Symptoms occur in three stages, although in some people no symptoms are apparent.

Stage one: one to six months after initial infection

- flu-type symptoms
- fatigue and loss of appetite
- aching joints

INFECTIONS/DISORDERS CAUSED BY SEXUAL CONTACT AND NON-SEXUAL MEANS

HEPATITIS B (continued)

Stage two: jaundice stage, lasting two to eight weeks

- yellowish colouring of skin and whites of eyes
- dark brown urine and light-coloured faeces
- pain in the abdomen
- weight loss

Recovery stage:

- skin and eye colour return to normal
- urine and faeces return to normal

Treatment: rest and a healthy diet, excluding alcohol. Complete recovery may take several months. In some people there may be long-term liver damage.

INFECTIONS/DISORDERS CAUSED BY SEXUAL CONTACT ONLY

GENITAL WARTS

Cause: certain types of a virus called the human papilloma virus. It is passed through skin-to-skin contact with the wart, primarily through vaginal or anal intercourse. Once a person has been infected by the virus, it can take from two weeks to a year for the warts to appear.

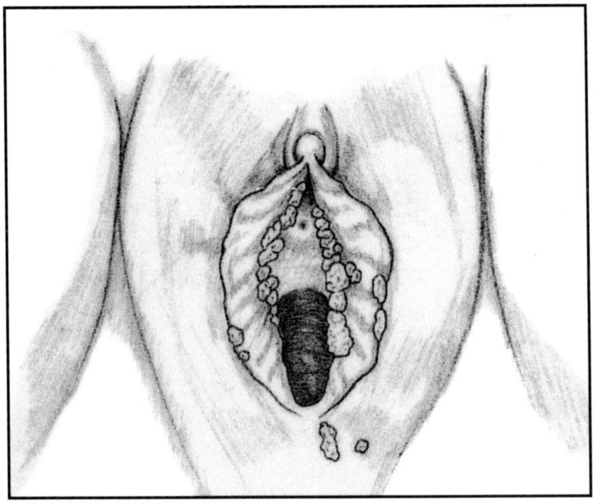

INFECTIONS/DISORDERS CAUSED BY SEXUAL CONTACT ONLY

GENITAL WARTS (continued)

Symptoms: the warts appear as fleshy growths of various sizes, on their own or in clusters. In women they are found in the vulva, vagina, cervix and anus, and have been implicated in cervical cancers. In men they are found in the penis, urethra and anus. They may itch but are seldom painful.

Treatment: usually by painting with a liquid

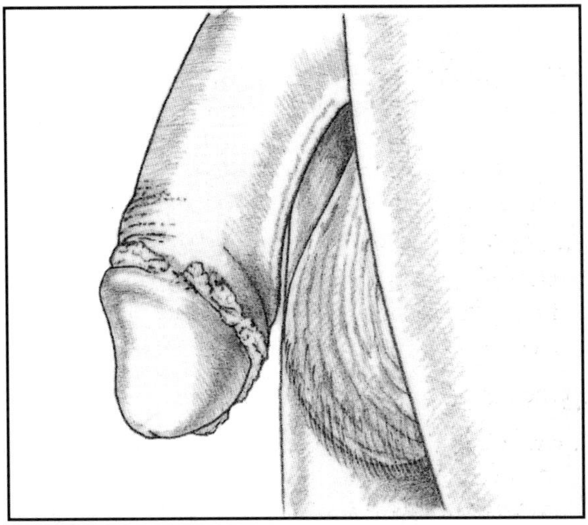

called podophyllin, several applications of which are necessary. They can also be frozen or cauterized.

TRICHOMONIASIS

Cause: a small parasite which infects the vagina. It is almost always passed through sexual contact. Men are only rarely infected, in the urethra. They can be carriers.

Symptoms in women are sometimes unnoticeable, but may include:

- a change in vaginal discharge, which becomes more watery or frothy, slightly yellow or green in colour, with a strong odour
- soreness and irritation in the vaginal area

INFECTIONS/DISORDERS SPREAD BY SEXUAL CONTACT ONLY

TRICHOMONIASIS (continued)

If untreated it can cause other infections such as non-specific urethritis (NSU) in men and vaginitis (inflammation of the vagina) in women. These are also curable.

Treatment: a course of tablets of the drug metronidazole for both partners.

CHLAMYDIA

Cause: a bacteria which infects the genitals and sometimes the eyes and throat. It is passed primarily through sexual contact, but can also be passed from mother to new-born baby, causing lung disease and eye infection. Chlamydia may lie dormant for some time before symptoms become evident.

Symptoms: there are usually no symptoms, and chlamydia often passes unnoticed. In women there may be vaginal discharge or pain on urinating. In most cases chlamydia is only noticed when it spreads elsewhere, in particular to the urethra where in men it is the most common cause of urethritis. In women it may lead to pelvic inflammatory disease (PID), which can cause infertility.

Treatment: a seven- to fourteen-day course of antibiotics.

NON-GONOCOCCAL URETHRITIS (NGU) (also known as non-specific urethritis or NSU)

Cause: NGU is an inflammation of a man's urethra, **NSU** an inflammation of a woman's sexual organs, caused by a number of different germs. The germs can be in the body for some time before any symptoms become evident.

Symptoms may include:

- discomfort or burning pain on urinating
- white, cloudy discharge from the tip of the penis

There may be no symptoms at all.

NON-GONOCOCCAL URETHRITIS (NGU) (continued)

Without treatment the inflammation can spread to the prostate gland and sometimes to the testes. This can be painful, and can even affect fertility.

Treatment: a seven to fourteen day course of antibiotics.

CHANCROID

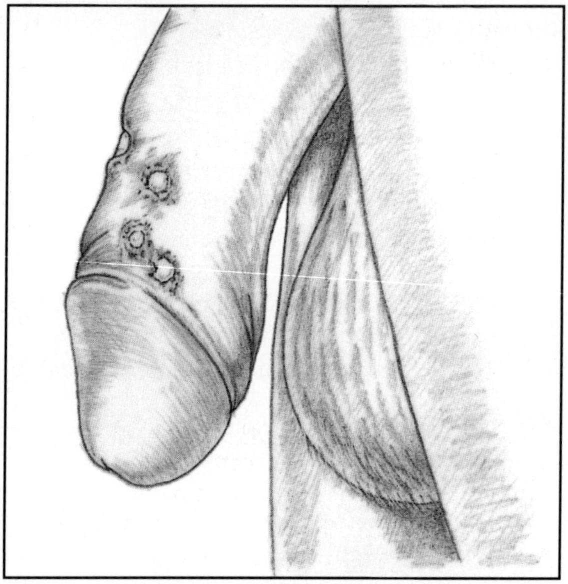

Cause: a bacterial infection which rarely occurs outside tropical and sub-tropical areas.

Symptoms: In men these appear about a week after infection, when a soft, inflamed ulcer appears on the genitals. It bleeds easily, and often spreads extensively, causing acutely painful destruction of the flesh. In extreme cases the foreskin and the head of the penis can be ulcerated away. Abscesses may also develop. Symptoms are seldom evident in women, as the lesions can be vulval or even within the vagina.

Treatment: antibiotics, sulphonamide drugs.

INFECTIONS/DISORDERS SPREAD BY SEXUAL CONTACT ONLY

GONORRHOEA

Cause: a bacterium called the gonococcus. It can affect the cervix, urethra, rectum, and occasionally the throat if it is passed by oral-genital contact. Its incubation period is usually two to ten days. It attacks the mucous membranes, causing inflammation and the production of pus.

Symptoms in men:

These are usually obvious and may include:

- discharge of white or yellow fluid from the tip of the penis
- burning pain when urinating
- discharge or irritation in the anus
- a sore throat

Symptoms in women:

These are usually slight and may even pass unnoticed. They can include:

- a change in the vaginal discharge, which may increase in quantity, become more watery, or turn slightly yellow or green in colour
- pain or discomfort when urinating
- pain in the abdomen
- discharge or irritation in the anus
- a sore throat

If untreated, in men gonorrhoea can lead to acute or chronic inflammation of the urethra, testes and prostate gland. These can cause difficulty in urinating and even sterility.

In women it can cause pelvic inflammatory disease (PID), which can lead to sterility. During childbirth it can be passed on to the baby as an eye infection.

Treatment: penicillin and other antibiotics are very effective in treating most cases of gonorrhoea, but early diagnosis is essential if the disease is to be cured completely.

SYPHILLIS

Cause: a bacteria called the treponema. This enters the body through tiny cracks in the skin or by penetrating mucus membranes, then lives and multiplies in the blood and other body fluids of the infected person. It is passed on by the fluid secreted from the characteristic sores or chancres.

Symptoms: the development of syphilis occurs in three stages. The symptoms are the same in men and women.

Stage one: Between one and twelve weeks after infection a hard, painless sore develops on or near the penis or vagina, or sometimes in the anus or mouth. It usually lasts two to three weeks.

Stage two: two to six months after infection a skin rash appears all over the body. It may develop to form pimples or pustules. Flu-like symptoms may also occur. This lasts for two to six weeks. Sometimes these first two stages are not even noticeable. Natural antibodies are also produced in the body, which in some cases are sufficient to cure the disease.

Late stage: this may occur long after the other symptoms have disappeared, many years after infection. If untreated the treponema can affect other parts of the body, and damage the heart and brain in particular. They can cause disfigurement and death, though nowadays this is rare.

Treatment: syphilis can be treated very effectively with penicillin if the disease is diagnosed early.

NOTICE

EFFECTIVE TREATMENT

MEDICAL HELP SHOULD BE SOUGHT IF AN INFECTION OR DISORDER OF THE SEXUAL OR REPRODUCTIVE ORGANS IS SUSPECTED. TREATMENT IS EFFECTIVE IN MOST CASES IF INITIATED IN THE EARLY STAGES OF INFECTION.

HIV AND AIDS

AIDS, the Acquired Immune Deficiency Syndrome, is caused by the Human Immunodeficiency Virus, HIV. In an infected person (someone who is 'HIV positive', or HIV+) HIV prevents the immune system – the body's defence mechanism – from working effectively. It does this by attacking the cells (known as CD4 cells) that co-ordinate the fight against infections. This makes the body vulnerable to potentially fatal infections that the immune system would normally destroy.

The Human Immunodeficiency Virus, HIV, the virus which causes AIDS.

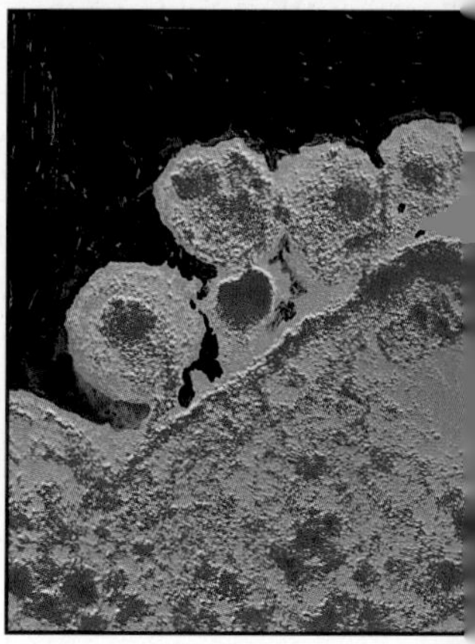

Defining AIDS

The precise definition of AIDS varies from one authority to another, and continues to evolve as understanding of the disease develops. Generally, a person is considered to have AIDS if they are suffering from one or more of a specific group of diseases associated with HIV infection, or if their CD4 cells fall from a normal count of 800 to below 200. Incubation periods ranging from eighteen months to ten years have been recorded, while some people never develop AIDS or any symptoms at all.

Warren Hills Cemetery, Harare, Zimbabwe. It is estimated that at the end of 1994, seventeen per cent of the adult population of Zimbabwe – 900,000 people – were HIV positive (World Health Organization).

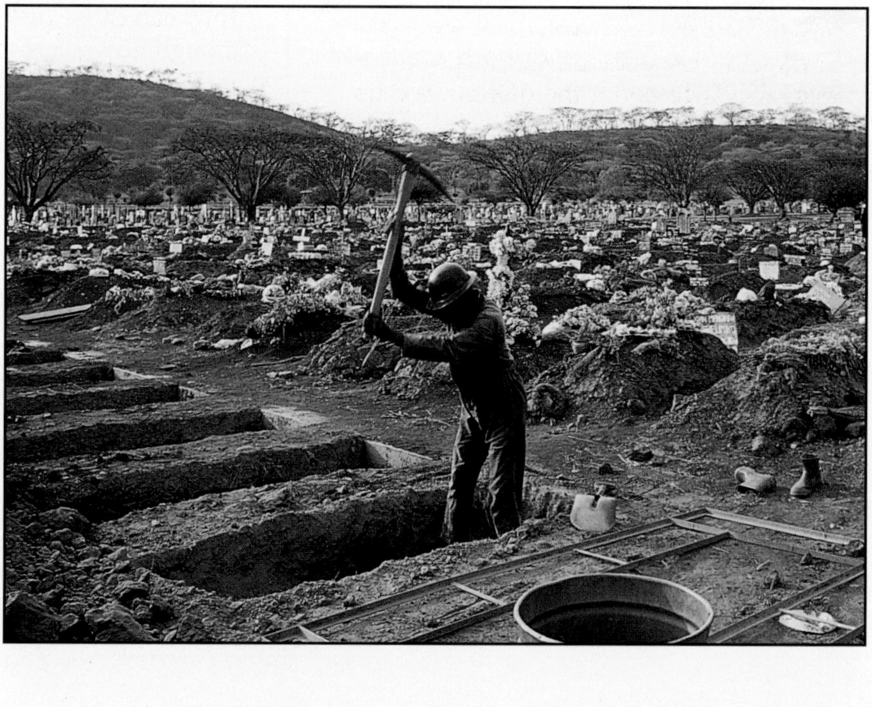

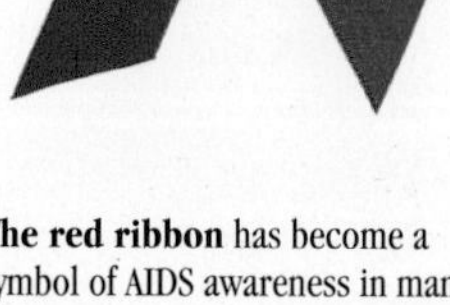

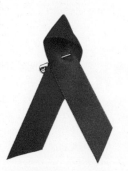

The red ribbon has become a symbol of AIDS awareness in many countries.

Symptoms

It is impossible to give an exhaustive list of symptoms of AIDS, as the forms taken by the disease are so varied. However, pneumonia, with shortness of breath, is the most common opportunistic infection and the often the first to appear. Other common minor symptoms, known as the AIDS-Related Complex (ARC), include weight loss, diarrhoea, fever, rashes, fatigue, coughing, insomnia, nausea and memory problems. Some of the other major symptoms of AIDS are recurrent herpes simplex, persistent generalized lymphadenopathy, a form of skin cancer called Kaposi's sarcoma, and cryptococcal meningitis.

The history of AIDS

AIDS was first diagnosed as a distinct syndrome in the USA in 1981. The disease was discovered as a result of an increasing number of unusual infections, primarily amongst the homosexual population, caused by a form of immune deficiency. It was only later that it was directly associated with other groups. Since that time the disease has spread to all sectors of society.

It was not recognized that the condition was caused by a virus until HIV was discovered in 1983. The main ways in which HIV is spread are now well understood (see next page). However, amongst the general public ignorance about the disease and its transmission is still widespread.

The origins of the virus remain unknown. It has been linked more strongly to Africa than other regions, but in reality there is little or no solid evidence to suggest where it came from or how it developed. It may have existed in humans for anything between twenty-five and a hundred years.

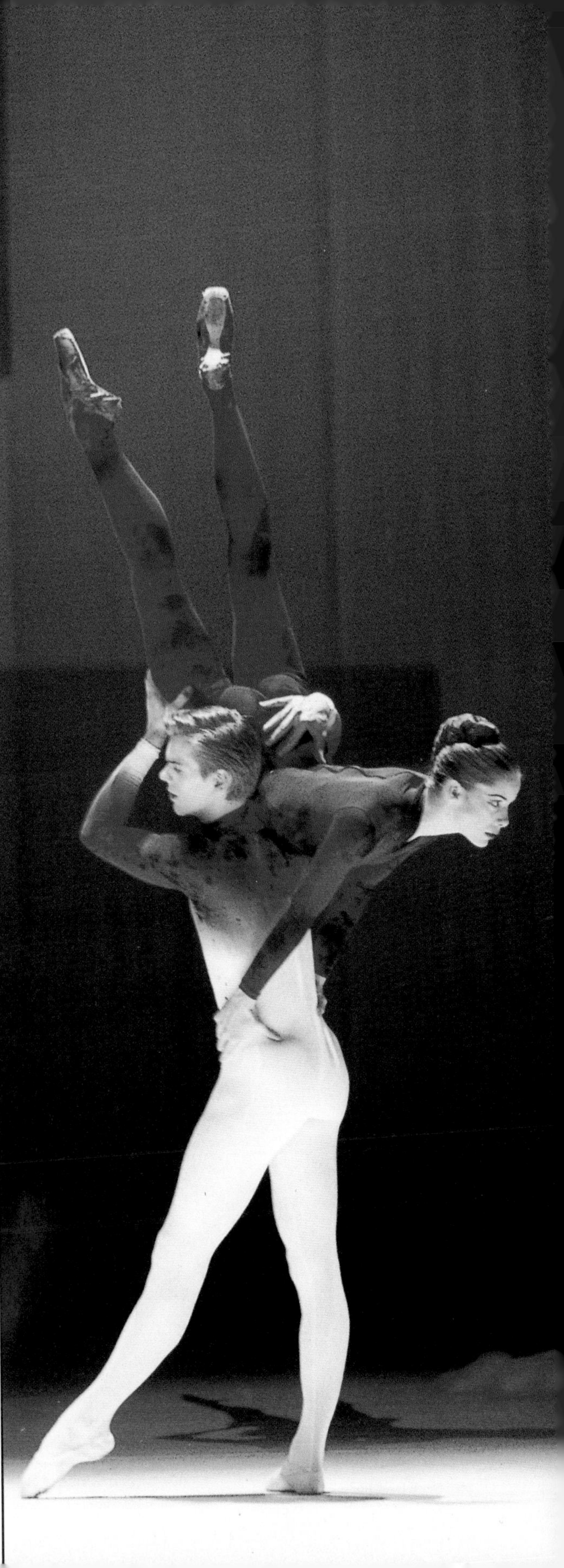

Dance with Death,
the ballet about HIV and AIDS,
choreographed by Mathew Hart
and performed by
The Royal Ballet, London, 1996.

Transmission
HIV is carried in various body fluids; in particular in blood and semen, vaginal and cervical secretions, and breast milk. It can be passed to another person through open wounds, broken skin or mucous membranes such as those in the urethra, vagina, cervix and rectum. There are four proven, substantial routes of transmission of HIV.

These are:
- unprotected sexual intercourse (vaginal, anal or oral – see under 'Safer sex')
- shared, unsterilized injection equipment in intravenous drug use
- blood transfusion or organ donation (thorough screening is now carried out in most countries to eliminate this risk)
- more rarely, from mother to baby in the womb, during childbirth or breast-feeding

Other activities which are potential routes of transmission include oral sex and sharing sex toys, as well as any activities which might involve shared blood, such as piercing and shaving.

Treatments
As yet there is no cure or vaccine for HIV. However, various medical treatments are available, functioning in a number of different ways, attacking the virus itself by reducing the speed at which it reproduces or by preventing it from fulfiling other functions.

These treatments include:
- AZT, a drug based on the building blocks of DNA and the first widely licensed treatment boosting the immune system inhibiting infectious co-factors
- preventing and treating opportunistic infections
- complementary and alternative therapies (i.e. non-scientific treatments such as homeopathy, acupuncture, massage and visualization) are also available, which may fulfil the above functions and help reduce stress, improve psychological health, and relieve pain.

In the meantime, research into the virus, its causes and possible cures, continues.

The International Display of the Entire NAMES Project AIDS Memorial Quilt, October 9 - 11, 1992.

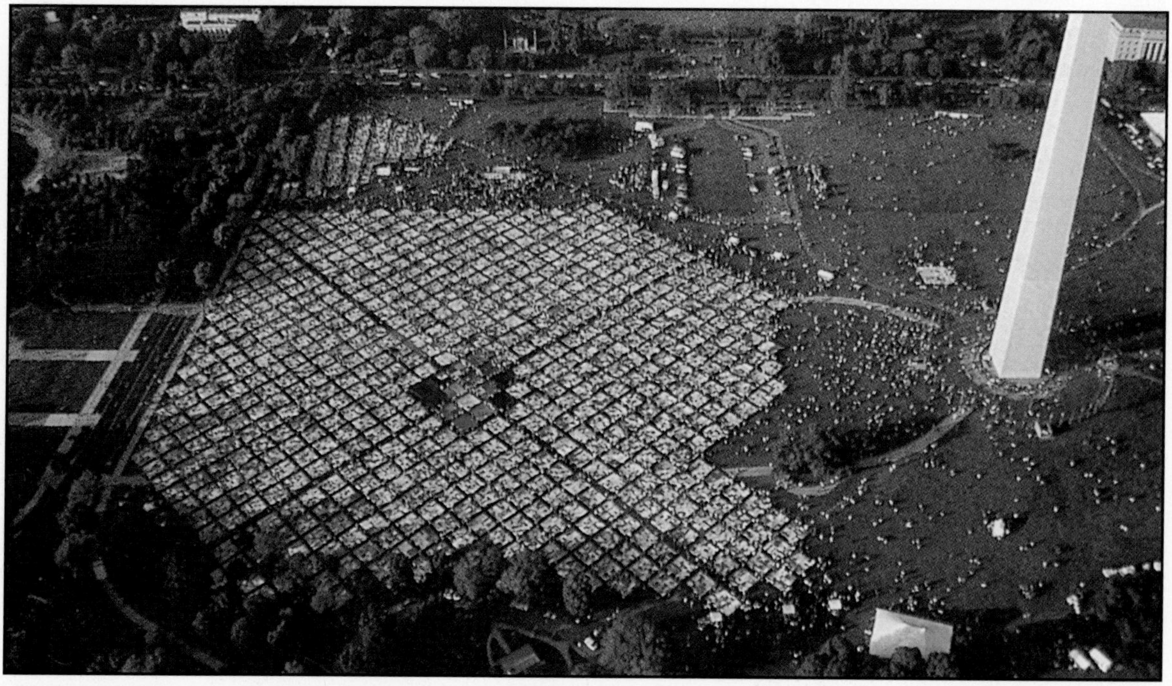

• **HIV** has not been detected in urine, faeces or vomit (except where these contain blood) or sweat. Only negligible quantities, insufficient for infection, have been detected in saliva, tears and blister fluid.

• **HIV** cannot be passed through casual acquaintance. Touching and kissing involve no risk provided that body fluids are not exchanged.

• **HIV** cannot be passed through shared cups, glasses, plates, cutlery, beds, baths or bed clothes.

• **HIV** cannot be passed on toilet seats, in swimming pools, or by sharing an office or classroom with an infected person.

• **HIV** cannot be passed by mosquitoes or other insects.

• **HIV** cannot be acquired by donating blood.

• **HIV** can only be passed during First Aid if substantial quantities of blood from an infected person come into contact with an open wound, cut or graze.

• **HIV** has never been known to be passed through mouth-to-mouth resuscitation.

It is particular behaviours that carry risk, not particular groups of people.

FACT: Various pre-1980s cases have been retrospectively (and controversially) diagnosed through descriptions of specific patterns of symptoms and stored blood samples. It is not known for how long the virus has existed in humans. It is thought that HIV might have escaped diagnosis in the pre-1940s period in the midst of the many infectious diseases in existence at that time.

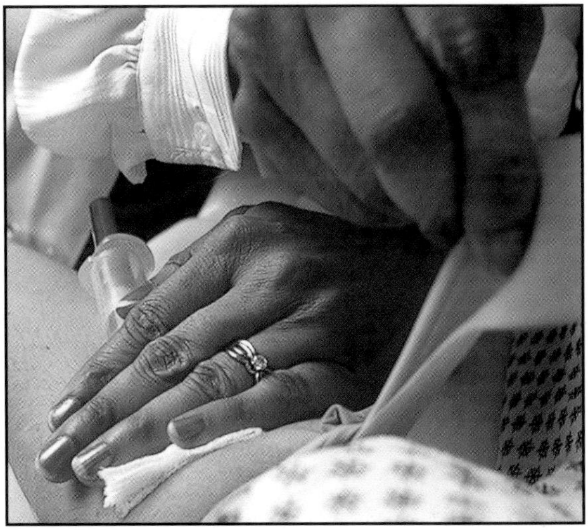

Testing
The HIV test is based on the detection of HIV antibodies in a sample of blood. Antibodies are substances produced by the body in response to a particular infection: the presence of the antibodies indicates the presence of the virus. It may be several months after exposure before the antibodies can be reliably detected, so it is often necessary to carry out two tests a few months apart. Testing on a regular basis may be advisable if a person is considered to be at risk.

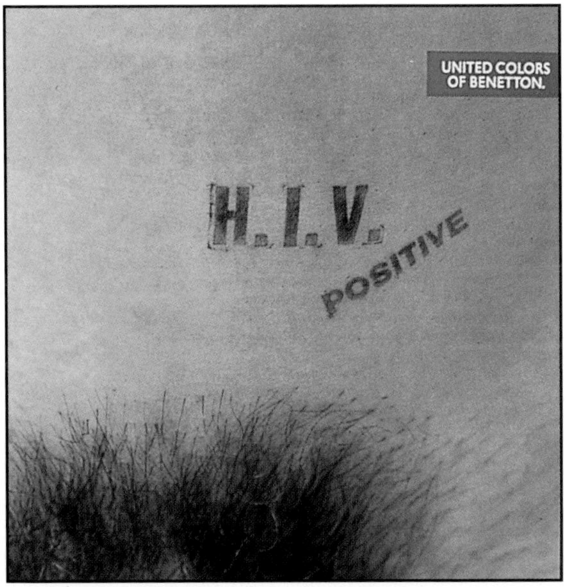

It is impossible to tell whether or not a person is HIV+ by their appearance.

SEXUAL HARASSMENT & ABUSE

Harassment

Sexual harassment is the use of sex to threaten or intimidate. It is the use of sex as a means of gaining power over an individual.

Sexual harassment can occur anywhere: at work, at home or in public places. It may come from strangers, acquaintances, colleagues, friends or sexual partners. It can include anything from wolf whistles to rubbing up against a stranger's body in a crowd, from obscene comments or phone calls to overt demands for sex: the key is that the behaviour in question is sexual in intent and that it is unwanted and unprovoked. Victims are usually women, but men may also be affected; in either case the harassor may be male or female.

The harm which it does is not physical, but psychological and emotional. In many societies and social groups sexual harassment is barely acknowledged, because there is no physical evidence or because the victim is seen as somehow responsible. This often has to do with the victim's class, race or social status: being seen as inferior in any way immediately damages credibility. In some countries sexual harassment in the work place is a criminal offence, but cases are notoriously difficult to prove as they tend to amount to one person's word against another's.

Child abuse

Sexual abuse of children is almost certainly the most disturbing form of abuse. While most children have some degree of sexual awareness, child sexuality is quite distinct from adult. A child may be aware of certain sexual issues but is rarely able to control them or make informed, mature decisions about them. Child abuse implies coercion and dominance, however subtle this may be.

Child abuse is sometimes divided into two types, incestuous and non-incestuous. Statistically, incestuous abuse is most commonly between father and daughter, although it has been suggested that this is less likely to occur where the father takes an active role in the day-to-day care of the child

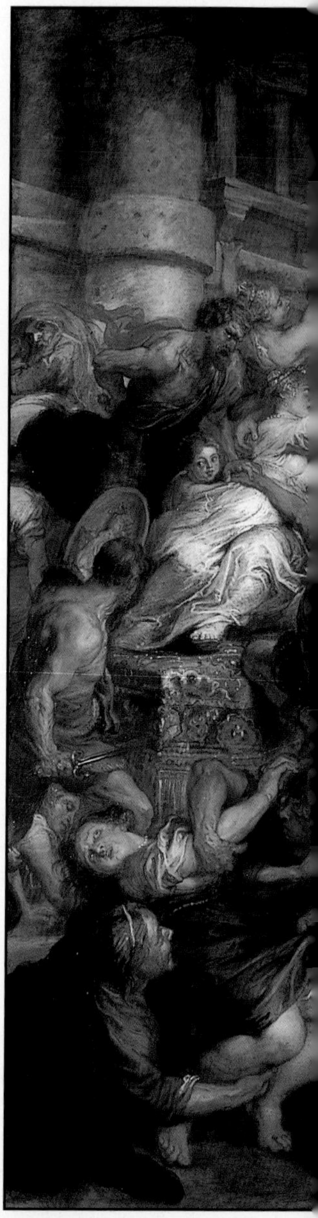

Sex crimes
Rape is forcing a person to have sexual intercourse against their will. Above: detail from a painting by Peter Paul Rubens (1577–1640) of the Rape of the Sabines.

or children. Incestuous abuse may also be instigated by an elder sibling or, more rarely, the mother; non-incestuous abuse may be perpetrated by a stranger, an acquaintance or a carer.

The immaturity of the victim complicates the issue of proving that abuse has occurred. A child cannot be relied upon to be able to tell truth from fiction, or to comprehend the importance of telling the truth. Children also tend to be more suggestible than adults. This becomes more complex still when members of the family are involved.

Victims of abuse often suffer long-term consequences, such as a difficulty in forming stable, trusting, loving relationships. If the abuse is incestuous it can affect the entire family. However, counselling is often extremely helpful, both for the victim and sometimes for the family as well. Many people are able to come to terms with their experiences and integrate them successfully.

Rape

Rape is forcing a person to have sexual intercourse against their will. Sexual assault encompasses all forms of forced sexual activity, including those which do not involve penetration of the vagina or anus with the penis.

Sexual assault involves extreme physical and personal violation. In many cases physical violence is used, but the victim can be forced into sexual activity by many other means, such as threats, fear, shock or exhortation. It has been linked to tolerance of other forms of violence, both in daily life and in the media, where physical violence can acquire a certain acceptability.

For the victim the effects can be devastating. Initial reactions can include anger toward the assailant, shock, fear, self-blame, shame and humiliation. There may be fears about HIV, other sexually transmitted diseases and pregnancy. There is also the question of how and whether to tell anyone. One of the greatest deterrents against reporting a rape or assault is that it may be suggested that the victim provoked the crime in some way. For a long time the idea that a woman's 'no' meant 'yes' carried some sway, while many rapists have suggested that their victim enjoyed the experience after initial resistance. The way a woman is dressed, her sexual history, whether or not she had been drinking, entering a bar alone, walking alone at night – all of these points have been mentioned in legal defence of alleged rapists. The victim's sexual history has also been considered relevant, although there are now laws against using this as evidence in some countries. Ultimately the only relevant question is whether or not consent was given for sex to occur. The term statutory rape may be used to refer to sex with someone who is below the age of consent, or who has been made unconscious or incapacitated by means of drugs.

Victims of rape can be male or female, of any age and social background. Statistics show the majority to be female, but in recent years more cases of male rape have been reported. Rapists are almost always male, although cases of sexual assault by women have also been reported. No conclusive psychological profile of a rapist has been produced. The majority of convicted rapists are not mentally ill and have nothing to distinguish them from other men. Their relationship to their victim can be as stranger, acquaintance, friend, family member, date, lover or long-term partner or spouse. It is estimated that at least fifty per cent of rapists know their victims.

Motives for rape are varied, circumstantial and individual. It may be an isolated act or part of a consistent pattern of abuse. No universal rules exist. However, it has been suggested that there is a link between the incidence of rape and sexual assault and the power relationship between the sexes. In some societies where women are subordinated – professionally, domestically, economically – rape seems to be more common. Certainly rape often involves a desire to overpower or dominate the victim.

2 SEXUAL FEELINGS & BEHAVIOUR

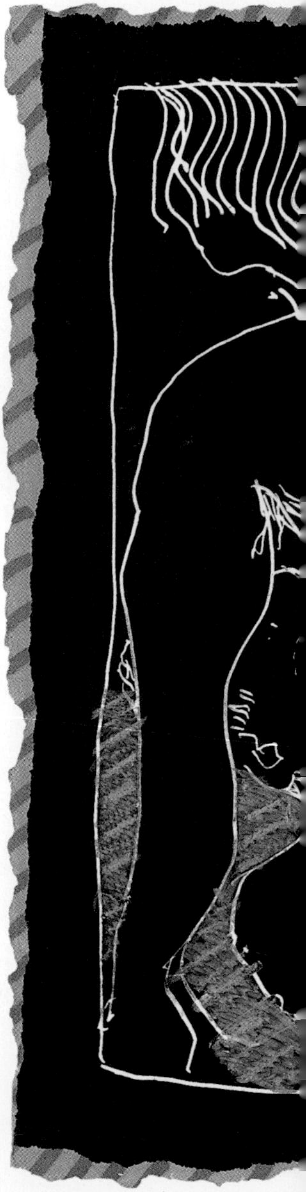

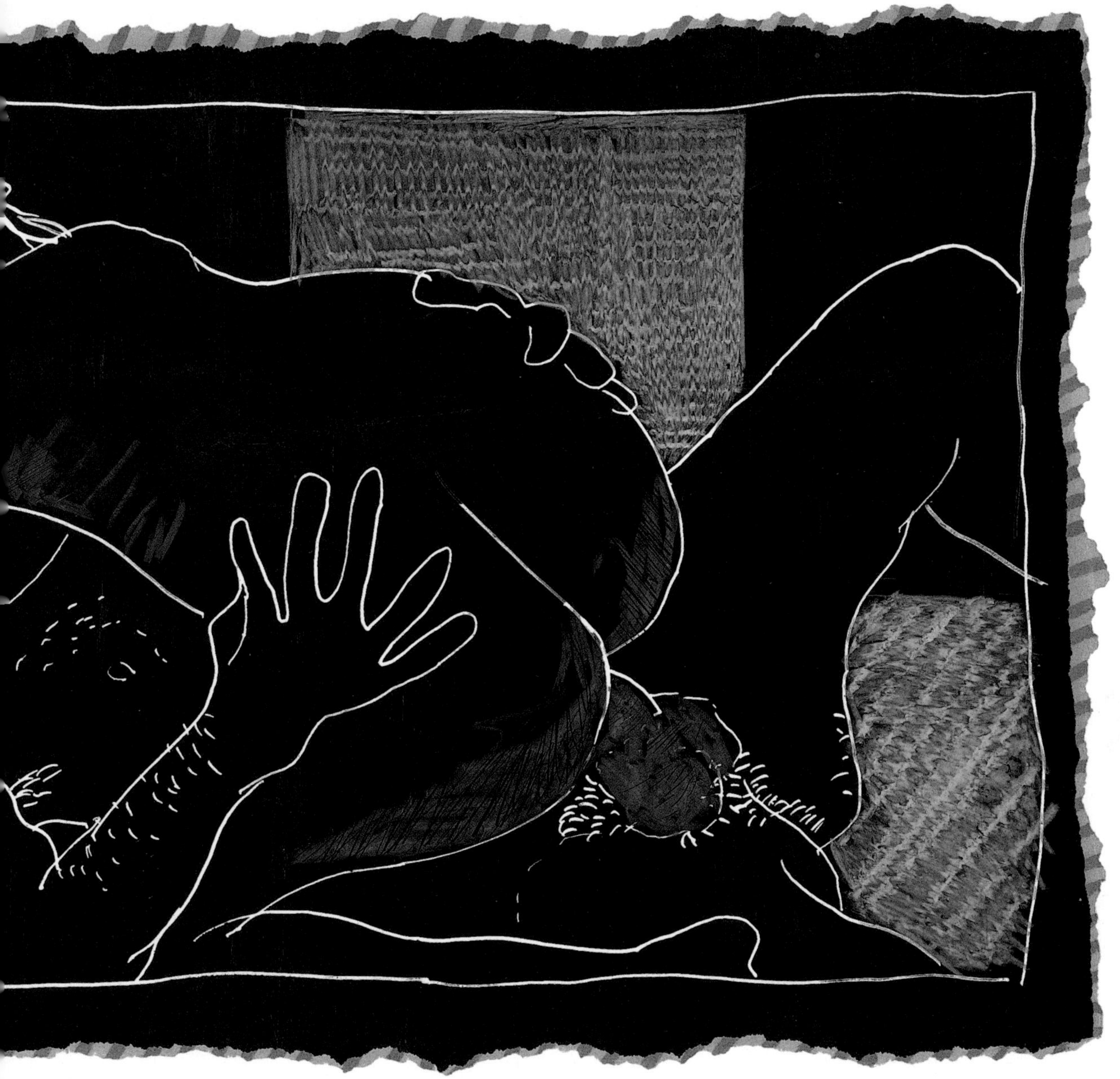

GENDER

The notion of gender goes far beyond the straightforward male/female distinction. Although based in biological differences, gender distinctions in humans incorporate innumerable social and psychological influences. Each person's understanding of gender identity affects every aspect of his or her life.

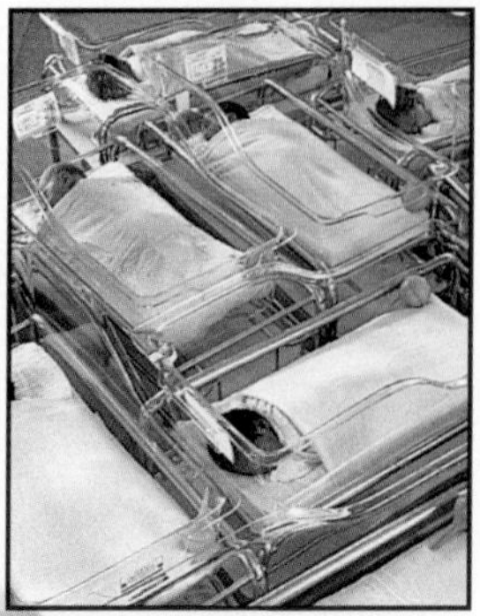

Sex is biologically determined at conception but **gender identity** develops between the ages of two and six years

What is gender?

Sex refers to the basic biological distinction between male and female, determined by sexual organs and hormones, the secondary sexual characteristics (that is, the distinctive, visible, physical features) and the chromosomes which determine them.

Gender is the associated sexual identity; it is the state of being male or female.

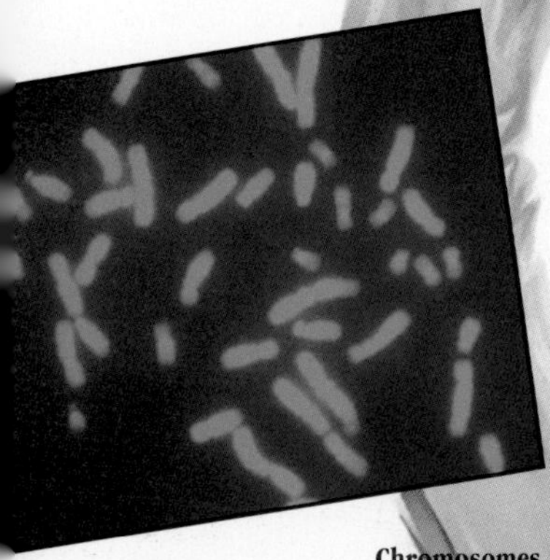

Chromosomes
XX for females
XY for males

Gender identity is the conscious sense of which gender one belongs to. This usually develops between the ages of two and six years, and involves recognizing one's own gender as distinct from or aligned to that of other people.

Gender role is the outward expression of this gender identity.

Observing the behaviour of parents or carers can be one of the main ways that children learn about gender identity.

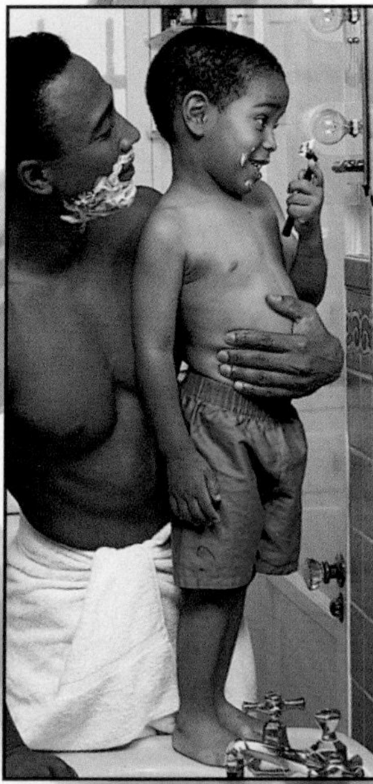

How does gender identity develop?

A person's sense of their gender identity is a central part of his or her psychological makeup. There are two major influences in its formation.

Firstly, and principally during childhood, there is the influence of parents and/or other gender role models. A child observes their behaviour and usually comes to associate particular activities or characteristics with each gender. He or she generally follows the example of their same-sex parent or carer, unless a conscious decision is made to reject it. Carers themselves also have an active role to play by encouraging or discouraging different kinds of behaviour in boys and girls.

Secondly, society and socially ascribed gender roles have their impact, as the child

See also:
conception to birth
sexual attraction
anatomy of sex
sexual feelings – male
sexual feelings – female

becomes aware of the norms of behaviour outside the home environment. This includes the ways in which gender identity is expressed and, more particularly, notions of 'masculinity' and 'femininity' or what is considered appropriate to each gender. This affects anything from attitude to the opposite sex to forms of dress.

Masculine and feminine

Certain personality traits have come to be associated with each gender. In many cultures men are expected to be active, assertive and tough, and women to be passive and gentle. Such criteria often form the basis of people's notions of masculinity and femininity.

These classifications may have a certain basis in biology, but they are also highly restrictive and in many cases completely unrealistic. For example, they preclude the possibility of female aggression and male sensitivity. In reality, masculinity and femininity cannot be defined in this way as there are few – if any – characteristics that can be seen as exclusive to men or women. In spite of this, many people feel obliged to fulfil such roles, to the point where they may experience a sense of failure or abnormality if they do not.

This also applies to sexual orientation. In many parts of the world, there is a sense that masculinity means being attracted to females and that females ought to be attracted to males. As in other assumptions about gender identity, in many cases this rule simply does not apply.

Gender anomalies

In some cases a genetic anomaly can cause a person's gender to be less clearly defined. This is often recognized at birth by the individual having genitalia which are not clearly typically male or female. The term most commonly used for this is 'hermaphrodite', but in fact true hermaphrodites are very rare. More common is the condition known as pseudohermaphroditism, which involves having one or more sexual characteristics which are not in common with the others.

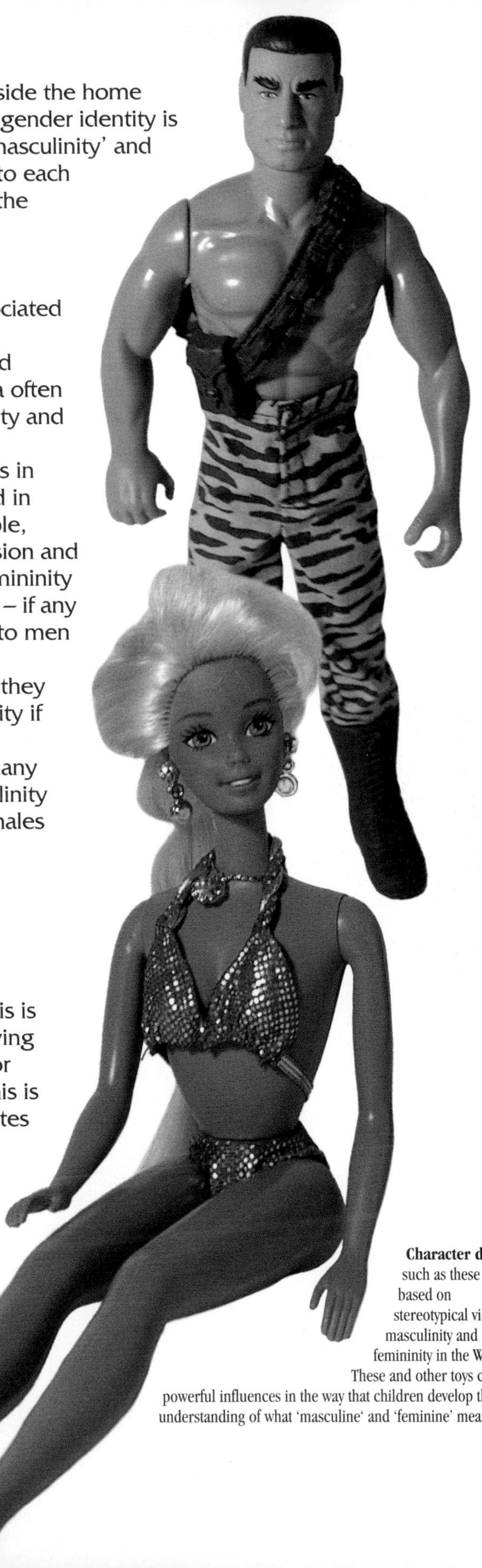

Character dolls such as these are based on stereotypical views of masculinity and femininity in the West. These and other toys can be powerful influences in the way that children develop their understanding of what 'masculine' and 'feminine' mean.

SEXUAL FEELINGS
FEMALE

SEXUAL FEELINGS

Endless generalizations have been made about male and female sexual psychology, many of them contradictory. The reality is that such contradictions are inevitable. Each individual's sexual psyche is determined and influenced by a unique combination of biological and psychological factors. Development begins before birth and continues throughout life, although gender role models in the early stages are important influences.

A common mistake is to assume that men and women are the same psychologically. There are basic similarities, but also fundamental differences.

"The great question ... which I have not been able to answer, despite my thirty years of research into the female soul, is 'What does a woman want?'"
SIGMUND FREUD

See also:
sexual attraction
clitoris
vagina
erogenous zones
sexual practices

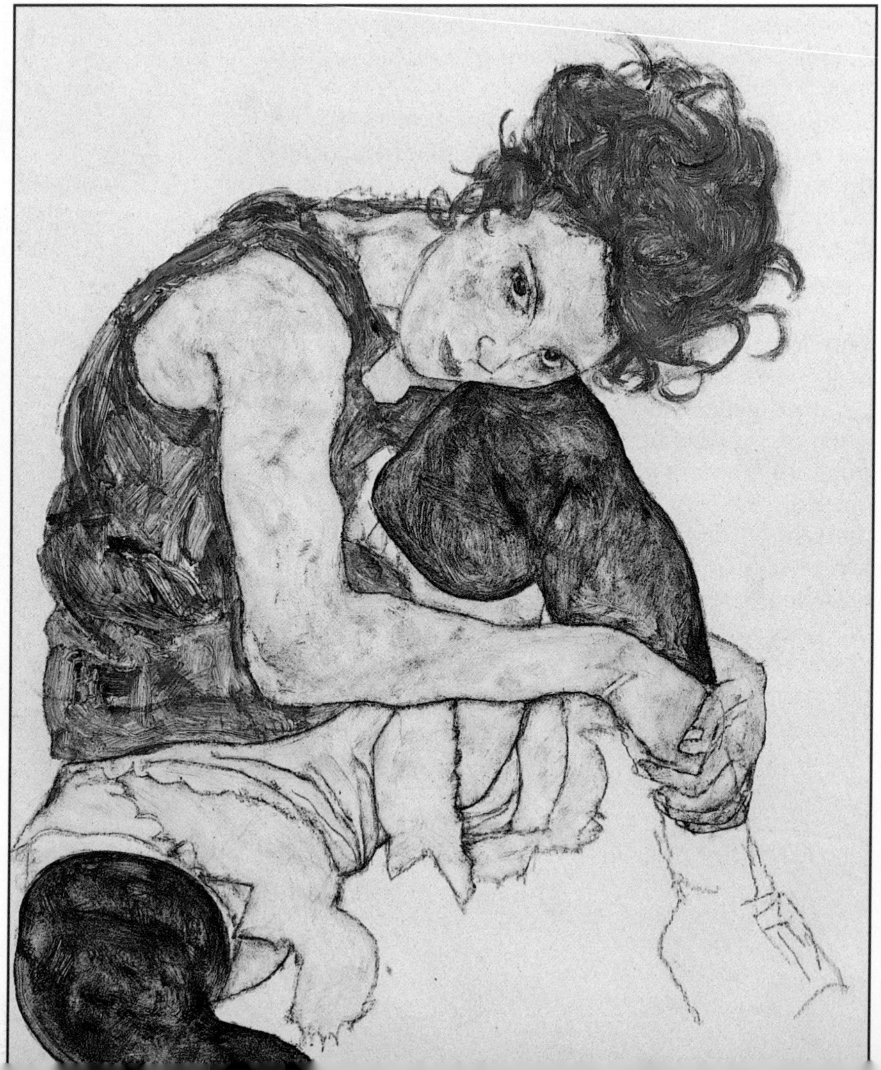

One man's vision of femininity – Egon Schiele's *Seated Woman with Bent Knee* (1917) (detail)

Biology and evolution
Each month a woman produces one ovum in contrast to a man's almost infinite supply of sperm; and women tend to lose their fertility (although not their sex drive) earlier in life. As well as this, they may be aware, albeit unconsciously, of their reproductive role. This has a profound effect on a woman's attitude to her partner. On a practical level, contraceptive measures mean that intercourse does not necessarily have to lead to offspring. However, it has been suggested that it is this natural instinct that accounts for women being, statistically, much less likely to engage in casual sex than men – and more likely to look for an on-going commitment. This sense of commitment may include a need for non-sexual signs of affection.

The sexual act
Sex roles may be influenced by the concept of vaginal intercourse as the basic sexual act. This may cause problems for the woman as well as the man. If the man feels under pressure to perform (see under 'Sexual feelings – male'), he may wish to take a dominant role while the woman remains passive. For some couples, or at some times, this may be ideal for both, but many women prefer to be the more active or dominant partner at least some of the time, just as many men may like to take a less active role. The sense of a man's dominance can also prevent him from expressing the tenderness and affection which his partner may need to feel. Some women feel under pressure to climax in sex which can lead to phenomenon of the faked orgasm.

Arousal
Sexual arousal for a woman tends to be more complex than for a man. The whole body can be an erogenous zone, with areas of particular sensitivity varying greatly from one woman to another. Visual stimuli are important but in a different way than for men, as women tend to respond more to atmosphere and situations. Hence the greater popularity of romantic novels among women than men. Women can also reach a higher state of arousal from fantasy than men.

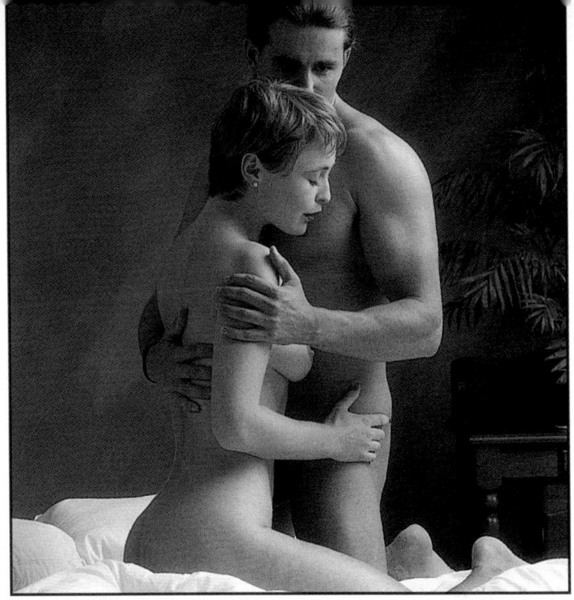

Notions of femininity
For a long time, ideas of femininity have been centred around a woman's appearance as the source of her attractiveness, above all in the West. Consequently, a woman's self-image is often influenced by how she feels about her looks and, in particular, her figure. Changing perceptions of women's place in society have had their impact here. Firstly, they have given greater value to a woman's sense of personal achievement. Secondly, while in the past women were seen as either 'sexy' and desirable or 'nice' and suitable for marriage, expectations are no longer so clearly defined.

Toilette of a Courtezan (detail), after Aubrey Beardsley

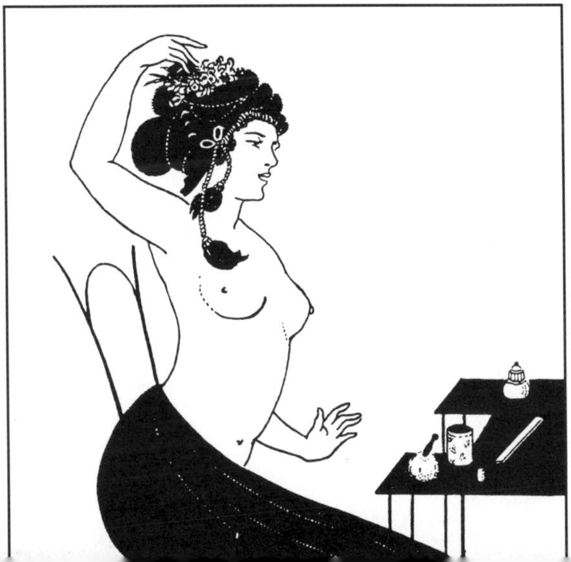

SEXUAL FEELINGS MALE

See also:
sexual attraction
penis
erogenous zones
sexual practices

Biology and evolution

The fact that a woman has only one ovum to fertilize each month while a man has an almost infinite supply of sperm may affect his attitude to his sexual partner, making him tend to be less bound by emotional commitment until he finally decides to settle down. Until this point he may feel no biological need of commitment. This may explain why, statistically, men are more likely to have casual sex and to be able to enjoy sex without an on-going commitment. Studies have shown that men tend to fall in and out of love more quickly and easily than women.

The sexual act

Popular culture puts great emphasis on the most basic sexual act, the vaginal intercourse necessary for reproduction. The widespread stress on this single aspect of sex puts great pressure on the heterosexual man. He feels that he has to have and maintain an erection and 'perform' in a dominant and essentially aggressive manner. Depending on his attitude to his partner, he may feel under pressure to make sure that she reaches orgasm every time. Many men are also concerned about the size of their penis.

The 'ideal' image of sex with its stress on vaginal intercourse and male performance is both unrealistic and, in many cases, undesirable, as it eliminates many of the more exciting and sensuous – as well as the more satisfying – aspects of sex play. It also excludes same gender sex.

Arousal

Male sexual arousal is – relatively speaking – direct and immediate. The erogenous zones are specific and men tend to respond to specific triggers. Both stimulation and arousal are focused more on the genitals. Visual stimuli also tend to be more important for men than they are for women, which may be why pornographic magazines and films tend to be more popular with and oriented toward men. Men tend to have stronger voyeuristic tendencies for the same reason.

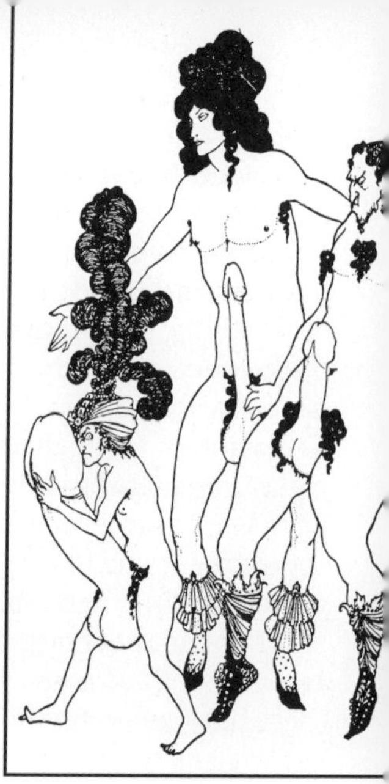

The Lacedemonian Ambassadors (detail), by Aubrey Beardsley, 1896 illustration for Aristophanes' *Lysistrata*. The penis – and penis size in particular – has always played an important role in the male sexual psyche.

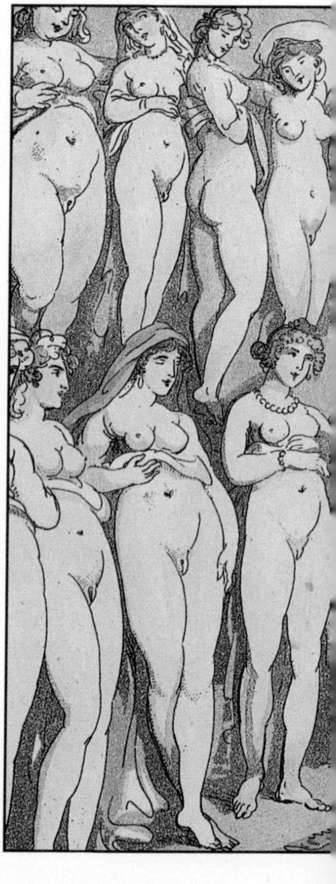

Notions of masculinity
Each man has his own idea of what it means to be masculine. This is determined both by cultural influences and by gender role models. The 'macho' man has long been a powerful image in the West. However, women's liberation has called out for men who are more in touch with the 'feminine' side of their nature, who are more sensitive and openly caring and not afraid to express their emotions. The balance between these two sides has left many men confused as to how they should behave, and in particular how they should behave toward a sexual partner of either gender.

The Harem, by Thomas Rowlandson. It has been suggested that men are biologically predisposed to have higher sex drives than women – they have a constant supply of sperm and their natural instinct is to make use of it.

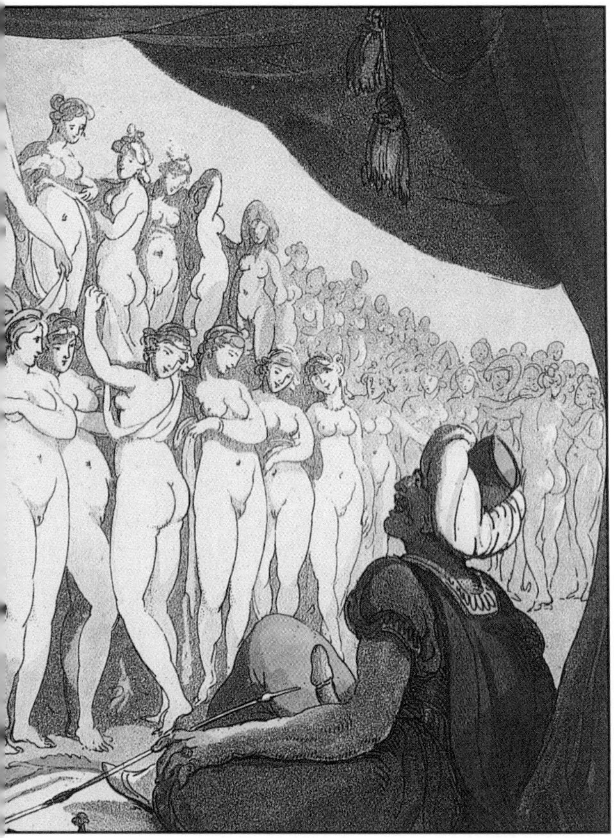

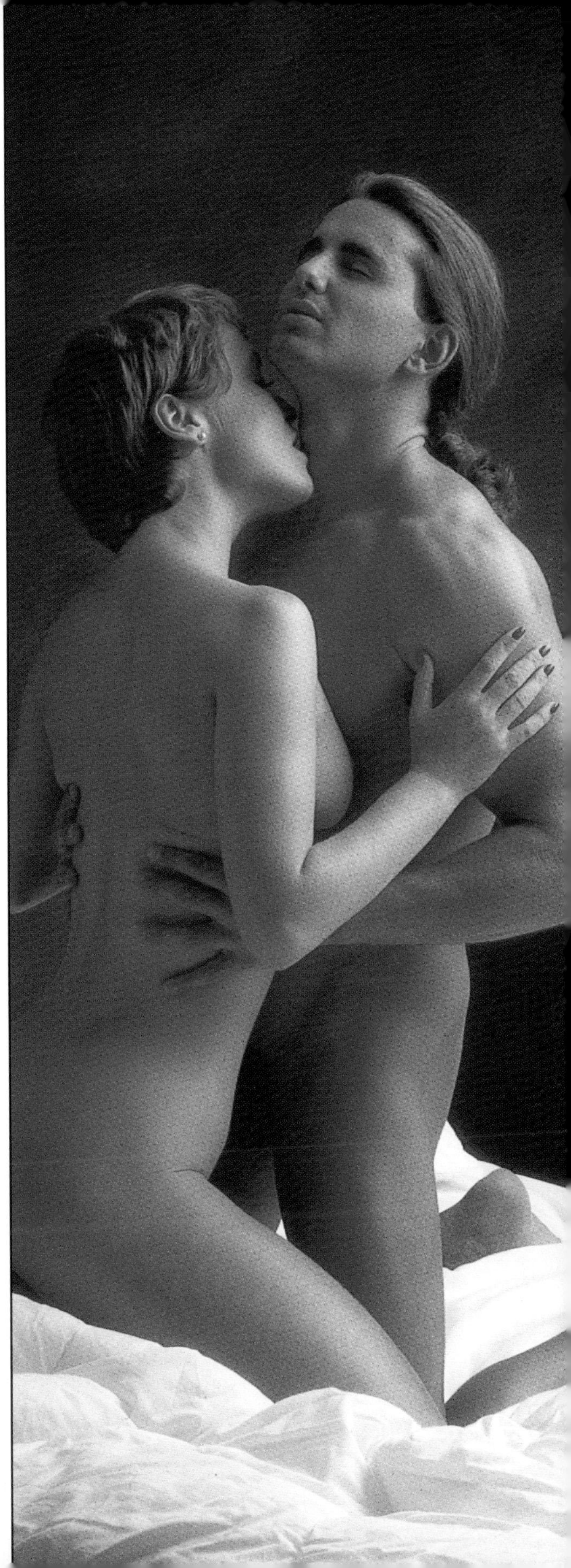

SEXUAL ORIENTATION

The terms 'homosexual', 'heterosexual' and 'bisexual' are commonly used to classify people in terms of their sexual orientation. However, the terms really refer not to people but to types of behaviour, and their use to classify people has lead to countless cases of misunderstanding and misrepresentation. Sexual orientation is not a simple matter: human sexuality cannot be divided into distinct groups. Understanding these terms and what they really mean can help people to express their own sexuality more completely as well as to understand that of others.

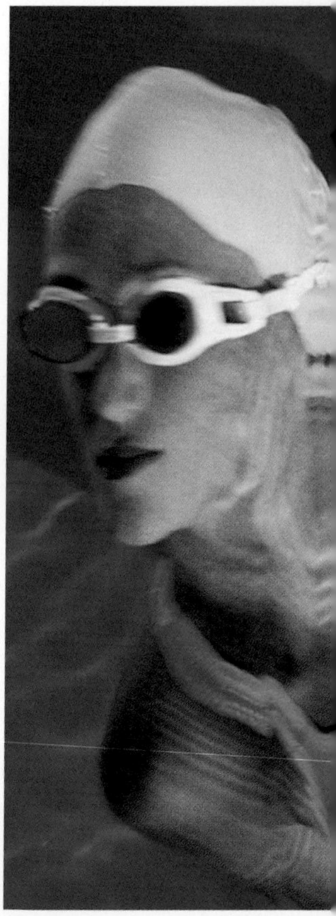

"I can't understand why more people aren't bisexual. It would double your chances for a date on Saturday night."
WOODY ALLEN

Describing sexuality

Homosexuality refers to sexual attraction to, or relations with, a member or members of the same sex; heterosexuality is with the opposite sex; bisexuality is with members of both sexes. Any of these behaviours can encompass everything from the occasional fantasy to full sexual relations.

Kinsey devised a seven-point scale from 0 to 6 to describe human sexual orientation more precisely: 0 represented people who were exclusively heterosexual; 6 represented those who were exclusively homosexual; and 3 applied to those who were equally attracted to men and women; 1, 2, 4 and 5 deal with all other degrees of preference, and take into account such factors as fantasies and isolated or one-off experiences outside a person's usual sexual preference. The system also deals with changes in preference throughout life. Many people are curious about other kinds of sexual experience and experiment at some time with different kinds of sexual activity. Ultimately, those who rate themselves at 0 and 6 are relatively few.

"My feeling is that we are all bisexual. I don't believe there is anyone who could honestly say at some point in their lives they have not been attracted to a member of the same sex."
KEN LIVINGSTONE, UK MEMBER OF PARLIMENT

See also:
sexual learning
pioneers of sexual reform
homosexuality and society

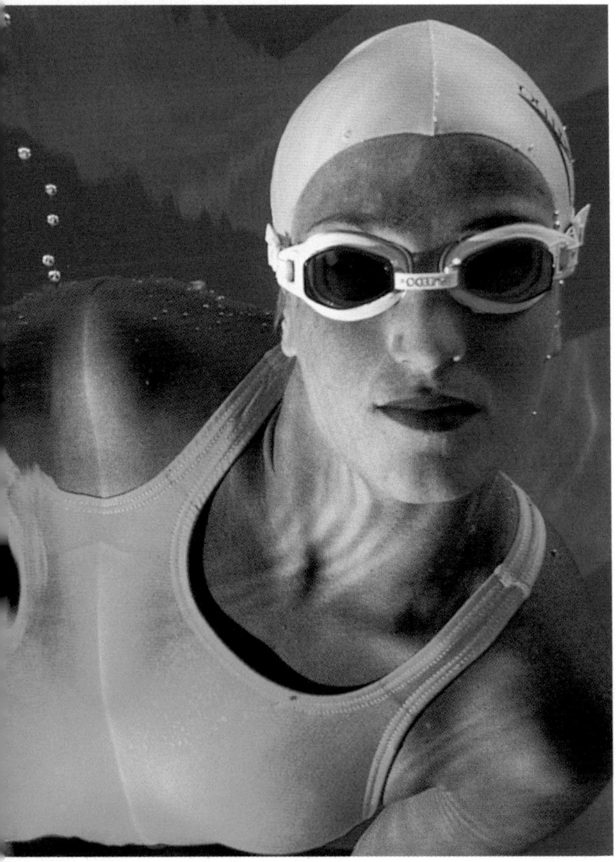

Which way?
It is increasingly believed that few, if any, people are exclusively homosexual or heterosexual. Human sexuality does not work within tight definitions or limitations – it can take many different forms and is fluid and flexible.

The facts

Kinsey's studies produced statistics suggesting that about thirty-seven per cent of males and thirteen per cent of females had some overt homosexual experience in the course of adult life, although his methods of gathering information have since been called into question. It is estimated that exclusively homosexual males comprise about five per cent of the adult population. The proportion of homosexual women is likely to be marginally less than this. A recent study in the U.K. indicated that 92.3 per cent of men and 95.1 per cent of women describe their sexual experience as 'only heterosexual'. It is also known that homo-erotic fantasy is common among people of all sexual orientations.

What determines sexual orientation?

There is a great deal of prejudice about sexual orientation. In most cultures such prejudice is a relatively recent phenomenon, as different kinds of attraction have always been part of human sexuality. There are a number of factors which suggest that non-heterosexual sexualities are natural consequences of biology and/or psychology.

- Records of homosexual activity have been found in all periods and a great many cultural groups. Even where it was not socially acceptable, it seems that it still occurred.

- Proportions of different types of sexuality seem to be approximately the same in all cultural and racial groups.

- Homosexual activity has been observed among other higher primates, including at times when opportunities for heterosexual activity were available.

- Various pieces of research point to a genetic basis for sexuality. Studies of identical and non-identical twins (identical twins have identical genetic makeups) show that if one twin is homosexual, an identical brother is much more likely to be homosexual than a non-identical brother. More recent research claims to have identified the relevant gene.

- Male homosexuality has also been linked to the number of male siblings: a study has shown that the greater the number of elder brothers that a man has, the more likely he is to be homosexual. The reasons could be biological or simply an effect of the treatment of younger siblings within the family.

- A lack of admiration for, or a lack of desire to be like, the same-sex parent has been linked to homosexual tendencies.

- Puritanical attitudes toward sex, if they lead to a deeply rooted fear of the opposite sex, may also encourage homosexual behaviour.

HOMOSEXUALITY & SOCIETY

Many people still consider homosexual behaviour – exclusive or occasional – abnormal or wrong, in spite of the research carried out into patterns of sexuality. It is still completely accepted in very few cultural groups. Homosexual activity continues to carry a social stigma, although there is some evidence that attitudes are becoming less dogmatic.

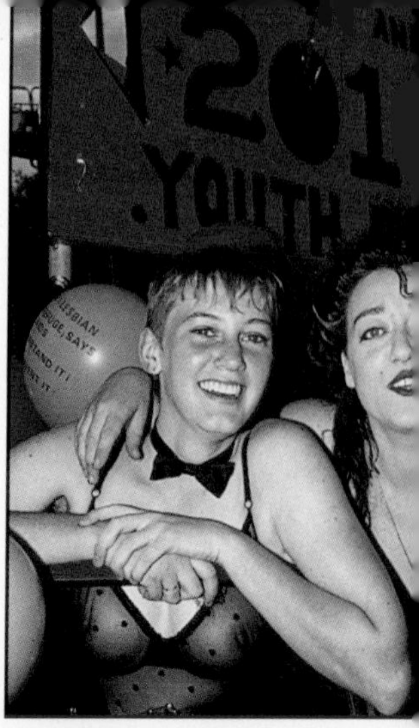

Gay rights have become an increasingly prominent social and political issue – and are frequently the subject of mass campaigns.

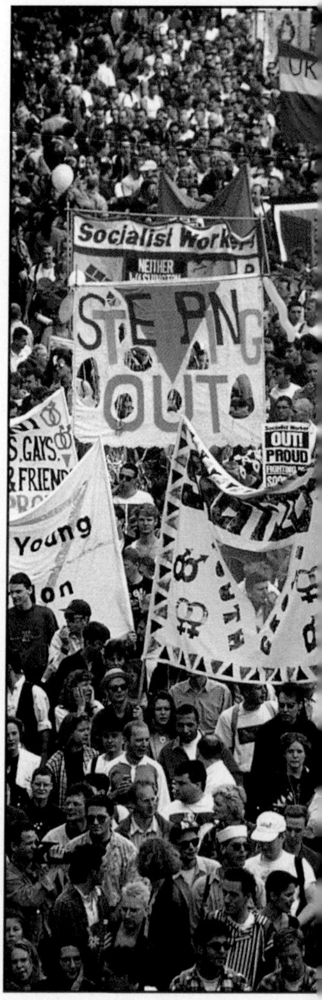

Them and us – some myths dispelled
The term 'homosexual' strictly applies to any kind of sexual behaviour – from fantasy to intercourse – with a member of the same sex, but it may be used to refer to a person who is exclusively or primarily attracted to or involved with same-sex partners. In many cultures there are strong taboos relating to all forms of homosexuality: these are largely due to misunderstandings and misconceptions.

The term 'gay' is frequently used to describe homosexuals, particularly men. The term 'lesbian' is used for homosexual women.

- It is not possible to identify a person as gay or lesbian by appearance. Some gay men and women play up 'camp' or 'butch' roles, but many do not.

- There are no specific gay or lesbian types: people who enjoy homosexual activity are as varied in terms of occupation, social class, dress, religion and education as anyone else.

- Gays and lesbians are no more likely to carry out sexual crimes than anyone else. Homosexual men are statistically less likely to abuse children than heterosexuals.

- Homosexual relationships are as varied as heterosexual relationships in terms of affection, physicality and commitment.

- Similarly, gay sex is just as varied, if not more so as heterosexual sex. Practices include kissing, touching, body-rubbing, oral sex, masturbation and – between men – anal intercourse.

See also:
sexual orientation
sexual attraction

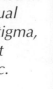

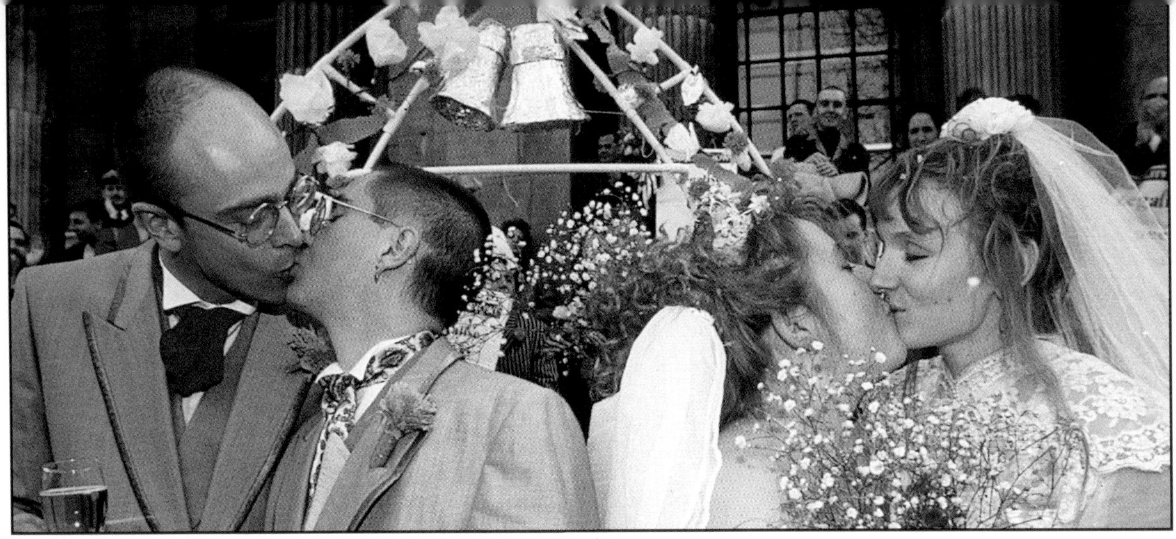

Double gay and lesbian marriage

Gay and lesbian culture

In many cultures social intolerance has forced homosexuality into a form of sub-culture. In Western society there are few places where people can be open about homosexuality, although acceptance tends to be greater where there are fewer religious restraints and in large, more cosmopolitan cities. In some societies homosexuality is illegal.

As a result, in many larger towns and cities gay and lesbian meeting places have been created. As for heterosexuals, some are for general socializing while others are intended specifically for finding partners, sometimes for casual sex. These venues include bars, restaurants, and occasionally steam baths and specific public lavatories.

In the present social environment the decision to 'come out', that is, to reveal one's sexual orientation can be difficult. While more and more people are coming to accept homosexuality, others react judgementally to overt homosexual or bisexual orientations. The fear of homosexuality is sometimes known as 'homophobia' and has resulted in persecution of gay men and lesbians. Some homosexuals believe they can strengthen their case and influence by 'outing', in other words, publicly revealing the sexual orientation of well-known and highly regarded gays or lesbians. This remains a controversial issue. Meanwhile, overtly gay themes in literature, film, drama, ballet and the visual arts are now accepted as part of mainstream culture in many societies.

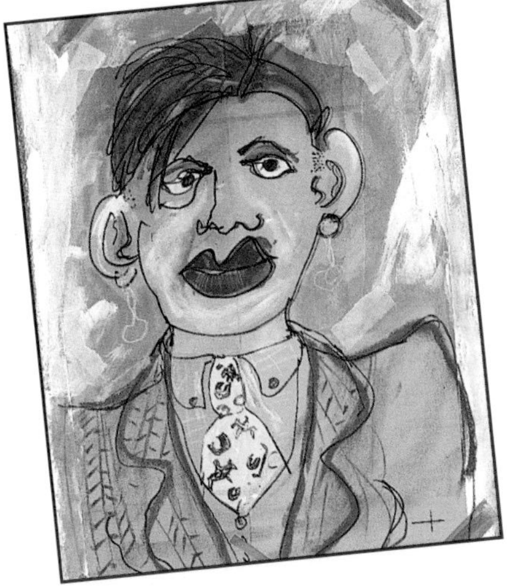

Slang terms

HOMOSEXUAL FEMALE

dyke, lesbian, bull dyke, butch dyke, deisel, radish, sapphist, gay, femme, Amy–John, bull dagger/bitch

HOMOSEXUAL MALE

faggot, fag, queen (closet, drag, wrinkle, chicken), dairy, fruit, pouf, nancy, poor, poorter, radish, daily, queer, quntie, Nellie, fem, belle, swish, latent, bender, woofter, brown-hatter, pansy

Adjectives: gay, bent, camp

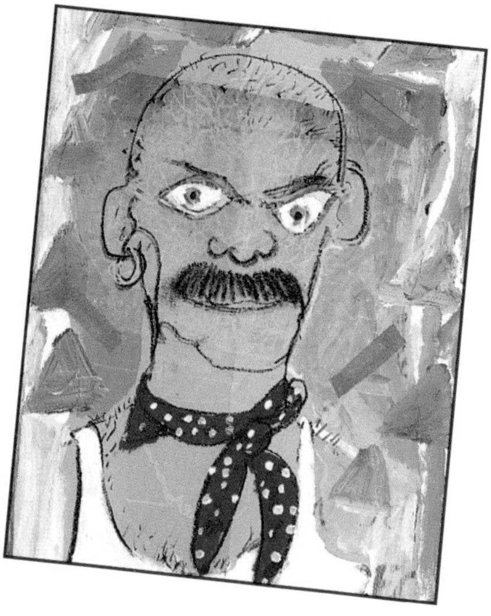

TRANSVESTISM

TRANSVESTISM AND TRANSSEXUALISM

Transvestism and transsexualism are two areas in which the gender boundary is blurred. Unlike hermaphrodites, both transvestites and transsexuals are born anatomically complete as one sex or the other. However, in a minor way in the case of transvestites and in a more fundamental way in the case of transsexuals, members of both groups are drawn towards living as the opposite gender.

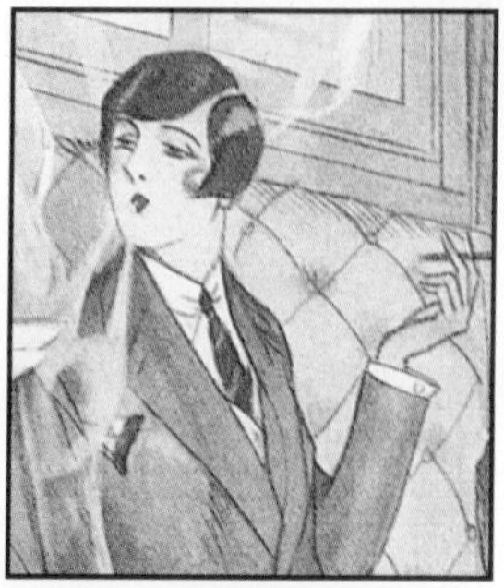

Females dressing in 'male' attire have rarely been seen as controversial. From an illustration in *La Vie Parisienne* (1926)

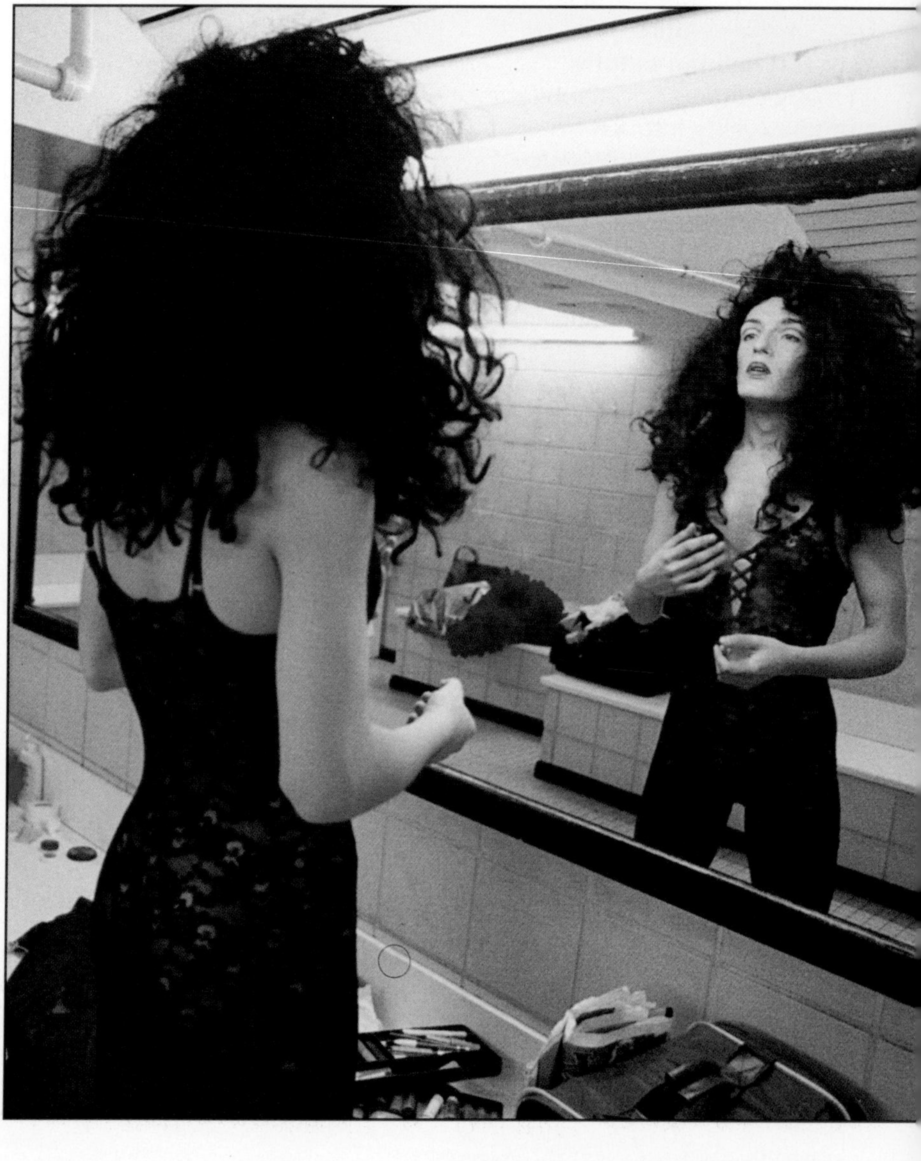

See also:
dressing and undressing
gender
bondage

Transvestism

Transvestites are men and women who like to dress in the clothes associated with the opposite gender, either occasionally or, in a few cases, all the time. Most transvestites are male and heterosexual; many are married with children.

In a high percentage of cases the motivation behind cross-dressing is a form of fetishism, with a sexual attachment to the clothing and accoutrements of the opposite sex. This may produce strong sexual arousal and even orgasm.

Other cases have to do with a man wishing to express the feminine side of his personality: women's clothing provides a sense of freedom and security, together with a release from the demands of the male gender role. This seems to be particularly common among homosexual transvestites.

The same behaviour may also be interpreted as a way of challenging the traditional gender roles ascribed by society, where many forms of dress and other aspects of behaviour are determined by gender.

Cross-dressing may be practised in public or in private, with or without the knowledge of a sexual partner. It is believed that it is usually carried out in secret and is thought to be not uncommon.

The term 'drag' is sometimes associated with transvestism. Homosexual transvestites are sometimes referred to as 'drag queens', particularly if their style of dress is very flamboyant. The term is also used in its original sense to mean men dressing up as female characters in theatrical productions.

◀ **Audition at Madame Jo-Jo's** – many of the more flamboyant transvestite men go to enormous effort to perfect their looks.

FACT: *Miss Vera's Finishing School for Boys who want to be Girls*, the first transvestite academy, opened in 1994 in New York. The academy's courses include 'What every girl should know about her five o'clock shadow' and 'How to prevent your evening gown being ruined by a bulging penis'.

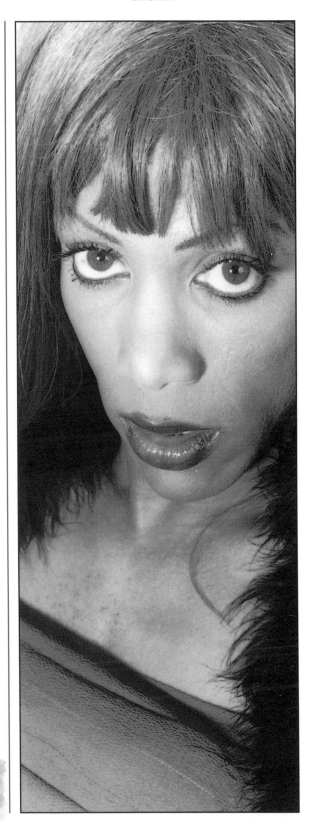

TRANSSEXUALISM

Transsexualism is quite distinct from transvestism – it is more deeply-rooted and more complex, and widely misunderstood. However, society at large is increasingly coming to understand, and ultimately to accept, this relatively rare condition.

Transsexualism or gender dysphoria
Transsexualism is a rare condition. Being transsexual means having an overwhelming sense of having been born with the body of the wrong sex: the biological sex and the gender identity are opposed. Transsexuals may cross-dress, but their attitude to their body and in particular their genitals is completely different from that of a transvestite. Transsexuals tend to wish to disassociate themselves from their bodies, even to the point of having their physical sex reassigned by means of surgery.

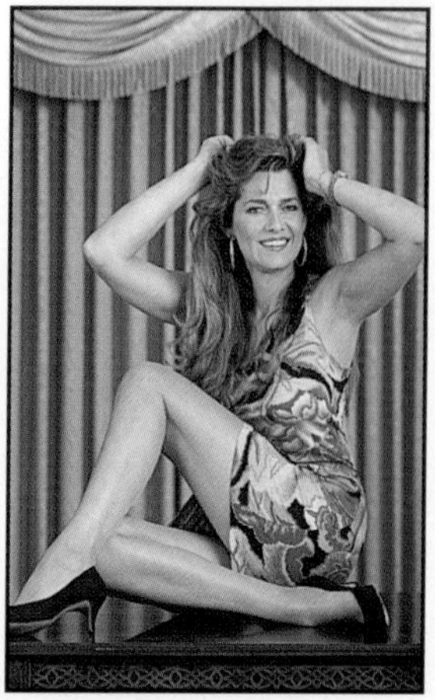

Male-to-female transsexual

Female-to-male transsexual

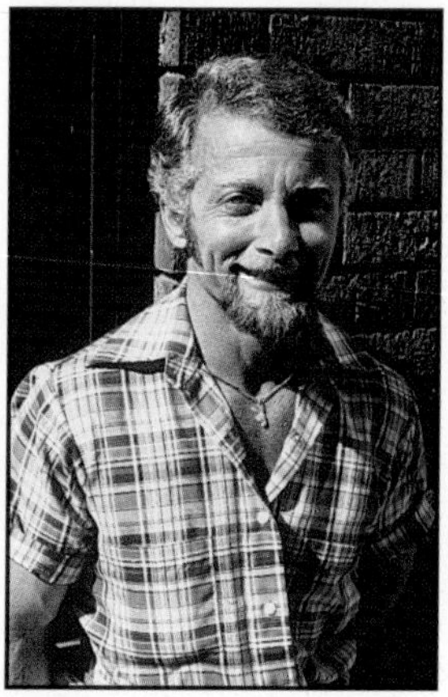

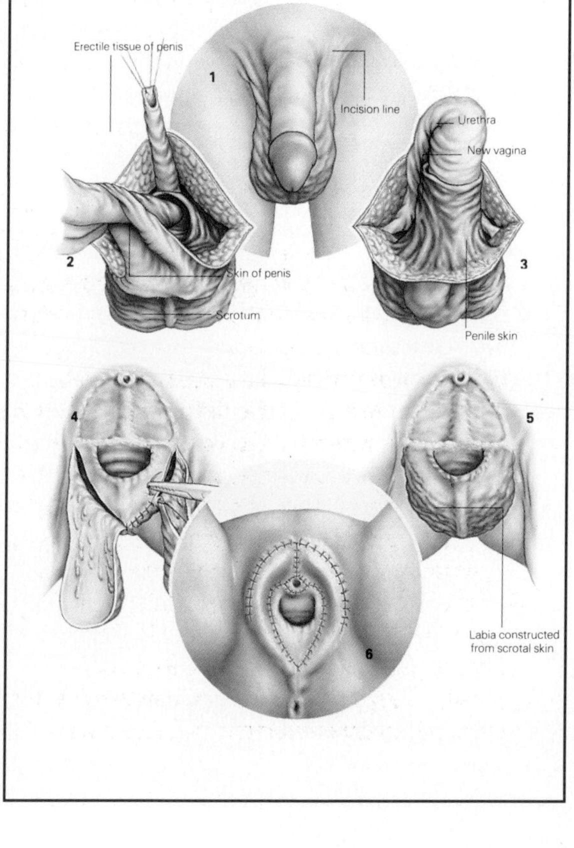

The male-to-female gender reassignment operation
A cut is made at the base of the penis (1); the skin is peeled back and the main body of the penis is removed (2). The penile skin is used to line a vagina, made in the region of the perineum (3). A cut is made in the scrotum (4) and the testes are removed, the scrotal sac being used to form the labia (5). Lastly, the urethra is moved to just above the vagina (6).

FACT: The first male-to-female gender reassignment surgery was performed in Denmark in 1952.

See also:
gender
sexual feelings – male
sexual feelings – female

Transsexuals are often very conservative with regard to perceptions of gender roles, seeing male and female roles as quite distinct. They tend to see themselves as heterosexual, being attracted to members of the opposite sex in terms of their sexual identity even though this is the same biological sex, although there are bisexual and homosexual transsexuals.

Once a person is convinced that he or she is transsexual, there are various courses of action open to them. For most, the ultimate goal is to have surgery to bring their body into line with their sexual identity: this is known as a sex change or reassignment. There are a number of less severe measures which can be taken, and which are usually obligatory as preliminary steps before the final operation on the genitals. These can include removal of body hair or hair transplants, silicone implants to change the body shape, and treatment with male or female sexual hormones (affecting the secondary sexual characteristics). Before the operation is carried out, transsexuals are expected to have lengthy counselling and assessment and to live as the chosen sex for at least a year.

The reassignment operation for male-to-female transsexuals consists of removing the testes and using the skin of the scrotum to line a surgically-created vagina. For female-to-male transsexuals the breast tissue is removed and a hysterectomy is performed, removing the internal female reproductive organs. In some cases, a penis is created with skin and muscle tissue taken from another part of the body. It will not contain the urethra, but in some cases implants can be included to make vaginal penetration possible. In both cases, sexual sensitivity may or may not be preserved.

While the law in many countries permits and acknowledges the process of sexual reassignment, few Western countries recognize a person's new alignment and he or she will seldom be permitted a legal marriage or a passport appropriate to the reassigned sex. However, in other parts of the world such people are accepted and identity respected. In parts of the Middle East and some Latin countries they may be popular as sexual partners and are not uncommon among sex workers; they may be employed to teach young girls how to please their husbands in bed and are often invited to weddings to bring good luck.

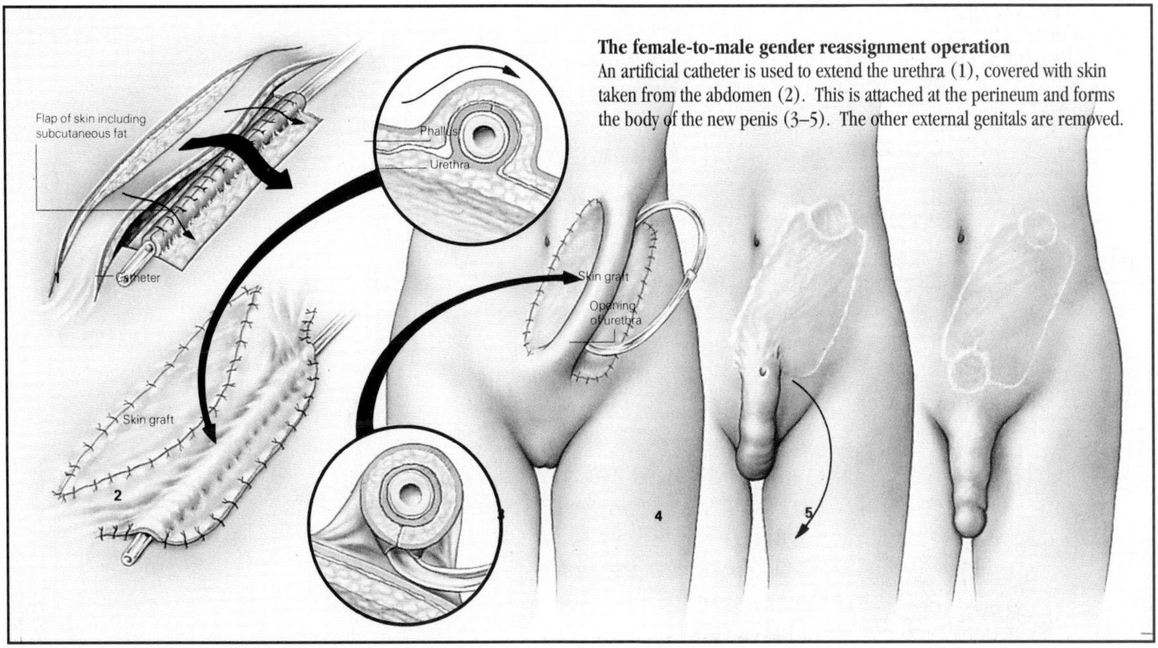

The female-to-male gender reassignment operation
An artificial catheter is used to extend the urethra (1), covered with skin taken from the abdomen (2). This is attached at the perineum and forms the body of the new penis (3–5). The other external genitals are removed.

SEXUAL LEARNING

SEXUAL AWARENESS IN CHILDREN

It is often thought that humans become sexually aware only when they reach puberty. However, sexual consciousness – both physiological and psychological – begins at or even before birth, and infancy and childhood are crucial stages in its development. In spite of this, infant and childhood sexuality continues to be surrounded by ignorance and embarrassment.

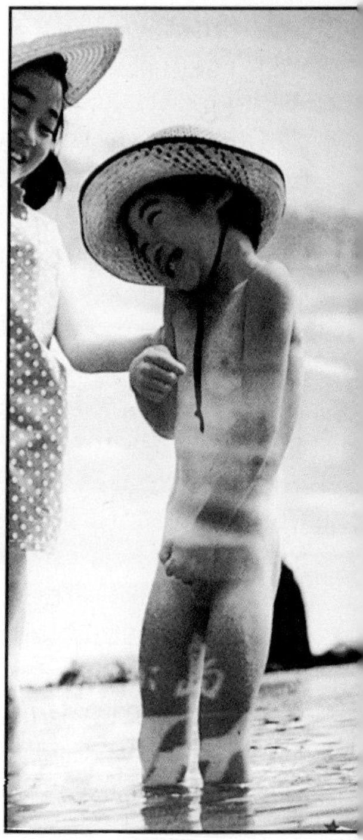

Childhood sexuality is more openly accepted in some cultures than others. This detail of a poster advertisement for Sadoga-shima shows kids enjoying themselves. That the boy is holding his genitals is not seen as shameful or something to be hidden, but is a symbol of innocent fun and joyousness.

Pre-birth and infancy

It is now known that male foetuses have erections, in many cases frequently, for some time before birth. This continues after birth, when vaginal lubrication in females has also been observed.

The extent of unborn or newborn children's consciousness of this activity is not known, but it is certain that their awareness of their body develops rapidly from birth. The earliest stages of learning are based on two things: exploration of the body and senses, and interaction with other humans. It is these same things that form the basis of sexual awareness.

An infant rapidly starts to take interest and pleasure in his or her body and bodily processes. Freudian psychoanalysts point to three early stages of development of physical awareness, described in terms of oral, genital and anal 'fixations'. Feeding and excreting are of obvious and immediate interest, but so too, it appears, is genital sensation: between the ages of six and twelve months most infants show interest in their genitals by fondling or exposing them.

Basic elements of infant care, such as rubbing, stroking, patting and breastfeeding, are important in creating physical awareness and a sense of security and intimacy with carers.

Loving relationships between parents, family members, other carers and children are an important basis for security in relationships and the ability to form loving attachments.

See also:
growth and change
gender
masturbation

Childhood

Much sexual learning takes place with peers. While girls usually learn to masturbate on their own, many boys learn with their peers. By adolescence, nine out of ten boys are masturbating; it is less common among girls. Many boys and girls are curious about the genitals of the opposite sex, although penises seem to attract more attention among both sexes.

Mutual kissing and fondling are common, as are pelvic thrusting, simulated intercourse and mutual masturbation. Intercourse is more rare, but has been known to occur. Activity may be heterosexual or homosexual, but the choice of partner or orientation is unlikely to be significant at this stage. It may be spontaneous or it may be imitative, influenced by sexual activity seen on television or intimacy between parents or other adults. Surveys suggest that as many as eighty-five per cent of adults recall some sort of sex play with peers between the ages of six and twelve. Personal, romantic attachments before the age of six are not uncommon.

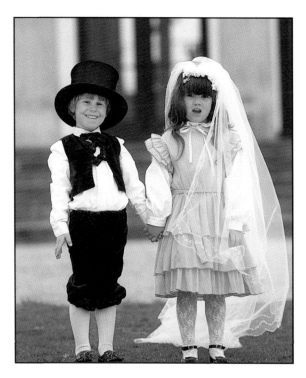

Children become aware of relationships – and the social practices affecting them – while still very young.

Sexual learning begins during childhood as children learn to interact with each other – and even seem to flirt here, playing doctors and nurses. In spite of this, they are still a long way from puberty and full sexual awareness.

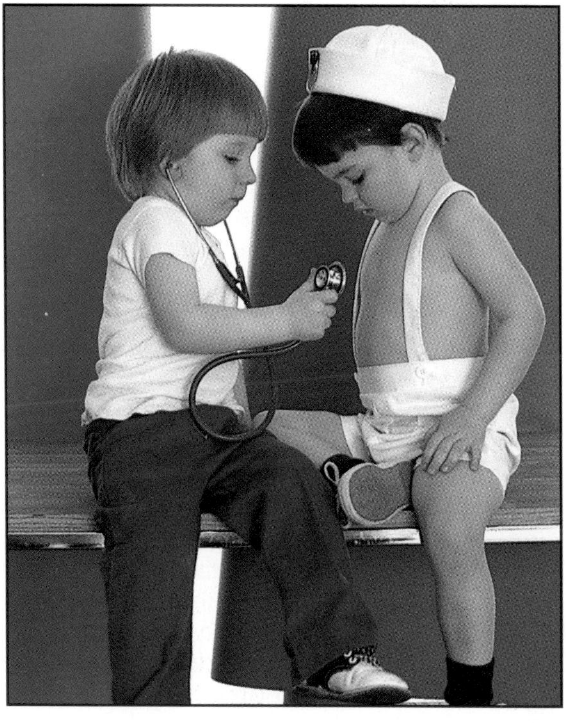

Attitudes to childhood sexuality

In many cultures childhood sexuality is either ignored or repressed. Those in which it is openly accepted as natural and healthy are relatively few although tolerance does seem to be increasing. Certainly, Western societies have progressed from the days when children were often forcibly restrained or punished for innocent masturbation. In a few cultural groups, sexual activity is actively encouraged from an early age.

The attitudes of parents and other carers to children's sexuality can be very powerful. Children learn from them how they ought to behave and if they are taught that sexual feelings are dirty or shameful this impression often remains with them for life. A parent or carer who is comfortable with his or her own body and sexuality will pass on this message to the child, who will learn that sex is natural and to be enjoyed without guilt or shame at an appropriate time.

SEXUALITY IN ADOLESCENCE

Adolescence is a time of change – physical, emotional and psychological. The physical changes are the most immediately noticeable, but they bring with them the need for psychological and social adjustments. It is often a time of intense confusion but it can also be exciting, heralding the change from childhood to the challenges and opportunities of adulthood.

Adolescence has been described as the second stage of the process of individuation. The first stage occurs in infancy and childhood and is based on an individual's relationship with his or her family, or carers and companions, and immediate environment. At this stage individuation is likely to be entirely unconscious. However at adolescence the individual is likely to be acutely – even painfully – conscious of some of the changes which are occurring, even if other changes are dealt with instinctively.

What is adolescence?

Adolescence begins with puberty, when the adult hormonal cycles are set in motion, bringing with them the range of physical and psychological changes that herald the development from child to young adult.

Physical changes

Puberty usually lasts between three and five years, from the ages of nine to thirteen in girls and ten to fifteen in boys. Some studies have suggested that the age at which puberty occurs is gradually getting lower worldwide. Puberty sees the development of the secondary sexual characteristics differentiating male and female, and is marked by the menarche or first menstruation in girls and the first ejaculation (spermarche) in boys.

It is usually at puberty that young people start to become sexually aware and/or active. Watersheds such as a girl's first menstruation or a boy's first ejaculation can be exciting or traumatic, depending on the kind of attitudes and information which the girl or boy has experienced. The development of other physical characteristics also has its impact. Physical awareness increases, as does a sense of personal and sexual attractiveness which may acquire a disproportionate amount of importance at this time. Adolescents who do not consider themselves attractive may find it harder to relate to their peers.

Social and psychological changes

Adolescence includes the development of identity, both personal and sexual. It is a time for developing personal, social and sexual self-confidence and learning to relate to prospective partners.

Adolescence also signifies a shift away from the family for emotional support and personal influence, in favour of peer groups and other, non-familial role models. An enormous variety of influences are experienced, and young adults has to choose between them as they forge their own identity and attitudes. This is part of becoming more individual and independent.

At the same time, sexual identity, attitudes and values are also forming. Adolescence is often a time of experimentation as people try out different gender and sexual roles until they find one with which they are comfortable. It is often a time for experimenting with different kinds of sexual orientation; transsexuals may also become acutely aware of their condition at this stage. This search for identity may continue until much later in life: social pressures may prevent a person from exploring their identity and sexuality, particularly at this delicate stage of development and, above all, if the kinds of identity in question are perceived as outside the norm in the cultural group.

Attitudes to adolescence

In many cultures, children are expected to assume adult roles before puberty. This may be a question of tradition or sheer necessity, as when children are expected to rear

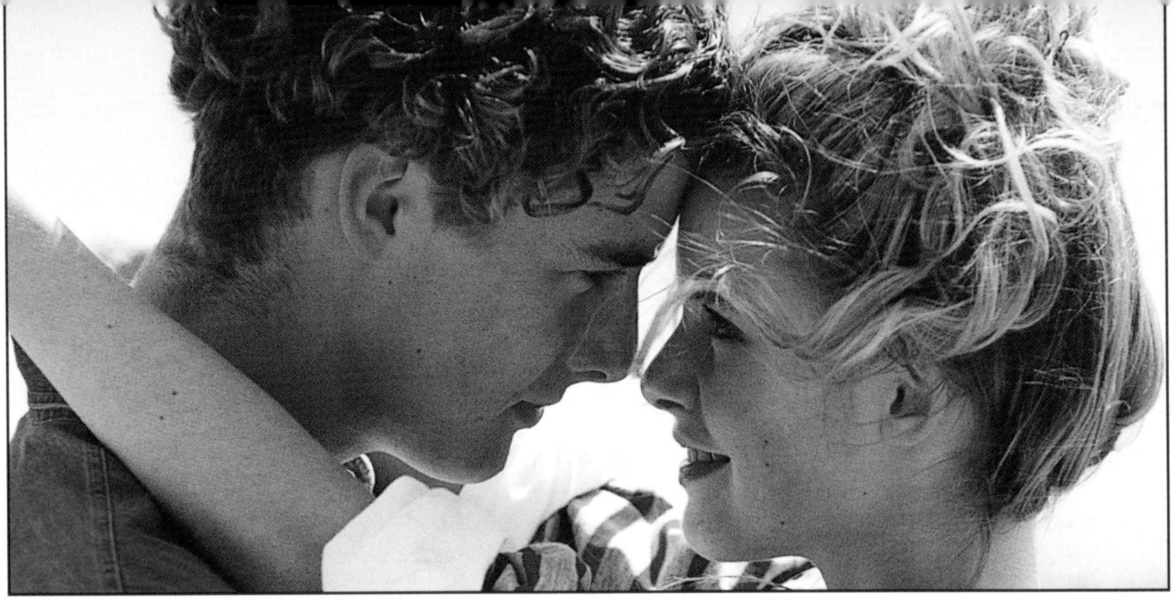

Adolescence can be a crucial time for exploring and developing sexual identity.

younger siblings or work to augment the family income. The situation in the West is very different, as the transition to adulthood has become prolonged to the point where a strong, independent youth culture has developed. This can influence anything from changing trends in fashion and music to attitudes to sex and sexuality.

Most cultures have some sort of formal rite of passage, to mark the beginning of adulthood before the social group, usually peers and/or elders. In the West these may include entering military service or being old enough to vote, buy cigarettes, drive or have sex legally, but practices vary greatly from one culture to another. Many involve some sort of trial of skill or strength: men having to climb a ladder of knives in parts of China or women enduring ritual scarification in many parts of Africa. Some are more overtly sexual, as in the practice of circumcision, which may be carried out on adolescents without any form of pain relief as a test of strength and endurance. Many cultures celebrate a girl's first menstruation with great ceremony, as in Bali and Nigeria, while cultural beliefs among the Etoro of Oceania and the Karaki of New Guinea dictate that young males must engage in certain forms of sexual activity with adult males in order to become fertile later in life.

These practices signify formally that the child has become an adult, although in many cases the greatest challenges are yet to come.

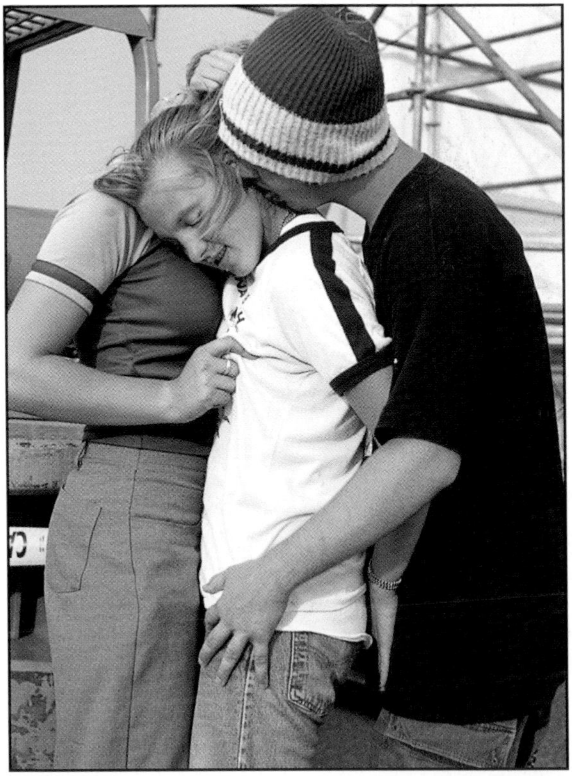

See also:
growth and change
sexual attraction
gender
sexual orientation

LEARNING ABOUT SEX

Learning about sex is a fundamental part of human development. What people learn about sex as children may influence them for life. People learn about sex at all ages and from a variety of influences. However, in some cultures it is almost a taboo subject. Attitudes to sex education can be one of the clearest indications of a culture's attitudes to sex in general.

What is sex education?

The term 'sex education' can refer to anything from the first discussion of human reproduction with a young child to the provision of clear, broad information on sexual practices and techniques for adults. It can come in the form of conversations with parents, siblings or peers, specific sex education classes, as well as all kinds of books, magazines, problem pages and telephone helplines, videos and, more recently, CD-ROMs. In many countries there are also adult courses or encounter groups dealing with sexual issues.

The importance of sex education

At first, sex education for children can explain the differences between the sexes and the processes of human reproduction. As puberty approaches, it helps young people to recognize and adapt to the changes in their bodies and emotions, and may prepare them for different kinds of interpersonal relationships. At later stages, it is important for developing knowledge, skills and attitudes in all areas of sexuality.

At all stages, sex education can provide a broad understanding of the whole range of human sexuality. It entails personal and social education as well as information about health issues. It can include:

- the mechanics of reproduction: intercourse, conception, pregnancy, childbirth

- all aspects of sexual health: sexual hygiene, infections and diseases, unintended pregnancy, contraception and safer sex, abortion, sexual abuse

- aspects of sexuality: gender roles, sexual orientation, giving and receiving sexual pleasure, masturbation, sexual practices, notions of normality and individuality

- aspects of relationships: sex, love and commitment, casual sex, sex and relationships, sexual technique, sexual responsibility

- attitudes to sex: religious and cultural beliefs, one's own and other people's personal beliefs

Sex education for young people sometimes focuses simply on the mechanics of sex and the potential dangers, with comparatively little attention paid to personal relationships, love, sexual attitudes and sexual pleasure. It may be riddled with euphemisms, failing to deal with issues clearly and frankly.

Adult sex education has existed for a long time in many cultures, in some cases as an art form. In the East, in particular, the art of loving has long been taken very seriously, and is the origin of such works as the *Kama Sutra*, *The Perfumed Garden* and many Taoist and Tantric works. In the West, such material has been scarce, and generally frowned upon. It is only relatively recently that high-quality, frank adult sex education material has become available.

The importance of sex education is seen most clearly where it has been inadequate. Poor sex education has been shown to be directly related to higher incidence of STDs, unintended pregnancies and abortions. It can also produce a fear of sex and other relationship problems. Certainly, there is no evidence that sex education increases early sexual activity or promiscuity. Finally, ignorance is very often the source of prejudice, with regard to sexual orientation and HIV in particular. Sex education not only helps people to enjoy sex and form positive relationships, but it can also build consideration and respect for others.

Attitudes to sex education vary enormously from one cultural group to another. While this particular form, as depicted by the eleventh century Chinese artist Su Shih, may be taking liberal attitudes to an extreme, the importance of sex education for people of all ages cannot be underestimated.

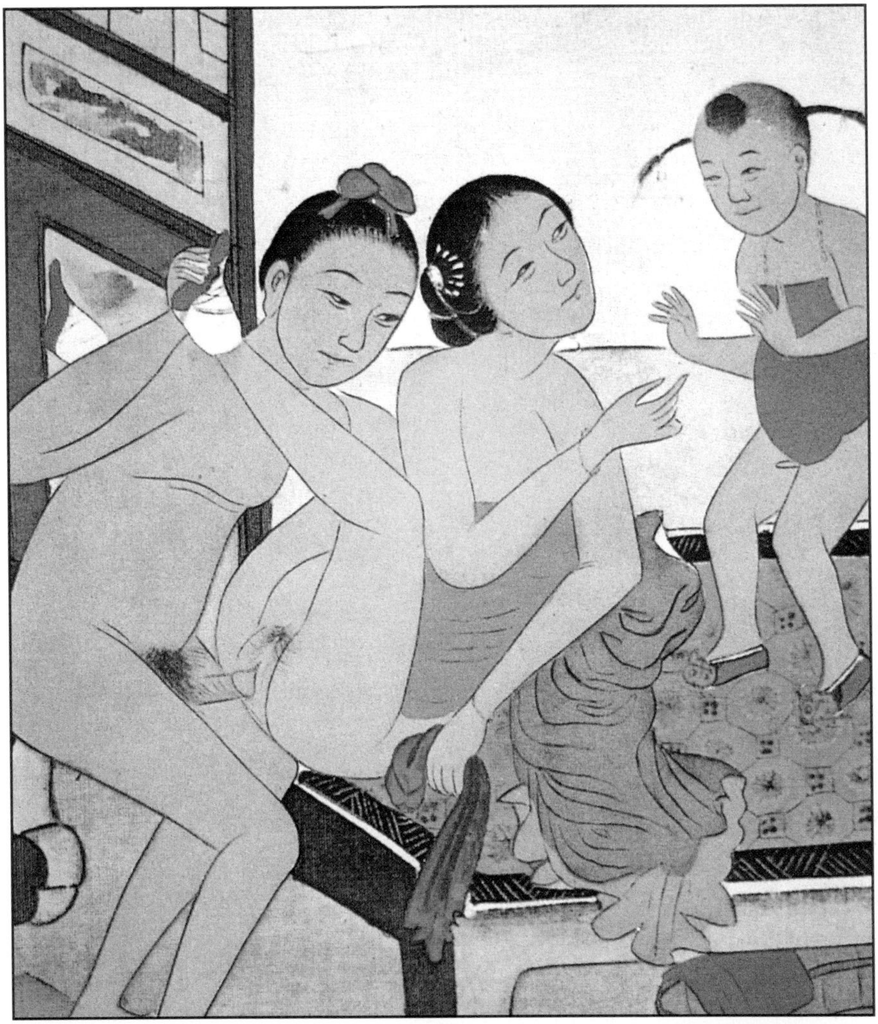

Sex education is now taught in schools in many countries, although the issue remains controversial. The young people themselves are, on the whole, enthusiastic, but feel that most sex education is 'too little, too late'.

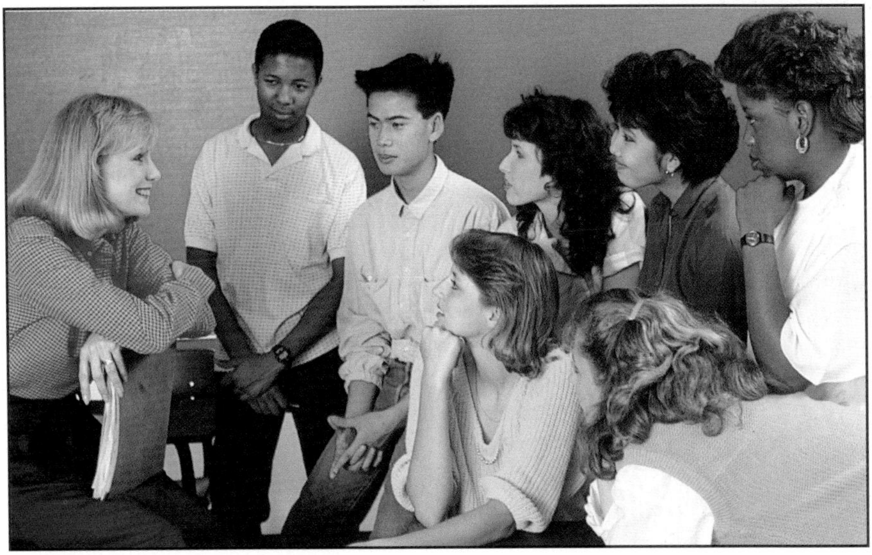

See also:
growth and change
masturbation
sexuality
health and hygiene

SEXUAL ATTRACTION

The essence of attraction between individuals remains the most elusive of all aspects of human relationships. Authors, poets, artists and philosophers have devoted their attention to it for centuries. More recently they have been joined by anthropologists, psychiatrists, psychologists and sociologists, gossip columnists and advice columnists, not to mention most socially or sexually active people. Still, it continues to evade identification, in spite of lying at the heart of sexual relationships. That unidentifiable spark of attraction, that complex cluster of responses, is the key to our interaction as sexual beings.

PHYSICAL ATTRACTION

This is the most immediate and superficial level of attraction. It dominates our first impressions and, if a sexual relationship develops, may continue to be a powerful force.

First impressions

The power of physical attraction is most significant in first impressions. Consciously or unconsciously, we make fundamental decisions about a person's suitability as a sexual partner within the first four minutes of meeting them – even within the first few seconds. These decisions are based entirely on physical criteria, although as relationships develop many other factors come into play.

Why is a person's appearance so important? Almost all people mention 'good looks' as something that they look for in a potential partner. Men in particular – regardless of sexual orientation – consider physical attractiveness to be essential: statistically the vast majority of men point to good looks as the most important attribute of a sexual partner.

Research carried out in Europe and the USA has pointed to a number of possible explanations for this. They include:

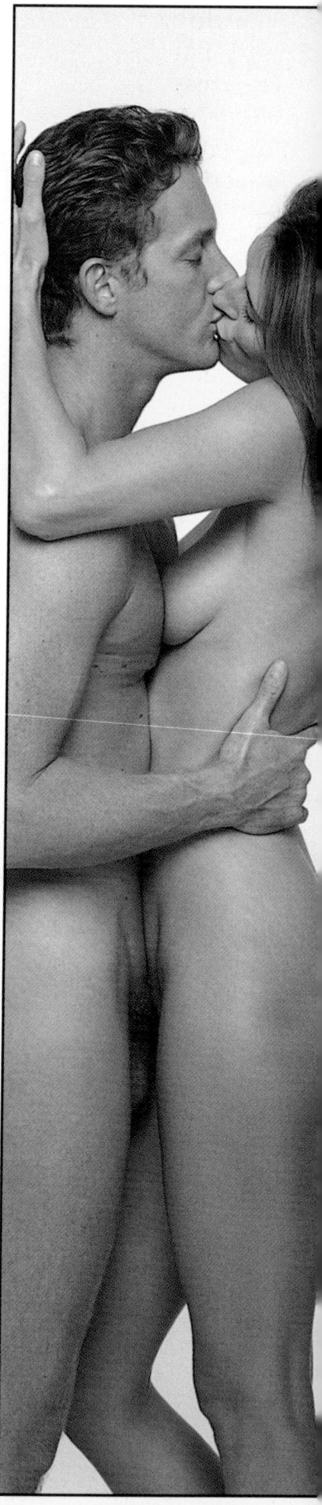

The essence of attraction remains the most elusive facet of human relationships.

● biology and evolution, incorporating the idea that the instinct to reproduce is a response to a series of physical signals

● the impression created in particular by the advertising, magazine, television and film industries that the best relationships are formed with a physically attractive person

● the association of good looks with a good personality. This impression may originate in children's literature, in which evil characters such as witches tend to be described as ugly and beautiful characters are generally virtuous

● the idea of an attractive partner being seen as a status symbol

Cross-cultural comparisons
Focusing on Western, developed countries with few cultural differences makes certain generalizations possible, but with regard to other cultures, less data is available. There may be some truth in Darwin's theory that people are attracted to the physical characteristics that they are most used to. He gave the example of beards being greatly admired in populations in which there is a genetic tendency towards hairiness. However, many ideas of attractiveness seem to be more socially rooted, in what certain particular attributes signify to a certain social or cultural group. The power of this kind of social conditioning is seen in the range of attitudes to physical build. For example, in some cultures, body fat is seen as an indication of health and high social status or wealth, while in others it suggests quite the opposite. In several distinct cultures fatness is seen as a sign of endurance and vitality during sex. Meanwhile, amongst the pre-World War Two Jews of Eastern Europe, pallor and extreme thinness were admired in men as evidence of studiousness and spiritual dedication.

In every case the distinct ideals of physical attractiveness are deeply rooted in the individual culture. Without understanding a particular culture, many of its peculiarities will be written off as 'oddities', such as the preferences for cross-eyes (Mayans), flattened heads (Kwakiutl), black gums and tongue (Maasai), black teeth (Yapese), joined eyebrows (Syrians), absence of eyebrows and eyelashes (Mongol), enormously protruding navels (Ila), pendulous breasts (Ganda), gigantic buttocks (Hottentot), fat calves (Tiv) and crippled feet (Chinese). To understand the origins of these preferences is to understand the cultural background of the people who hold them.

Male teenager from Wodabe tribe, Nigeria
Notions of attractiveness, including those relating to notions of masculinity and femininity, vary greatly from one culture to another. In this tribe, painting the body and face – as well as other forms of body decoration – is an important aspect of male attractiveness.

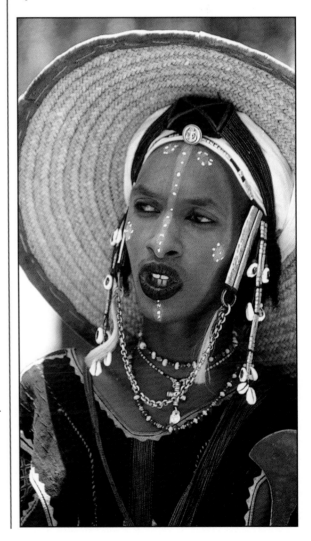

Western stereotype: what women look for in men

In surveys, women frequently point to height, well-muscled upper bodies and small, firm buttocks as attractive features in men. This echoes the patterns of choice of mate followed by our most distant ancestors, the females of which had to look for a mate who would provide healthy offspring, protect them, especially during pregnancy, and hunt for food. Consciously or not, and regardless of women's changing role in society, the attributes which women tend to seek in prospective partners suggest that they look for a mate who can be relied upon in all these aspects. They are attracted to men's bodies more for what they represent in terms of this 'reliability' – power, protection, security – than for the bodies themselves. For this reason, a woman may be attracted to a man of any kind of build, depending on what particular physical features hold these associations for her. At the same time, this theory may account for the fact that many women are also strongly attracted to non-physical attributes such as occupational success and power, or personality traits such as confidence, assertiveness or independence.

"I require only three things in a man: he must be handsome, ruthless and stupid"
DOROTHY PARKER

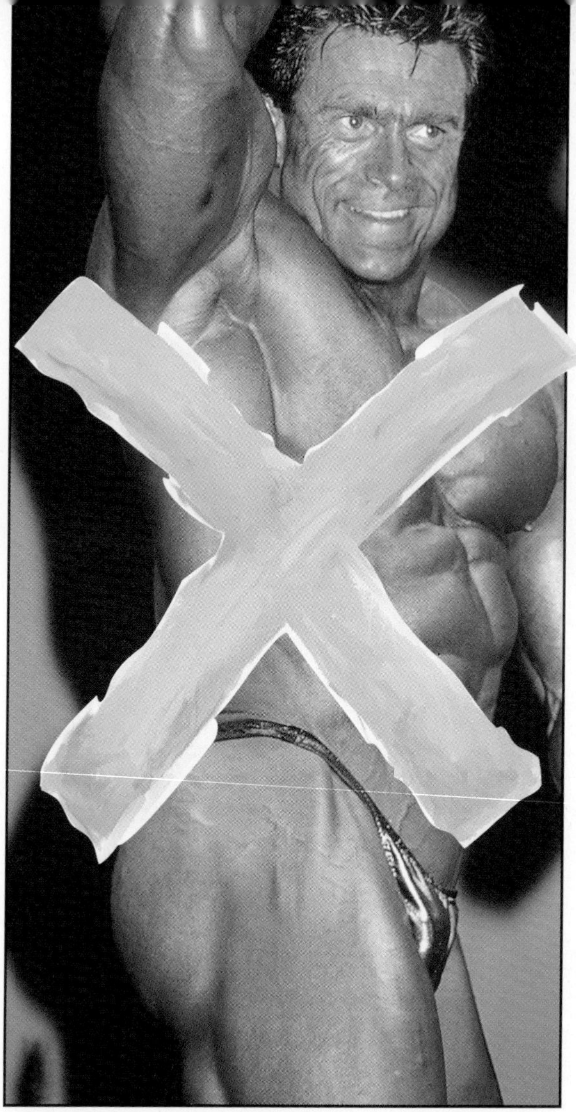

This body builder seems to have got it wrong – generally speaking, women are more interested in non-physical attributes in partners.

Survey of attraction

ATTRIBUTES VALUED IN MEN, BY WOMEN:

1 Intelligent
2 Sense of humour
3 Successful
4 Good in bed
5 Reliable
6 Physically attractive
7 Sensitive
8 Kind
9 Handsome
10 Similar interests

Notions of attractiveness in the West

It may, ultimately, be impossible to generalize about what people find attractive. In particular, when a relationship is formed a great many other, non-physical factors influence people's attitudes. However, a great many surveys have been carried out in Europe and the USA with regard to what physical features people find attractive in prospective partners. From these, certain trends emerge, many of which can be explained by the influence of evolutionary patterns.

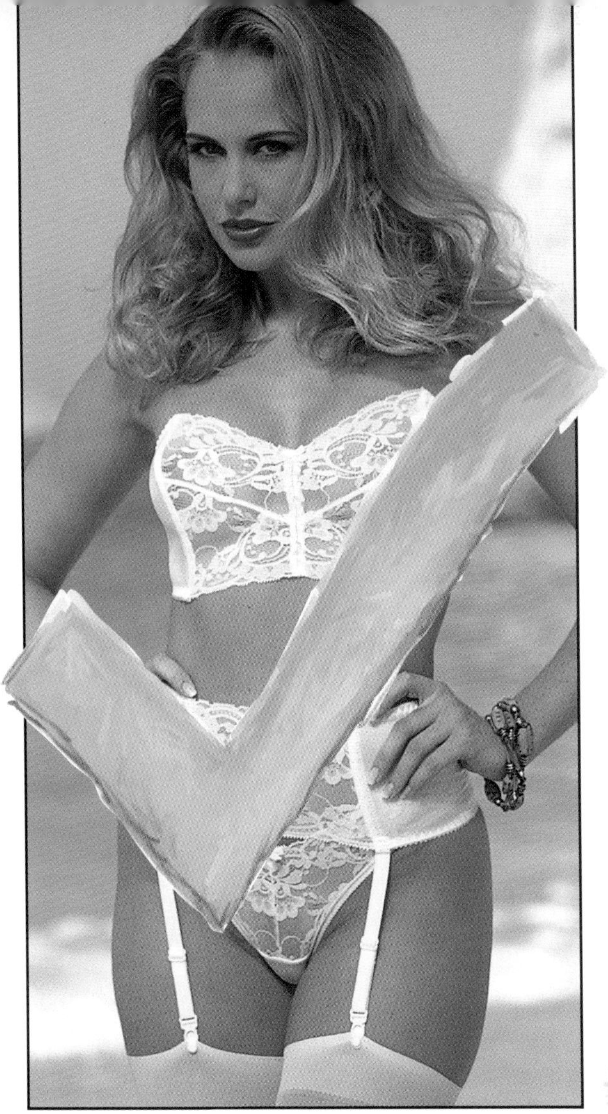

Men, on the other hand, tend to be much more orientated towards the physical – even though the specific type of looks or body that a particular man finds most attractive is entirely a matter of personal preference.

Western stereotype: what men look for in women

Evolutionary patterns also seem to dictate men's choice of partner, in that purely physical attributes – including youth – are considered much more important, as they search for a child-bearer. Again, an impression of health – suggesting fertility – is often considered attractive. However, the film, television, fashion and advertising industries have led to the perception of a fairly narrow stereotype as the ideal of female physical beauty. But in the same way as many, if not most, women are not over-preoccupied by penis size, a woman with blonde hair, long legs and large breasts is not the ideal for all men. For men, physique is a priority, but the nature of that physique is much more a question of personal preference. In many cases men will describe themselves as 'breast', 'bottom' or 'leg men'. It has even been suggested that sporty, extrovert men tend to prefer large breasts while intellectual introverts prefer small breasts.

"Being a sex symbol has to do with an attitude. not looks. Most men think it's looks, most women know otherwise"
KATHLEEN TURNER

It is often said that 'opposites attract'. While in psychological terms it is increasingly thought that we are attracted to people similar to ourselves, when it comes to physical attraction the differences play a key role. The biological differences between the sexes – women's softer skin and more rounded bodies, for example, and men's firmer bodies and greater body hair – can be fascinating to a member of the opposite sex.

Survey of attraction

ATTRIBUTES VALUED IN WOMEN, BY MEN:

1 Physically attractive
2 Beautiful
3 Kind
4 Sensitive
5 Sense of humour
6 Intelligent
7 Similar interests
8 Reliable
9 Sporty
10 Successful

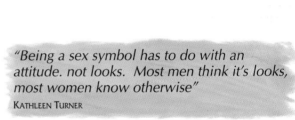

SEXUAL ATTRACTION AND SMELL

Smell is possibly the most evocative of human senses, possessing an emotional potency that the other senses may not. Smell can affect mood, stir memories and evoke fantasies.

Experts now believe that smell can be as important as appearance and personality in determining choice of partner. Within seconds of meeting someone we draw intuitive sensory conclusions about him or her; if they possess the 'right' smell, a process of 'olfactory bonding' may occur at a conscious or unconscious level.

The mechanisms of smell

Human beings can distinguish more than 10,000 different 'odorous chemicals'. However, each person's sense of smell is completely unique. Smell is learned by association and based on personal experiences.

The sense of smell functions in a part of the brain that controls learning, memory, appetites and basic emotional states such as fear, hate, love and sexual arousal. All smells have a chemical shape that fits like a key and locks into smell receptors inside the nose. The smell message is then passed directly to the brain, triggering an immediate signal in the centre of moods, emotions and long-term memory patterns.

Humans possess some three million scent glands. Most are found in the armpits and genitals, with others in the navel, nipples, scalp, mouth and eyelids. Musky smells are contained in armpit odour along with scents which are linked to sexual attraction. These may produce unconscious erotic responses or memories of certain events in the past. Human bodies are among the most sophisticated smell-producing systems in the animal kingdom and each person's personal smell is as individual as their fingerprints or DNA makeup.

Provocative perfumes

The secret of any strong sensual appeal in a perfume has always been ascribed to the 'animal base notes' in it and consequently humans have plundered the animal kingdom for its precious scents for centuries. The best perfumes contain ingredients which produce erotic responses. One group of smells which are arousing to humans are odorant secretions released from the skin around the sexual organs. From the animal world these include musk, civet and castor. Ambergris, the 'pearl of the whale', has a smell similar to human hair. All of these substances are used in the manufacture of provocative perfumes. In high concentrations, the odours of musk and civet resemble human sex-attractant smells.

Some plant scents have much the same impact on the human sexual response as animal ones. Frankincense resembles the body oils of dark-haired people and myrrh that of fair-haired people. Gum resins have a musky smell, henna blossom has the odour of semen and vanilla that of warm, human skin. Costus and mace are the only two plants which are actively erotic to humans.

Pheromones

Pheromones are chemicals emitted from the skin's surface, conveying messages which produce responses, often sexual, in others. In the animal kingdom pheromones are widely used in communication and can be turned on and off at will. A female silk moth can sexually excite every male for miles around by emitting one type of pheromone.

That pheromones exist in the human world is undisputed. They fall into two categories, attractants and primers. Primers cause biological changes in women and account for such phenomena as menstrual synchrony among women living together. Attractants can cause sometimes overtly sexual personal attraction between individuals.

It is now suspected that there are as many as forty or fifty human sex pheromones. These are produced by the face, genitals and armpits and can stimulate attraction and desire in others. A leading expert on the science of smell, Dr George Dodd, has suggested that pheromones have an exact counterpart in aphrodisiac scents. These 'sexual scents' can be divided into families, each of which corresponds to familiar scents. They include the soft, warm fragrance of sandalwood and musk and the human equivalent of the wild boar's sex pheromone. Luxurious, odiferous foods such as caviar, oysters, game and champagne make up the remaining families of the sexual scents. Dr Dodd has now produced a body spray containing manmade pheromones combined with the seven sexual scents, which may boost a person's sexual attractiveness.

However powerful a human pheromone or a particular scent is, it is unlikely that it will produce an instantaneous and involuntary, blind response of passion and sexual receptiveness, as it can in the animal kingdom. Instead, in a species as cognitively advanced as humans, pheromones and provocative scents are likely to work as part of a much broader and more sophisticated picture.

"Scents are surer than sights and sounds to make your heartstrings crack."
RUDYARD KIPLING

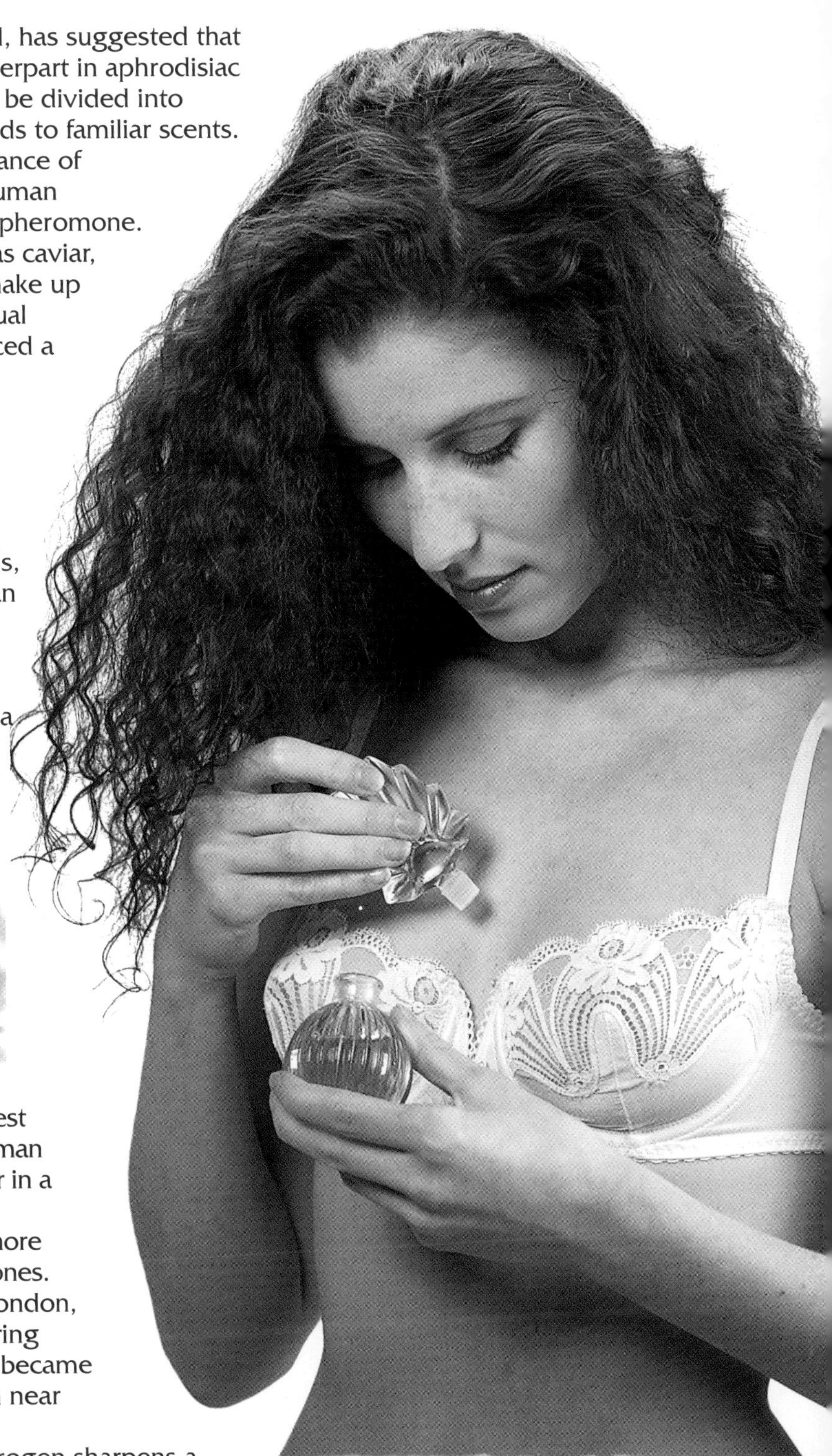

Facts

Experiments have been done to test the effectiveness of one of the human attractant pheromones. One chair in a waiting room sprayed with the pheromone was selected much more frequently than the non-sprayed ones.

Staff at Basildon Zoo, North London, England were banned from wearing perfume as some of the animals became 'embarrassingly lascivious' when near perfumed people.

The female sex hormone oestrogen sharpens a woman's sense of smell, making it keener than a man's. The scent women are best able to detect is musk, associated with the smell of male bodies.

"One should wear perfume wherever one expects to be kissed"
COCO CHANEL

ATTRACTION: PSYCHOLOGICAL FACTORS

The nature of attraction is hard to identify even in terms of relatively straightforward physical criteria, but it becomes more complex still when the innumerable psychological factors are taken into consideration. These include the obvious elements such as common interests, but also other factors which influence our choice of partner. Although we may be completely unaware of them, these may be the more powerful influences.

> *"Love looks not with the eyes, but with the mind"*
> SHAKESPEARE, A MIDSUMMER NIGHT'S DREAM

Personality

It is impossible to define universally attractive characteristics of personality. An impression of vitality, a positive outlook, humour or enthusiasm are often considered appealing, if for no other reason than that they suggest health and energy. These characteristics can be linked to the influence of evolutionary patterns as we are, if heterosexual, probably subconsciously searching for a mate who will provide healthy offspring. Sensitivity is also often mentioned as being important for both women and men. However, it is more likely to be the more individual characteristics, the idiosyncrasies and mannerisms, which attract us to a particular person.

Social and cultural pressures

There are various psychological factors of which we may be only partially aware. These include a range of social or cultural pressures, varying from one population group to another, such as the socioeconomic status or the religion of a prospective partner.

The role of the imagination

There is also a less practical side, in which the imagination plays a key role. This is seen in the idea of attraction based on previous sexual experience, real or imagined. According to this theory, we have in our subconscious a particular 'image' of attractiveness to which we unconsciously relate our current experiences. The role of film, television, literature and other media is fundamental here. As love and sex feature so frequently in the media, we are regularly presented with examples of all kinds of views about what constitutes attractiveness and what constitutes the ideal relationship.

Attraction and childhood

This takes us into the realms of unconscious influences, and brings us to one of the oldest and most researched theories of attraction: that of the influence of childhood and the family. Cases of people feeling sexually attracted to members of their immediate family appear in the Bible and in much Classical literature. The common terms for sexual attraction to a parent of the opposite sex, the Oedipus complex and the Electra complex for boys and girls respectively, are taken from Greek mythology. These complexes, and many other links between family relationships and sexual identity, were first investigated by Sigmund Freud at the turn of the twentieth century. Freud was the first to recognize sexuality as the source of human will and to infancy as the source of sexuality.

The idea that what attracts us to a potential sexual partner may be linked to certain characteristics of our parents is still widely accepted. Many theorists now believe that it is not only our parents who influence our choice of partner, but also the whole family structure. Tests have consistently shown that even before speaking to one another, people are attracted to those whose families have a similar structure. This can be in terms of levels of affection, strictness of discipline, parental expectations, or significant changes or losses at particular ages. Whether we wish to copy or to escape the characteristics of our families in our own relationships, the influence of the family background may be as inevitable as it is pervasive.

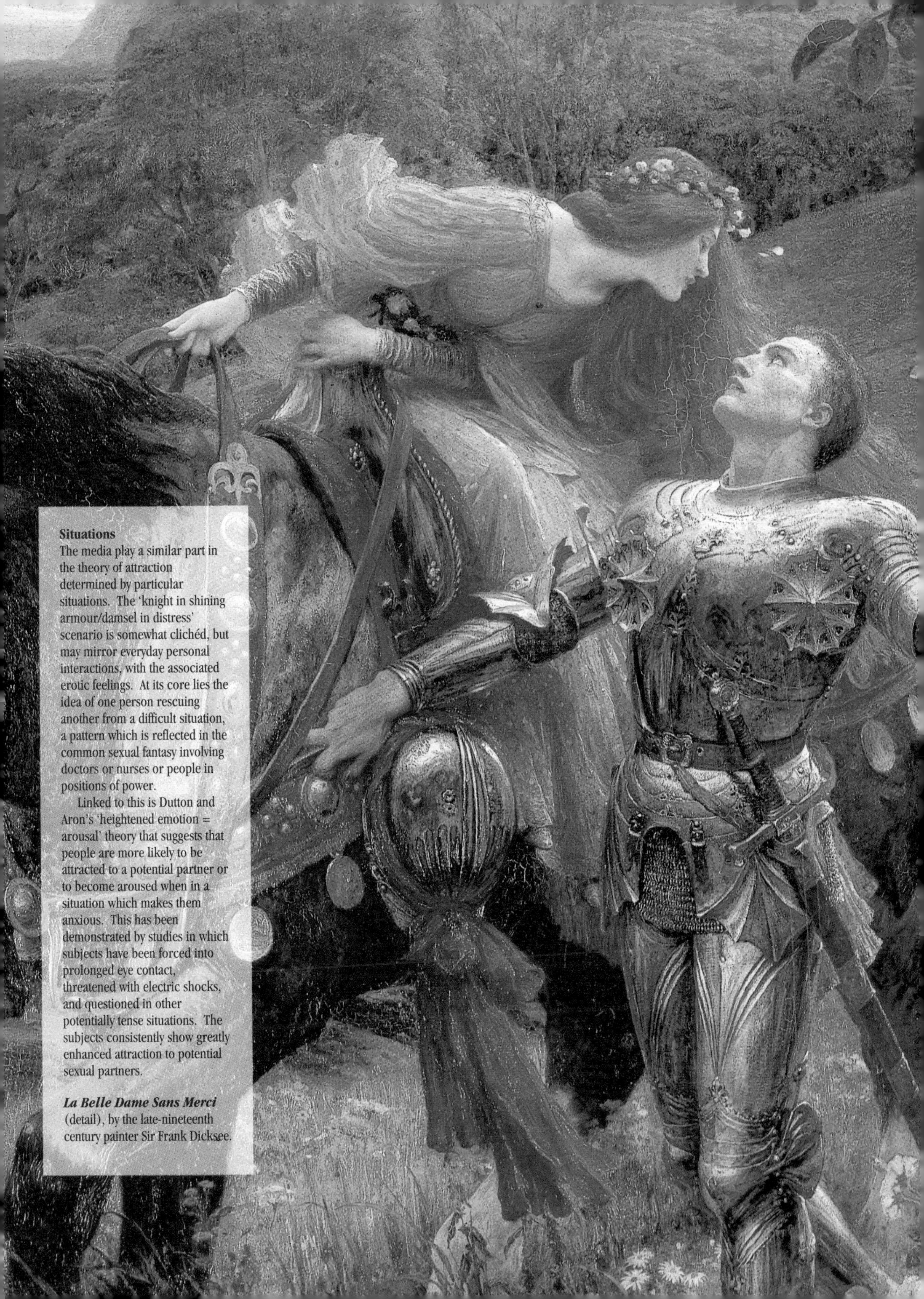

Situations

The media play a similar part in the theory of attraction determined by particular situations. The 'knight in shining armour/damsel in distress' scenario is somewhat clichéd, but may mirror everyday personal interactions, with the associated erotic feelings. At its core lies the idea of one person rescuing another from a difficult situation, a pattern which is reflected in the common sexual fantasy involving doctors or nurses or people in positions of power.

Linked to this is Dutton and Aron's 'heightened emotion = arousal' theory that suggests that people are more likely to be attracted to a potential partner or to become aroused when in a situation which makes them anxious. This has been demonstrated by studies in which subjects have been forced into prolonged eye contact, threatened with electric shocks, and questioned in other potentially tense situations. The subjects consistently show greatly enhanced attraction to potential sexual partners.

La Belle Dame Sans Merci (detail), by the late-nineteenth century painter Sir Frank Dicksee.

BODY LANGUAGE

The spoken word accounts for only a small percentage of our communication with other people. Most of our communication is through what is known as body language, the facial and bodily movements which – consciously and unconsciously – express our thoughts and feelings.

Just as the meaning of a single, isolated word is limited, an independent gesture or movement may reveal relatively little. However, combinations of words form sentences and combinations of movements may be even more expressive. An understanding of the way the different aspects of body language function can make us more aware both of the way people react to us and of the way we appear to them.

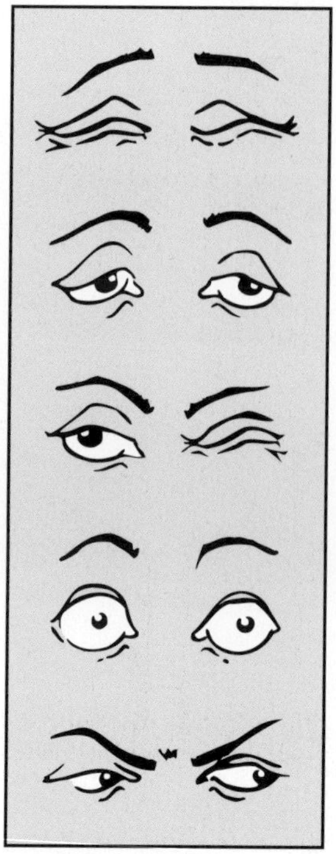

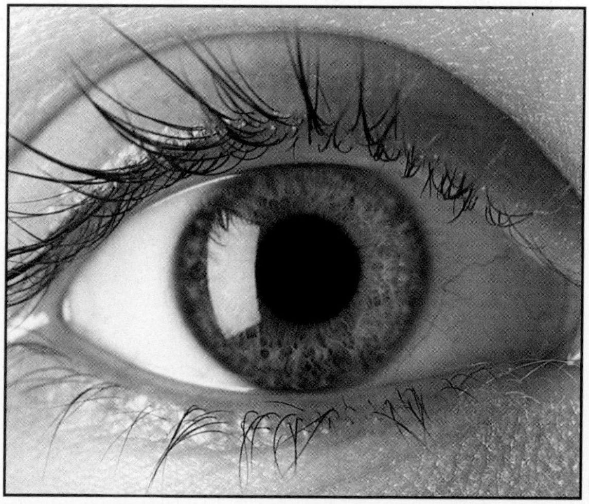

"They heard the wave's splash, and the wind so low, And saw each other's dark eyes darting light Into each other – and, beholding this, Their lips drew near, and clung into a kiss."
BYRON, DON JUAN

"The eyes are the windows to the soul."
JOHN BUNYAN

"Drink to me only with thine eyes, And I will pledge with mine."
JONSON

"Speech happens not to be his language"
ATTRIBUTED TO MME DE STAEL (on being asked what she found to talk about with her new husband, a hussar)

Eye contact

In surveys on notions of attractiveness, time and time again people mention the eyes as the most important facial feature, and often (particularly among women) as the most important attribute of the whole person. This is more than merely part of a physical assessment. Our eyes are frequently more eloquent than our voices, and can reveal more than we intend or realize.

See also: touching communication

The eyes can be a clear indication of emotion in the very earliest stages of any relationship. They are often the best way of establishing initial interest or rapport: hence the well-worn clichés of 'love at first sight' and 'eyes meeting across a crowded room'.

Generally speaking, when they talk, people look at each other for no more than two-thirds of the time, their eyes meeting for barely a second at a time. People who like each other maintain more eye contact, and if they are attracted to each other, eye contact is greater still. Games may be played, as two people try to catch each other's unguarded gaze. Men tend to look for longer and more openly, although if women do the same it may sometimes be interpreted as a blatant sexual signal. Women tend to look away then back at a person in whom they are interested. In both cases, eye contact can establish a sense of openness and sexual attraction.

When a person looks away to break his or her gaze the direction to which they turn can also be significant. It has been said that looking downward indicates strong inner emotion; looking up suggests an active imagination; looking sideways can imply rehearsing or recalling words or thoughts.

Attraction may also be betrayed by the appearance of the eyes themselves. With sexual attraction they tend to widen and the pupils dilate. With sexual arousal the pupils remain enlarged but the eyes may narrow and become less focused. This may be considered a strong sexual signal – a fact recognized by Italian courtesans in the sixteenth century, who used small quantities of the drug belladonna to dilate the pupils. The drug acquired its name at that time as the word belladonna means 'beautiful lady' in Italian. Eye decoration has been common in many cultures.

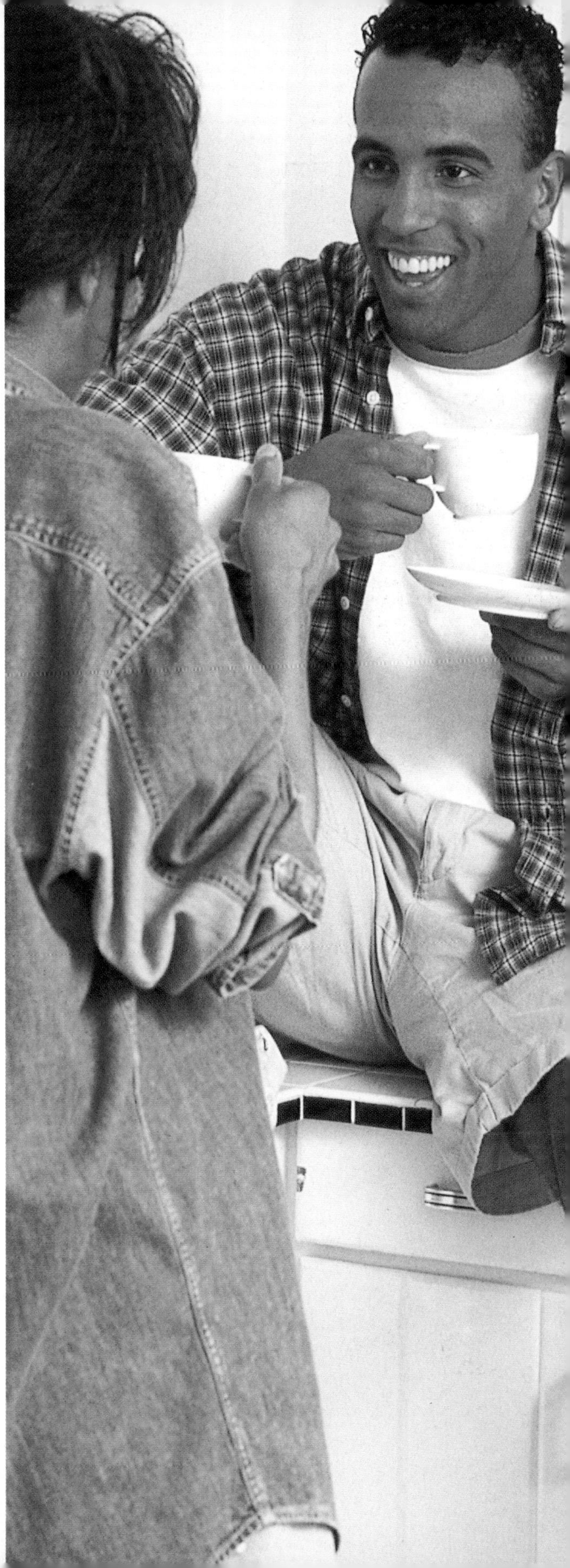

Eye contact can be a powerful way of conveying feelings – these people are clearly enjoying each other's company.

Personal territory
Research into people's reactions to the proximity of other individuals in specific situations has led to the classification of four zones of personal space.

● THE PUBLIC ZONE: OVER 4 METRES
This zone relates to public performances. This may be in the context of the theatre, the Church or education. 'Audience' and 'performers' are separate and defined and any interaction between the two can be disconcerting, as when actors move into the audience, or a single member of the audience is singled out by a performer.

● THE SOCIAL ZONE: FROM 1.2 TO 4 METRES
This is the zone occupied by strangers and distant, professional acquaintances. It may include shopkeepers and domestic workmen with whom interaction tends to be on a formal level.

● THE CASUAL OR PERSONAL ZONE: FROM 0.5 TO 1.2 METRES
This is the zone in which we operate at social gatherings and in offices. It allows casual interaction enabling people to get to know each other with no sense of threat or invasion.

● THE INTIMATE ZONE: UP TO 50 CM
This is the zone to which only lovers and close friends, associates and relatives are admitted. If anyone else tries to enter this zone it can seem hostile and invasive (see also 'Touching'). The body reacts to this degree of proximity with a rush of adrenaline. This increases the pulse rate and blood flow through the body, preparing it to fend off or flee an invasion, or to respond warmly to the closeness of a loved one.

These zones vary from one person to another; for instance, the distances tend to be reduced between two women and increased between men. They also vary greatly from one culture to another. Movement from one zone to another can occur as situations change and relationships develop, but crossing a boundary too soon can be threatening. The movement from social to intimate zones can be eased initially with socially acceptable excuses such as lighting a cigarette, sharing an umbrella or dancing.

Posture, gesture and attraction
Posture and gesture can also form a strong indication of one person's feelings for another. This is another area where animal instincts come into play, as we preen

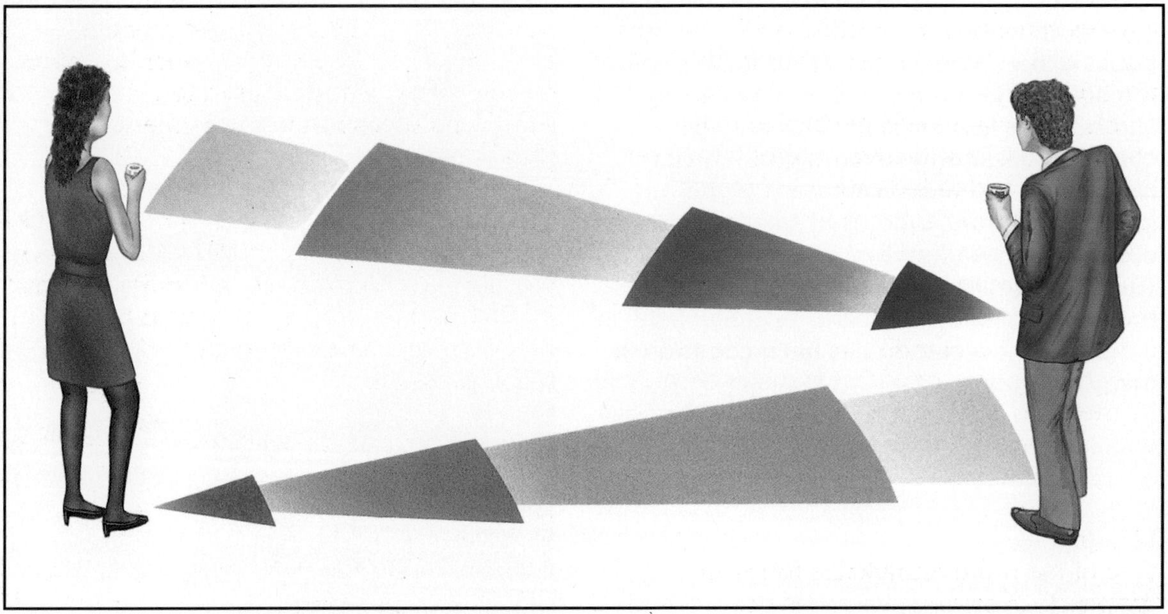

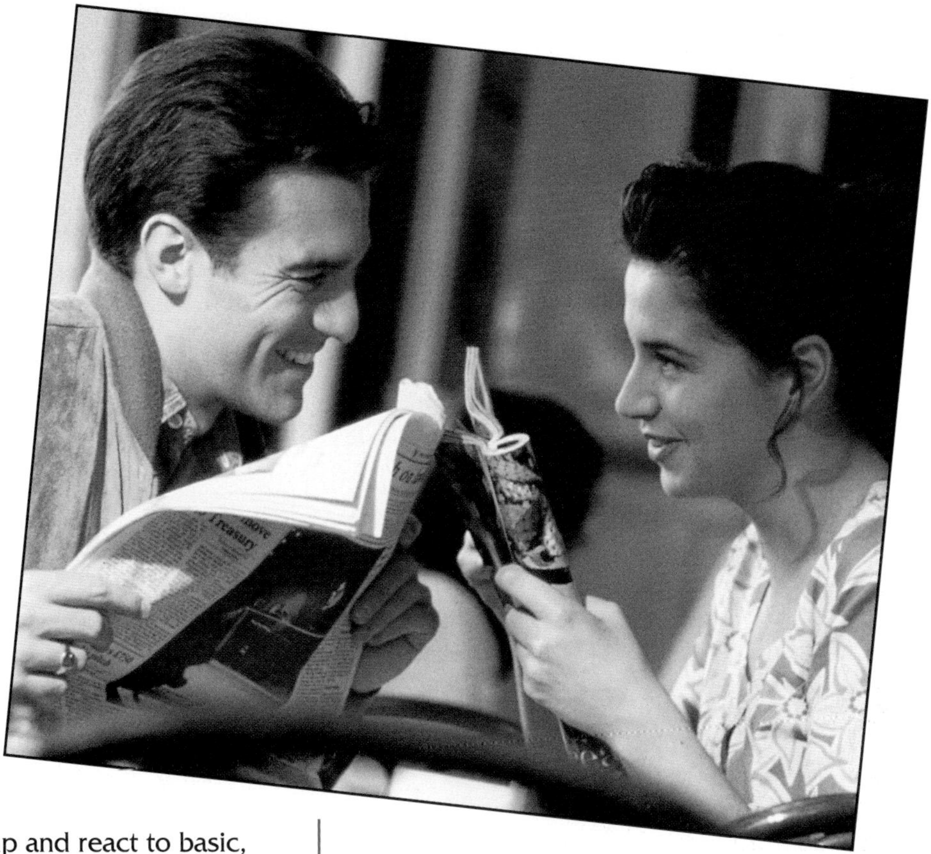

Actions speak louder than words – the posture of this man and this woman, and the echoing in the way they are holding their newspaper and magazine, clearly show warmth and attraction.

ourselves for courtship and react to basic, subtle sexual signals. Open body movements combined with sensitivity to other people's body language can be very attractive. Likewise, negative or 'closed' gestures can be surprisingly powerful and barriers can easily be created with a crossed leg or arm, a lack of eye contact or the turn of the body.

We use posture and gesture to make ourselves more attractive, to emphasize our best points and to indicate our interest in a specific person in a group by 'pointing' our body or just one foot toward the person in whom we are most interested, whether sexually or socially. We may also touch ourselves or each other. However, there are also specific uses of body language employed by men and women – consciously and unconsciously – to attract or to demonstrate attraction to a prospective partner.

Echoing

One of the more remarkable forms of unconscious communication is posture and gesture echoing. Research has shown that we tend to copy the body language of people that we like. The closer the relationship the more evident this behaviour becomes, as emotional and psychological rapport and trust develop. A conscious form of this echoing, subtly following a person's posture or gestures, can also be used to establish some kind of rapport with an otherwise distant or unfriendly person.

While this kind of echoing is generally quite unconscious, in an intimate relationship it can extend to bodily processes over which we have no control at all. It is quite common for lovers to develop synchrony in heartbeat, breathing rate, body temperature and even blood pressure.

"There's language in her eye, her cheek, her lip,
Nay, her foot speaks; her wanton spirits look out
At every joint and motive of her body"
SHAKESPEARE, TROILUS AND CRESSIDA

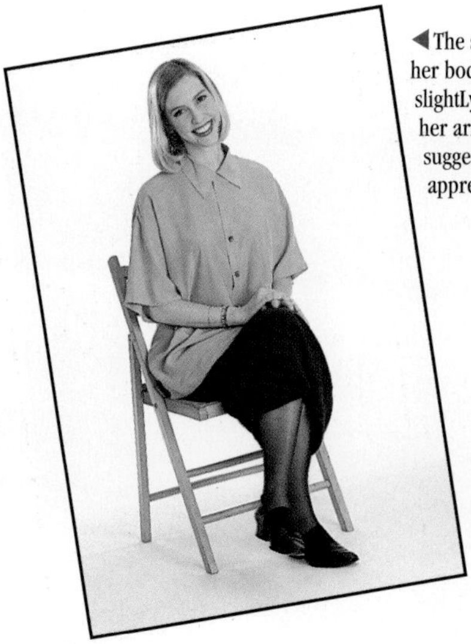

◀ The smile is friendly, but her body is upright and slightLy angled away, whilst her arms and legs are closed, suggesting that she is slightly apprehensive.

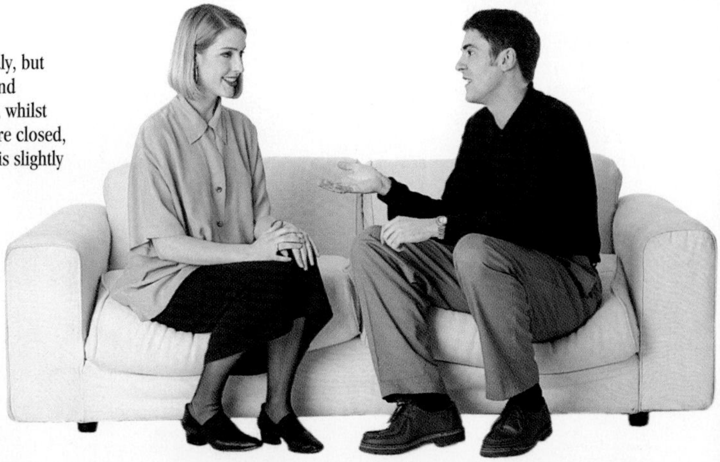

▲ **1.** He is making the first advances – his posture is relatively open, though the left hand shows he is slightly guarded. Her gestures are closed, but her smile inviting.

▶ 'Preening' – classic female courtship signals: the legs are crossed towards you, the head is tilted, and one hand is on the knee whilst the other 'preens' the hair, revealing the subconscious desire to look youthful and attractive.

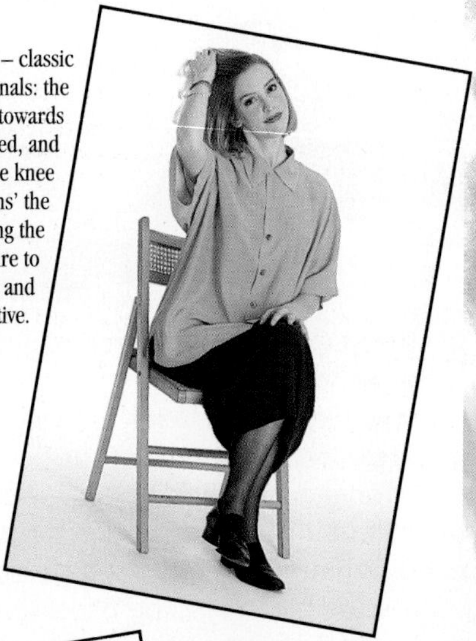

Female courtship gestures

The woman will want to make a good impression, but her gestures may be more subtle that the man's and she may be hesitant to make the first moves. General appearance, body language and the use of voice and touch are all significant.

If she is attracted she may:

- cross legs towards the person to whom she is attracted, or cross and uncross them.
- straighten her body, drawing attention to her breasts
- touch or stroke her hair during conversation and tilt her head
- look briefly at the person then look away again
- lean forward with interest during conversation
- lower and soften her voice
- smile warmly and open her eyes wider
- touch the person, sometimes by brushing something off their clothing

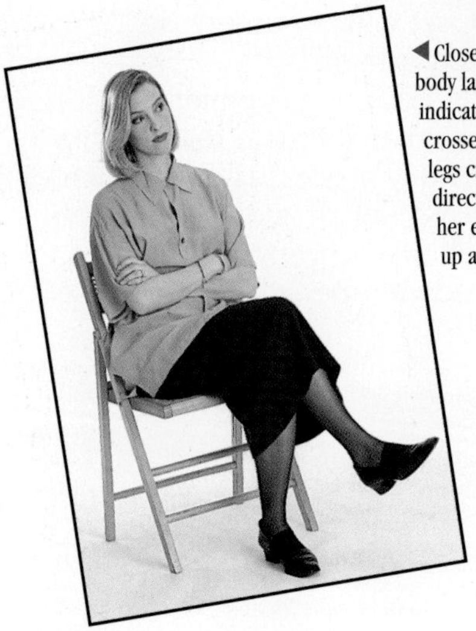

◀ Closed, disinterested body language is indicated by the firmly crossed arms, the legs crossed and directed away, with her eyes looking up and away.

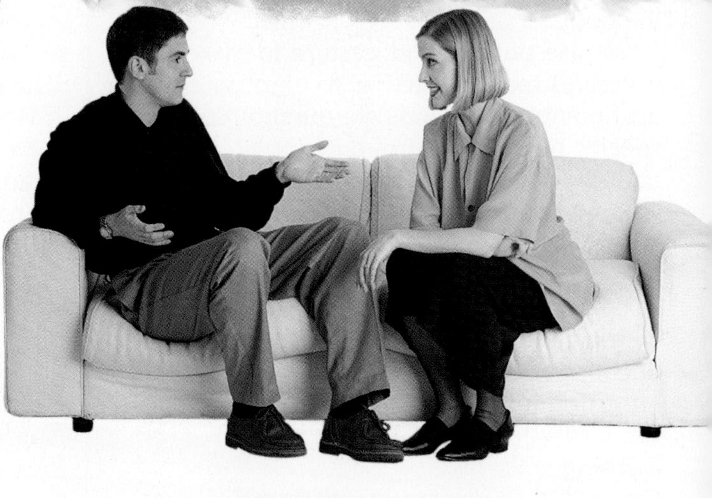

▲ **3.** His gestures are open but he is leaning away. She is angled towards him and her raised eyebrows intensify eye contact.

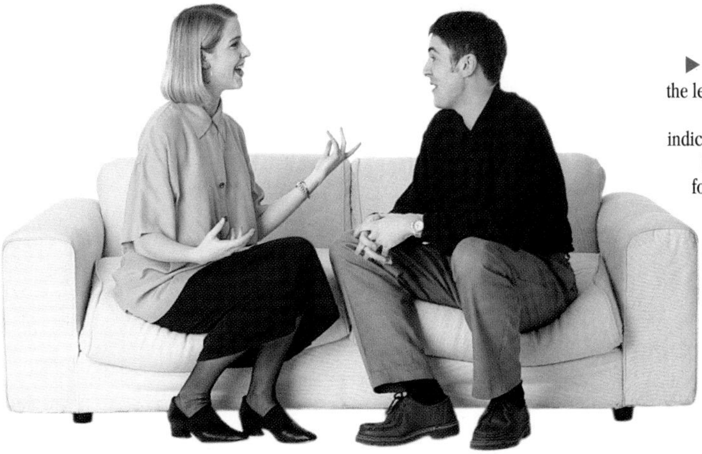

▲ **2.** She is opening up her facial expression and hand gestures, turning her hands and wrists upwards and angling her body further towards him, whilst he is angled closer towards her – the ice is breaking.

▶ In a female, a hand on the leg would be a come-on, but in a male, it is a indication of stubbornness. His outer arm and leg form a barrier to close interaction.

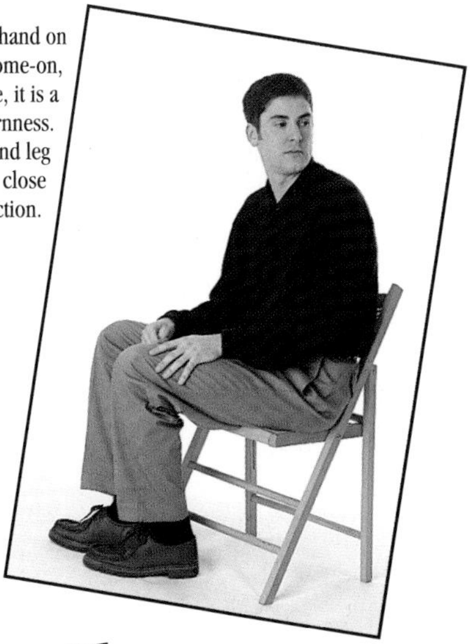

Male courtship gestures

The man will want to make a good impression. That impression will involve general appearance, body language and tone of voice as well as actual spoken words and touch. It may also include specific preening gestures.

If he is attracted he may:

- smooth his hair or clothing
- flatten his abdomen and stand tall
- thrust his hips and chest forward, sometimes with hands on hips
- maintain eye contact
- lower and soften the voice
- touch the person he is attracted to, perhaps with a hand around the shoulders or on the elbow
- sit with his pelvis tilted upwards and legs apart
- smile warmly and open the eyes wider

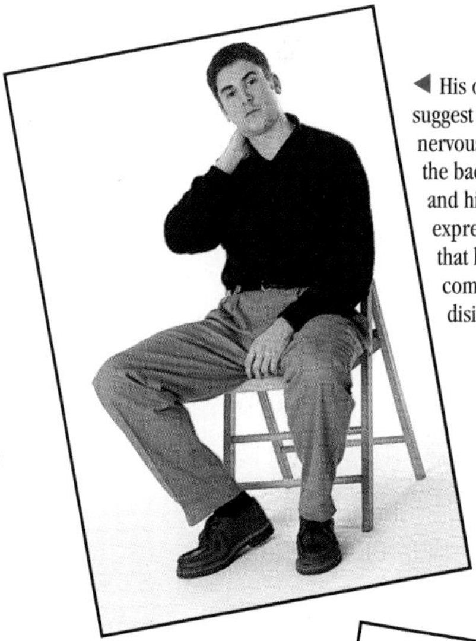

◀ His open legs suggest that he is not nervous, but rubbing the back of his neck, and his closed facial expression, indicate that he is completely disinterested.

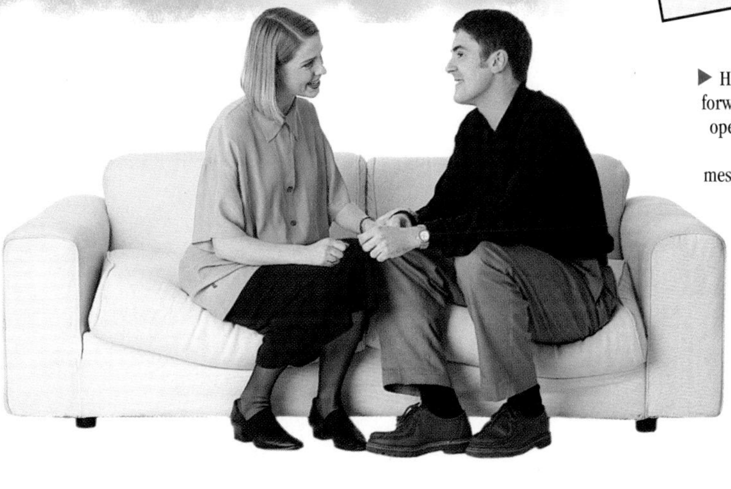

▲ **4.** Their bodies are open and turned towards each other. Eye contact is strong, and they have bridged the gap between them with their hands.

▶ His exposed palms, forward-angled body, open legs and smile all give a strong message of interest.

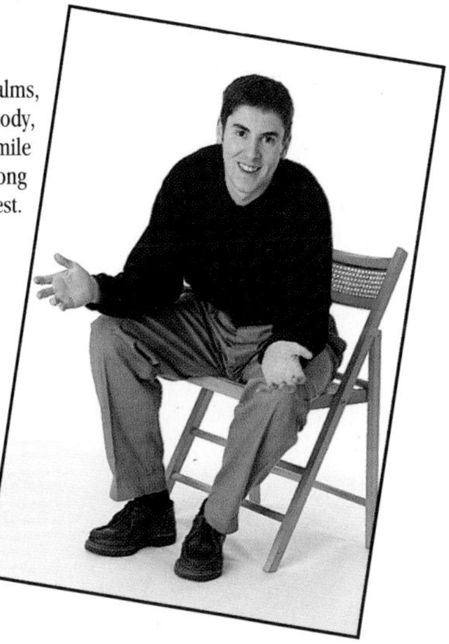

TOUCHING

Touching is one of the most basic forms of communication. As newborn babies, we first come to know our environment and form bonds with other people through touch. Touch – or the lack of it – continues to be a significant aspect of all our relationships.

In terms of where and how we touch another person, different kinds of touching are appropriate in different situations. Above all, this is determined by the nature of the relationship between the people concerned. Completely distinct kinds of touching may take place between, for example, close relatives, business associates and lovers. In some cases the distinction may be less clear, for example between lovers and close friends. However, there is a boundary between the two, the nature and location of which vary from one person to another. This boundary must be respected. Even allowing someone to come close to it is a gesture of trust. If the boundary is crossed in the wrong way, or at the wrong time, it can seriously damage a relationship. But, if both people feel comfortable with the boundary being crossed, it can take the relationship to a whole new level of intimacy.

***Touching** ... stroking, scratching, pressing, pinching, rubbing, tickling, smacking, feeling, squeezing, patting, caressing, massaging*

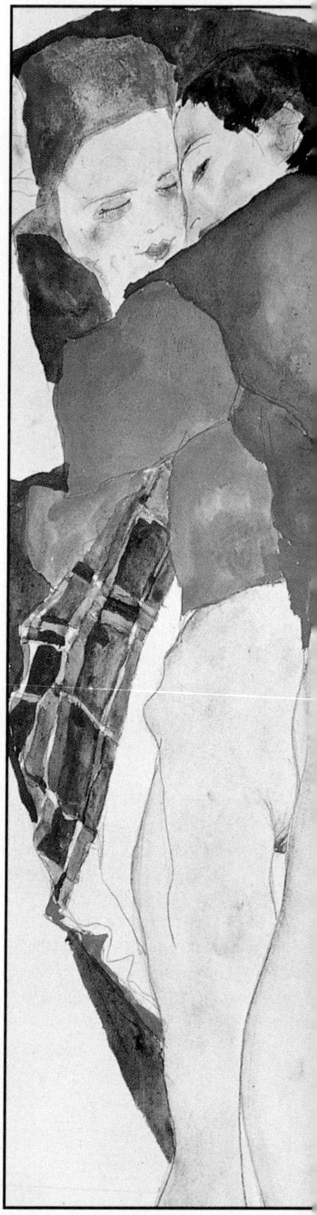

Lovers (detail), by Egon Schiele (1911)

Types of touch

The various kinds of touch may be classified into five levels of progressive intimacy. These help to define what kinds of touch are acceptable in specific situations.

● LEVEL 1 – the touch of professionals, including teachers, beauty therapists and medical practitioners, dentists, oculists and physiotherapists. It may be soothing and reassuring, even sensual, as in the case of massage, or stressful, as in some kinds of medical examination.

See also:
sexual awareness in children
erogenous zones
body language
sex aids and toys
kissing

FACT: The skin of an average adult covers more than 2 square metres and weighs up to 4 kg. It contains millions of nerve endings which relay all kinds of sensory information to the brain. It is often considered to be the largest sexual organ.

● LEVEL 2 – touch in social situations, as in the many forms of greeting and farewell, some sixty per cent of which involve some physical contact.

● LEVEL 3 – any form of contact between friends, from a reassuring touch on the hand to an open and enthusiastic embrace. The amount of this kind of contact with which people feel comfortable depends largely on what they are used to: some families and some cultural groups are more tactile than others.

● LEVEL 4 – the more intimate touch which may be permissible between parent and child, close friends, and lovers. It is a clear demonstration of trust in the relationship, although it is also affected by cultural factors.

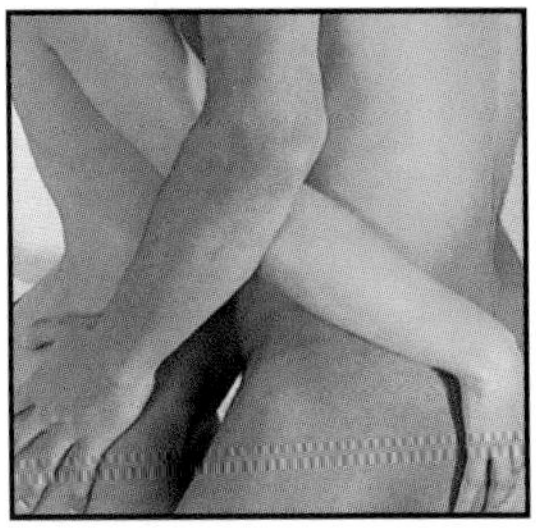

● LEVEL 5 – the sensuous touching between lovers as part of sexual arousal.

Touch in a loving relationship

As a relationship develops and trust is built up, the kinds of touch which are appropriate may move through these levels. Most relationships begin with the distant and formal social touch before moving on to friendly touch; only occasionally does this develop into the more intimate loving or sexual contact.

The movement from one level of intimacy to another often comes through trial and error. We try to interpret each other's body language before attempting any kind of physical contact; then, when we touch, we observe the person's reaction. Any kind of backing off shows that the person is not comfortable with our touch; a returned touch is a more positive signal. Any individual may have certain 'no-go' areas where they do not like to be touched for personal or cultural reasons. Excuses for touch – to test the water – can also be found, such as lighting a cigarette or passing something from hand to hand.

Once intimacy has been established, touch can take many forms and can be a fundamental part of any sexual relationship. It is largely through touch that we come to know our sexual selves. In the same way, touch can be the key to getting to know someone sexually.

Sexual touch

Sexual touch is distinguished from friendly or loving touch by where and how people touch each other. The significance of touching particular parts of the body may vary from one cultural group to another. For example, while in the West rubbing noses is something people in a close personal relationship might do for fun, in Polynesia it used to be a formal greeting. However, generally speaking, the more intimate the touch, the more intimate the relationship. People tend to start by touching the parts nearest to them, such as hands and perhaps shoulders or knees. Touching the face, or allowing another person to touch one's own face, is a powerful signal of affection and trust. Touching the thighs, the trunk of the body and anywhere near the breasts or genitals makes the gesture overtly sexual.

Erotic touch comes into its own when clothes are removed and skin-to-skin touch begins. This can take many different forms, and can develop as intimacy grows. Ultimately it can become a powerful and sensuous facet of lovemaking.

The skin responds to all kinds of stimulation and each individual has specific parts of the body which are particularly sensitive. Some seem to be gender-specific while others vary from one individual to the next. They may include anything from the fingertips to the genitals themselves. These are known as the erogenous zones.

Pressure, temperature, speed and rhythm can all be varied to produce an enormous range of sensations. Touch can be with the fingertips, the hands, the feet or any other part of the body. While the sensation of skin on skin can be highly arousing, different sensations can be produced by touching with other objects or materials, such as hair, feathers, fur, velvet, silk or satin, rubber or leather, water or ice or sexual aids such as a vibrator.

KISSING

A kiss is one of the most common gestures of affection. It can also be one of the most intimate and erotic.

Human beings are the only animals able to kiss in this way: the J-shaped muscles in the lips contribute to this purpose. This may be because evolutionary processes required the development of sexual signals on the front of the body when humans started to mate face-to-face. However, the origins of the practice of kissing mouth-to-mouth lie not in mating but in caring for the offspring, in mouth-to-mouth feeding. Many animals feed their newborn offspring in this way, making it one of the most natural gestures of trust and intimacy. Even now the sensual side of the experience of eating is often linked to, or combined with, more overtly sexual activity.

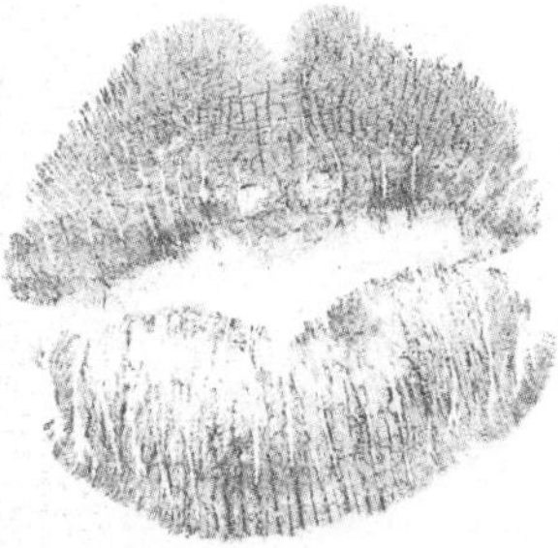

Kissing and relationships

Kissing on the cheek can mean many different things, depending principally on cultural factors. Social kissing by way of greeting is common in many areas of the former Soviet Union, and most Mediterranean and Latin American countries. It is more common between women but in some countries also occurs between men. English and American men rarely kiss as friends, except occasionally in moments of triumph on the sports field. Between two women or a woman and a man, it is largely a gesture of affection.

The first mouth-to-mouth kiss is generally taken as a specific sign of the beginning of an intimate relationship. Even after this stage kissing can continue to stand as an indication of the affection between the two people concerned. According to Relate, Britain's marriage guidance counselling organization, unhappy couples tend to stop kissing even before they stop having sexual intercourse. Many sex workers (prostitutes) refuse to kiss

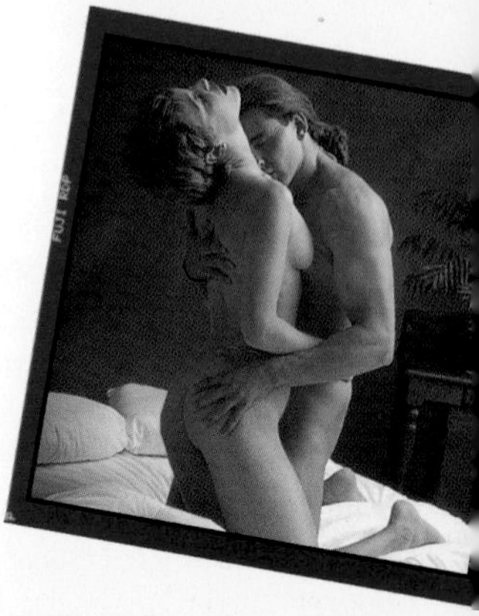

"A kiss can be a comma, a question or an exclamation point. That's basic spelling every woman ought to know."
MISTINGUETT

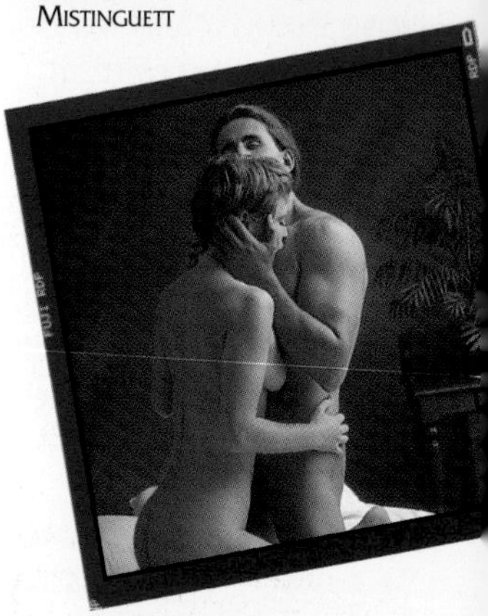

"The sound of a kiss is not so loud as that of a cannon, but its echo lasts a great deal longer."
DR OLIVER WENDELL HOLMES

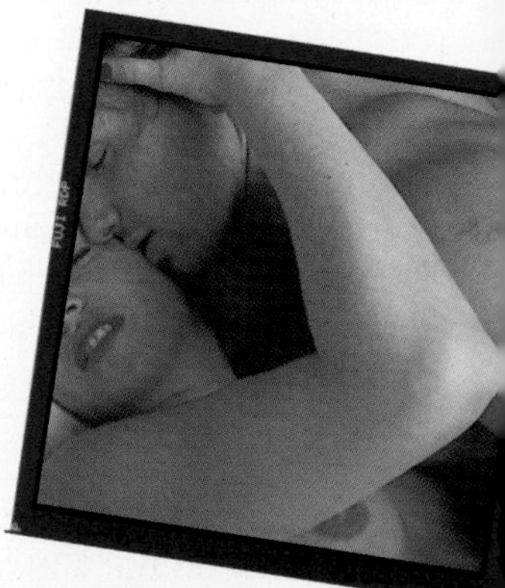

"... we did one of those quick, awkward kisses where each of you gets a nose in the eye."
CLIVE JAMES, UNRELIABLE MEMOIRS (1980)

See also:
oral sex
touching
erogenous zones

FACT: A passionate kiss can burn up as many as twelve calories

Ways of kissing
The mouth is a highly mobile and responsive organ, allowing for great variety in types of kiss. Kisses can be anything from soft and tender to deep, passionate and even rough. Kisses can mimic intercourse, the tongue 'penetrating' the mouth, ears or vagina. The entire body can be explored with kisses.

● EYES OPEN OR CLOSED? Men tend to be more visually stimulated than women and are therefore more likely to kiss with their eyes open. Statistically, ninety-seven per cent of women and only thirty per cent of men kiss with their eyes closed.

● LIPS OPEN OR CLOSED? Different kinds of kiss are appropriate in different situations. However, it has been suggested that certain types of mouth-to-mouth kiss may reveal certain character traits or attitudes to the relationships in question. For example, an unwillingness to kiss with open lips may suggest some kind of fear of intimacy, while kissing with closed lips then opening the mouth for more lingering kisses, indicates sensuousness and passion. Kissing with open lips and using the tongue may imply generosity or the desire to create a strong and intimate bond.

Other variations which make each person's way of kissing unique include the varying degrees of rhythm, speed, pressure and moisture, the softness or firmness of the lips and tongue and the amount of movement of the lips and tongue. Sometimes the teeth can be used and kissing can include nibbling or biting. Any part of the body can be kissed, in any way.

their clients on the lips. Clearly, for many people mouth-to-mouth kissing is even more intimate than sexual intercourse and may therefore be reserved only for the most meaningful relationships.

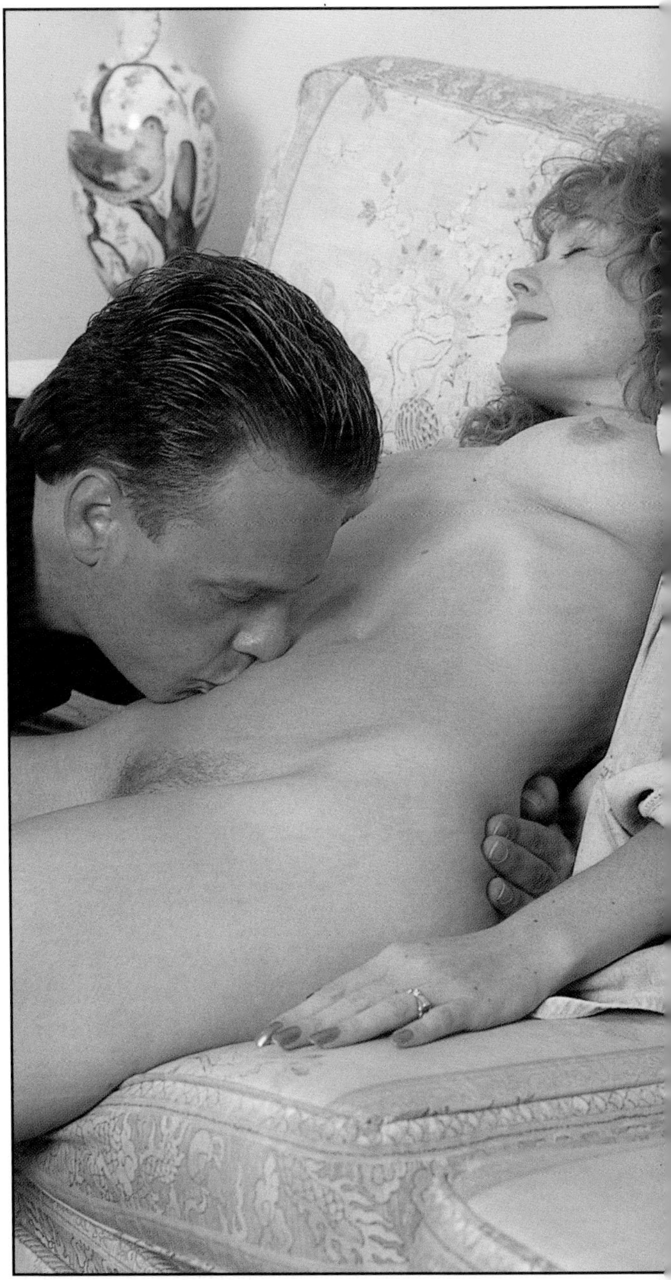

FACT: Kissing can be addictive. The glands at the edge of the lips and in the mouth produce chemicals which enhance and stimulate desire during kissing. The very action of kissing boosts the production of these chemicals.

EROGENOUS ZONES

Any part of the body can be sexual. Any touch can be sexually arousing, particularly when the people touching each other are emotionally involved. However, some parts of the body are especially sensitive. The genitals are the most obvious example, but other, apparently non-sexual parts of the body can be extremely erotic. These areas of high sensitivity are sometimes known as the erogenous zones.

Male and female

The erogenous zones in the male tend to be more clearly defined and more uniform from one man to another than they are in the female. The genitals are by far the most sensitive parts and male arousal tends to depend more upon genital stimulation than anything else.

For women, however, stimulation of almost any part of the body can be highly arousing. There is also considerably more variation from one woman to another. Some women have been known to come close to, or actually reach, orgasm through stimulation just of the breasts, mouth or even the earlobes. In spite of this the effects of arousal are still most strongly felt in the genital area, primarily in the clitoris.

The sensitivity of different parts of the body can also be governed by psychological factors. These may be influenced by past experiences and associations, or by culture-specific taboos. These may make a certain part of the body a 'no-go' area, or they may make it that much more sensitive and erotic.

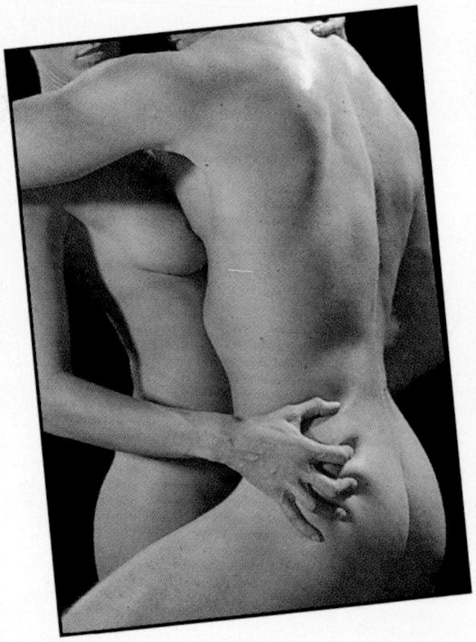

Female erogenous zones
All of the skin, but in particular:

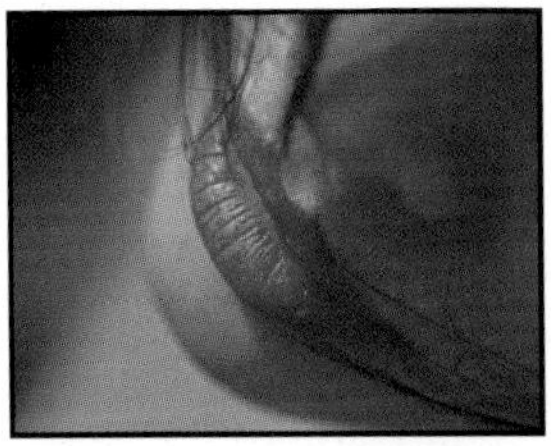

- face: mouth, cheeks, eyelids, eyebrows, forehead, hairline, temples, back of neck and earlobes

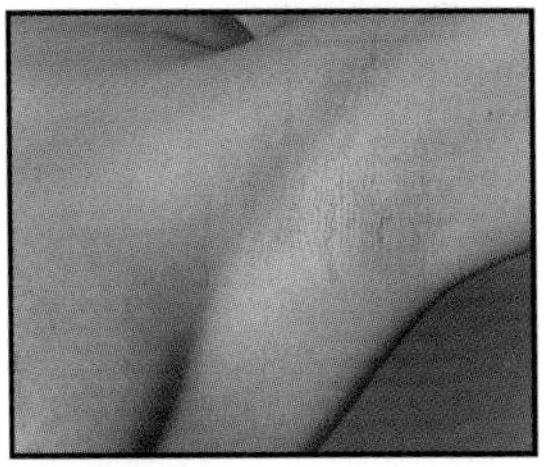

- arms, armpits, inside of elbow, hands

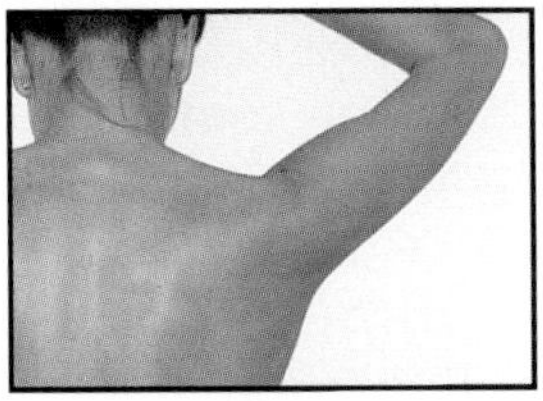

- breasts, nipples

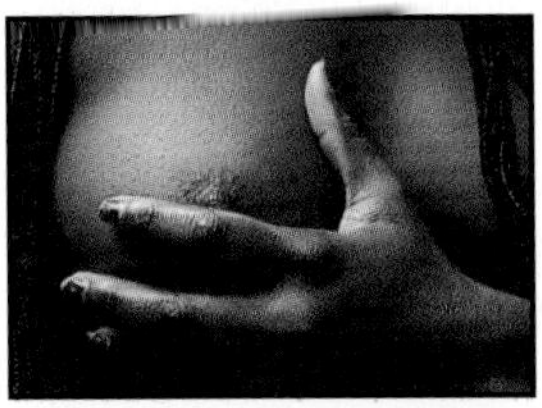

- abdomen, navel
- genitals: inner lips, clitoris

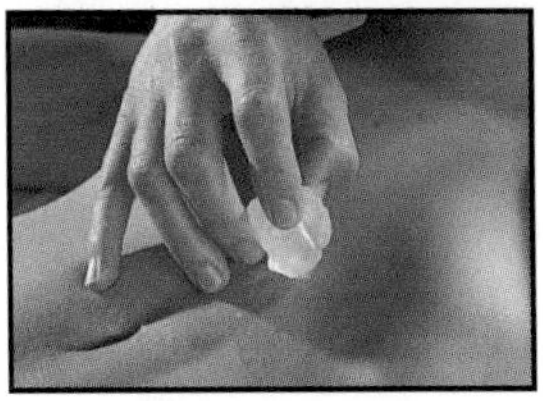

- back, base of spine
- perineum
- buttocks
- anus

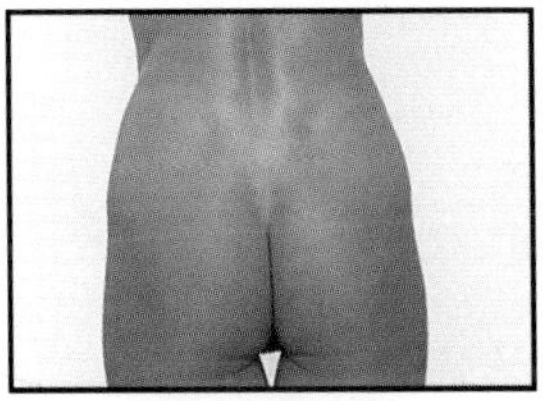

- feet and legs, inside of thighs, back of knees

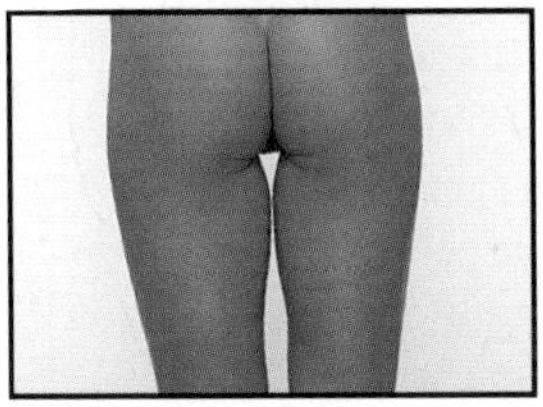

Male erogenous zones

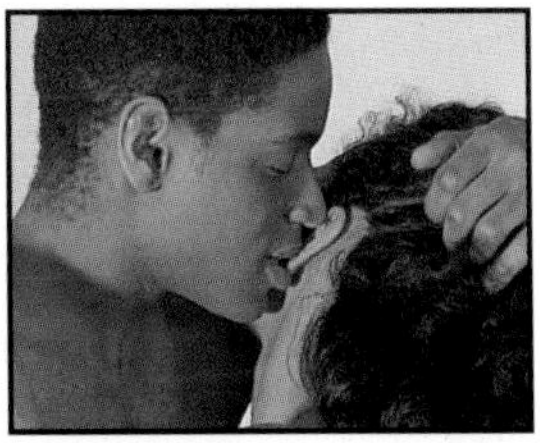

- face and neck, nape of neck, earlobes and lips

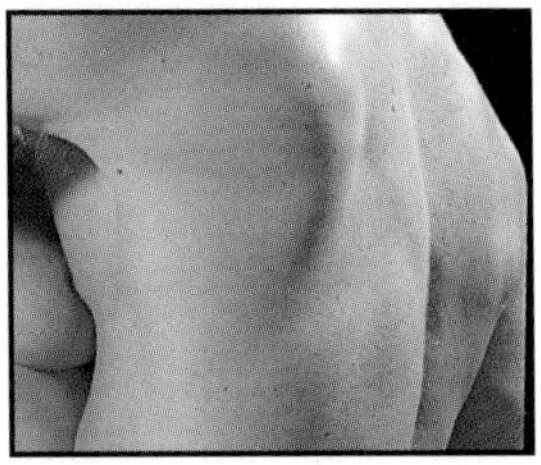

- back, shoulders and small of back

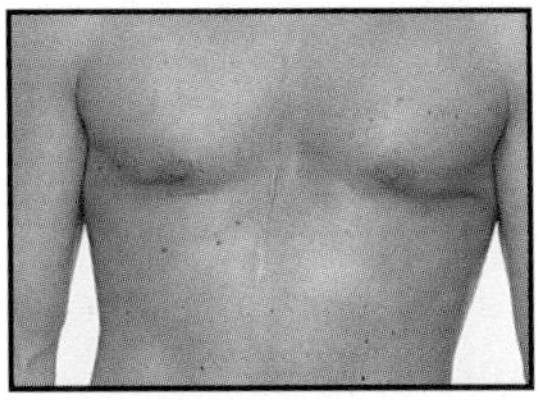

- chest, nipples

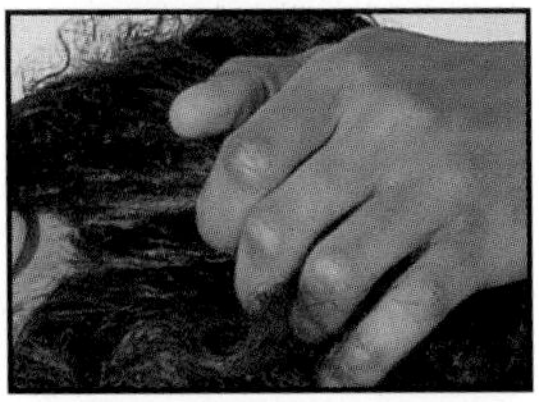

- hands, fingertips and palms

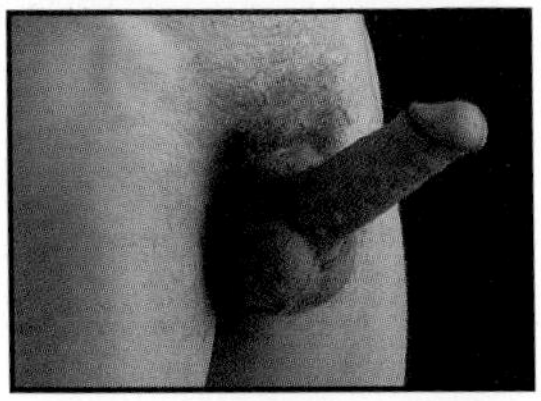

- genitals: perineum (area between penis and anus), testes, glans, frenulum of penis

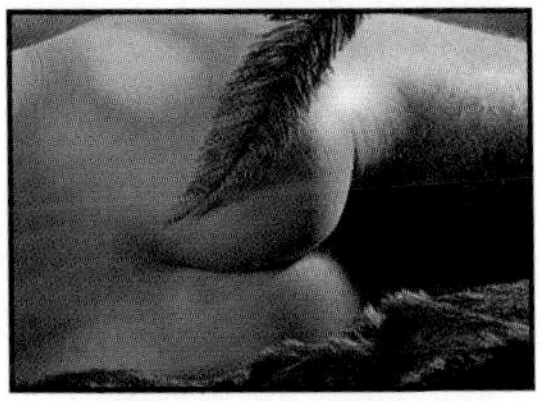

- buttocks
- anus

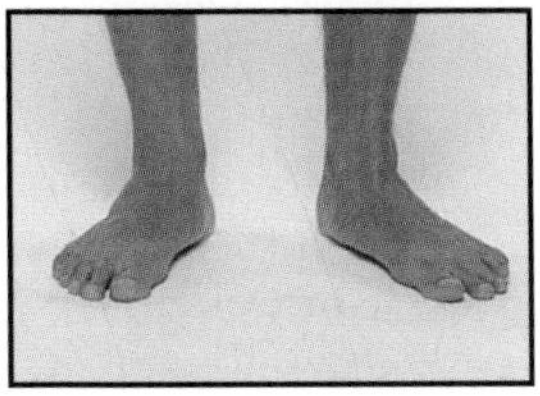

- soles of feet

SEX & DISABILITY

Disability is one of the last remaining taboos about sexuality. Those who have no major disabilities tend to know little about the issues of disability and sexuality; many know nothing at all. However, sex is a part of almost everybody's life and in most cases disability need not prevent a person from both enjoying sexual feelings and expressing them.

Historically, the media have emphasized certain aspects of sexual relations, creating the image of an unattainable and unrealistic ideal of attractiveness. The reality is that people are not perfect and everyone has some form of physical, psychological, emotional and/or social limitation or imperfection. Short- or long-sightedness, slight deafness, physical imperfections and personal problems and insecurities are all common, minor forms of disability, which can affect people's daily lives and their relationships. Severe forms of disability – such as visual or hearing impairment, paralysis, multiple sclerosis, muscular dystrophy, cerebral palsy, shortness of stature, learning difficulties, mental illness – are often treated differently by society. However, they are common (severe disabilities affect ten per cent of the population), they have an enormous impact on the way people live their lives and, like the more minor forms of disability, they do not reduce such basic human needs as self-confidence, independence and intimate personal relationships.

Learning difficulties
People with learning disabilities are not forever childlike. They mature physically and have sexual drives. Parents, siblings, teachers, carers and society in general sometimes find this difficult to accept and may also fear that the disabled person may be sexually and socially exploited. Sex education for those with learning difficulties and for others about learning difficulties has been shown to improve understanding.

See also:
sex aids and toys
sex positions
masturbation
oral sex
sexual learning

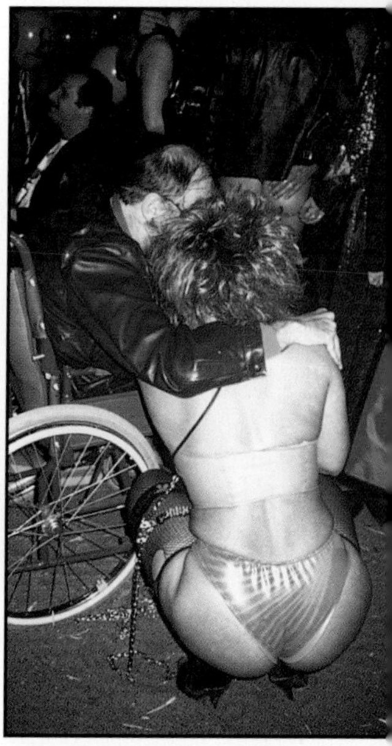

The UK's Sex Maniacs' Ball is in fact a charity event to support The Outsiders Club, which provides information and opportunities for integration for people with disabilities. Many people with disabilities attend...

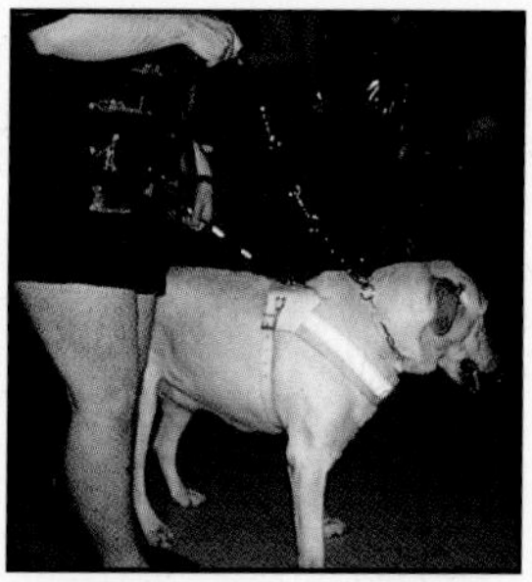

... even blindness did not stop this transvestite from attending the Ball.

Overcoming limitations
Relationships in general and sex in particular can be more difficult for those who have some form of disability. The difficulties range from the specific limitations imposed by the particular disability to broader issues of the way disability and sexuality are perceived by others. Very often it is these perceptions and attitudes that create the obstacles; although in many cases recognizing that obstacles exist can be part of the way to overcome them.

Social factors

● Many people seem unable to recognize those with disabilities as sexual beings. This can be acutely damaging to others' confidence and self-esteem.

● Even when people with disabilities are seen as sexual, assumptions regarding sexual orientation or preferences often come into play. People with disabilities are as likely to be homosexual or to have particular sexual preferences as anyone else.

● Having a relationship with a disabled person can mean taking on all the prejudices that society may have against disability. However, it can still be highly satisfying and exciting for both partners.

● Sex education for disabled children tends to be inadequate or non-existent. Disability also tends to limit opportunities for mixing with peers, which is the other main source of sexual learning among children and teenagers. Even editions of the media designed for the disabled, such as tape recorded newspapers for the blind, are usually edited and tend to take a cautious approach to sexual issues, once more restricting access to information about sex, although more and more organizations are starting to address this matter.

● Dating agencies, too, are often less than welcoming and helpful to people with disabilities, although increasing numbers of organizations now provide a specialized service.

● Many homes and institutions for people with disabilities are recognizing that their clients have sexual needs and are training staff to address this issue in a realistic way.

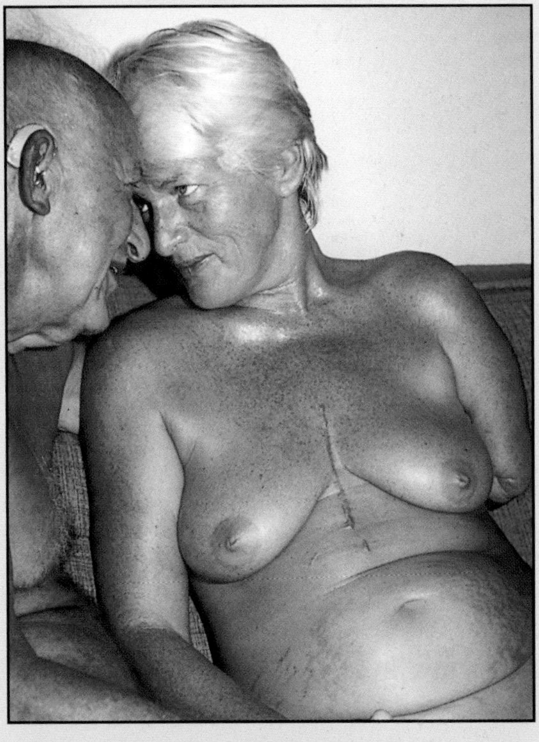

Physical factors

Sex is an important and life-enhancing force. It can be a source of health and healing as well as pleasure. If it is practised with due respect for the limitations imposed by a particular disability, it can ease pain, relieve anxiety and preoccupations and build confidence. After an accident that causes disability it can provide reassurance and aid recovery.

Physical disabilities can interfere with sex, but by being open-minded about sexual alternatives and communicating with partners, sex can become just as varied, sensuous, adventurous and intimate as for people with no form of disability. There is much more to sex than vaginal-penile penetration. Even where this is possible, experimenting with other options – while being realistic about limitations – can be exciting and rewarding.

● Loss of feeling in one part of the body can produce heightened sensation in other parts. Erogenous zones can often be transferred and new erotic sensations can be discovered. Where there is some feeling this can be enhanced with the use of sex aids such as vibrators which produce stronger stimulation.

● Adapting to a lack of mobility or strength can involve experimenting with different positions, which do not put strain on weak or painful parts of the body but make other parts accessible and give room for movement. Certain positions also require less energy, to help deal with fatigue or cardiac problems.

● Blindness and deafness do not inhibit the other senses, which can provide clear and intimate ways of communicating needs, pleasure or appreciation.

● Experimenting with positions can also ease difficulties with muscle spasm. In some cases, muscle-relaxants can help.

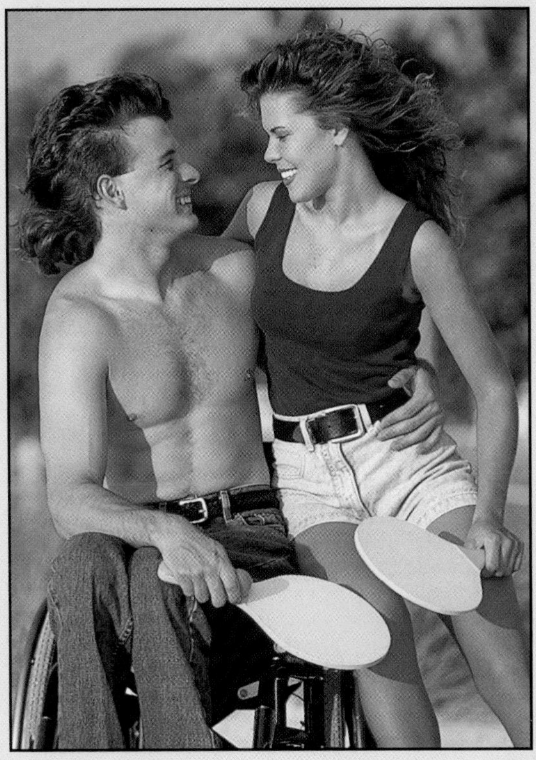

SEX POSITIONS

WOMAN ON TOP

The woman on top positions can provide intense pleasure for both partners. In addition, the woman can control much of the love-making. Deep penetration is possible, but can be regulated by the woman's feelings and desires. Lighter penetration may be desired. If the woman is pregnant, this position may be more comfortable. If the male partner is very heavy this may also apply. These positions allow for many parts of the genitalia to be stimulated (see diagram below).

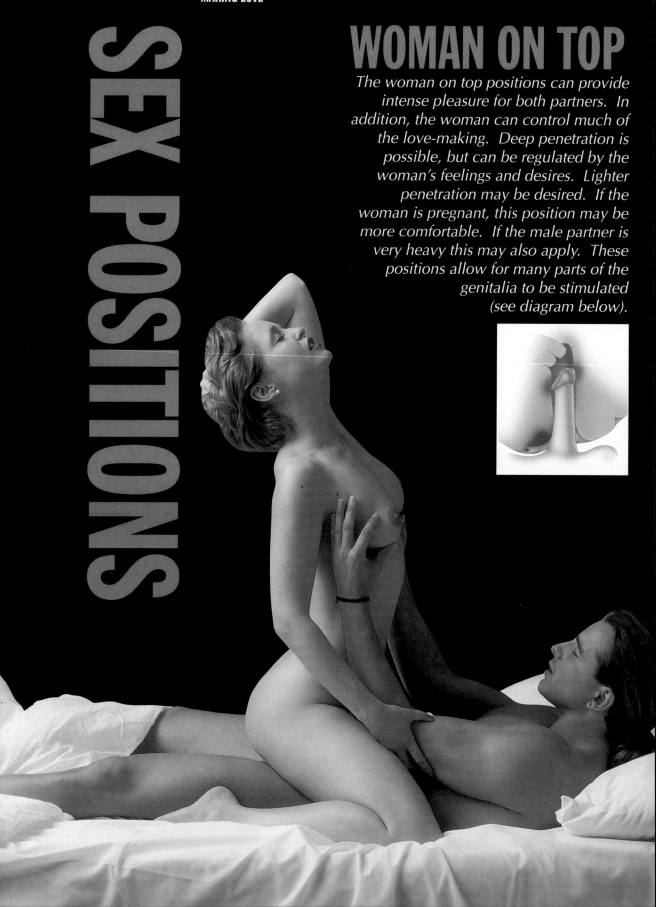

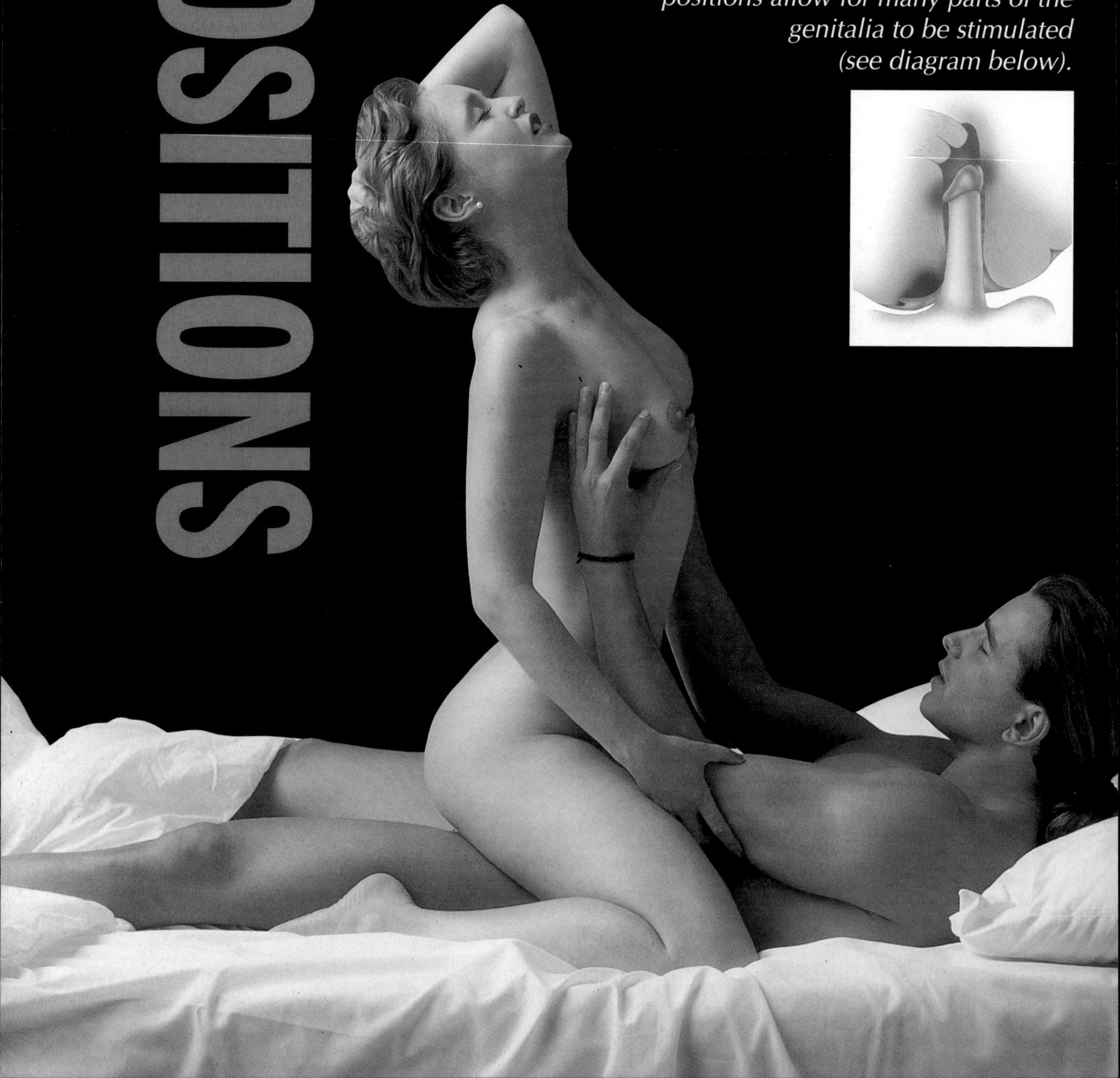

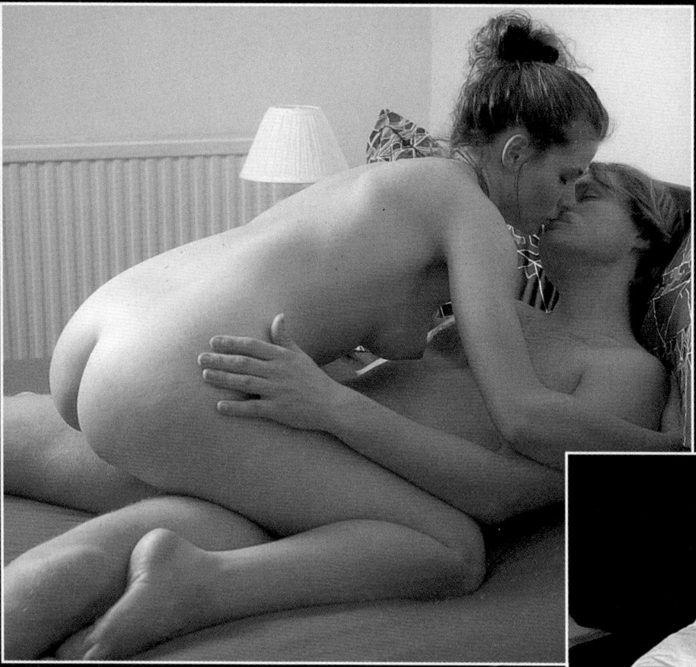

▲ This face-to-face position provides a strong sense of intimacy while the woman is on top. They can both reach her breasts and clitoris.

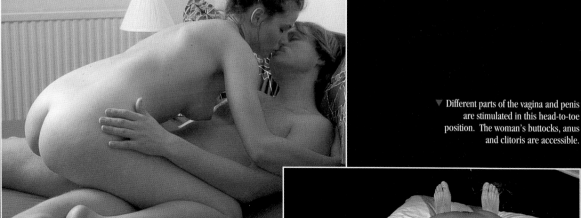

▼ Different parts of the vagina and penis are stimulated in this head-to-toe position. The woman's buttocks, anus and clitoris are accessible.

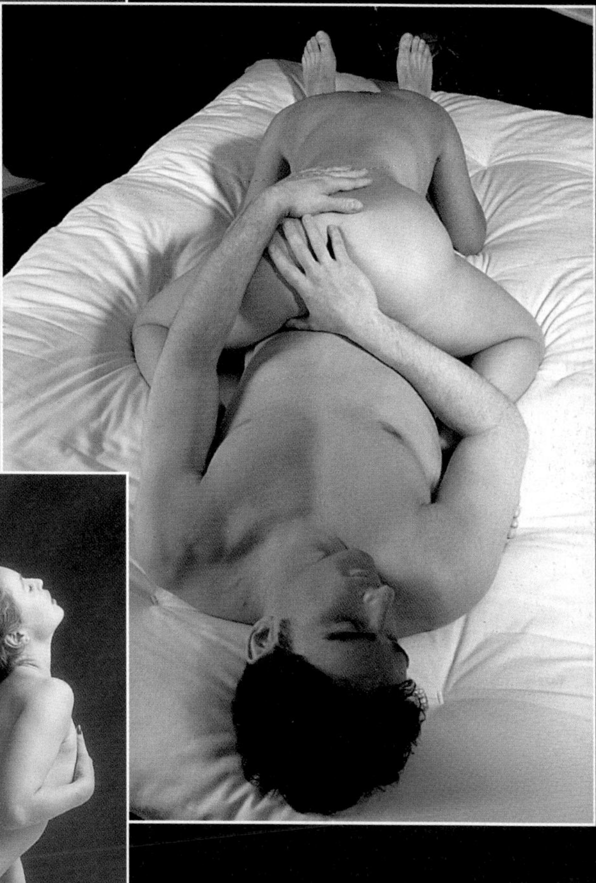

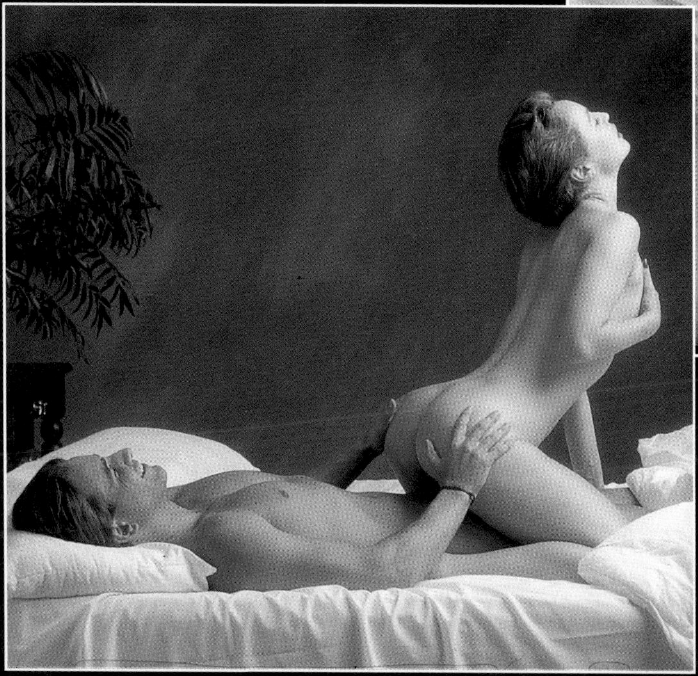

◀ The woman can stimulate the penis with controlled movements. Little exertion is required from the man.

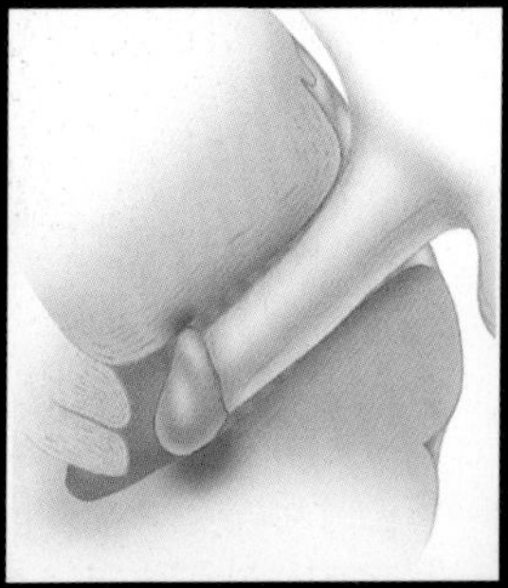

MAN ON TOP

The man on top positions, and in particular the missionary position, where the woman's legs are apart with the man between them, are traditionally the most common positions. The woman has less control and less ability to move sensuously, but variation is possible to increase the pleasure received by each partner. Deep penetration and stimulation of the penis and clitoris is possible in all these positions. Couples will need to experiment to discover which positions and actions give most pleasure. Generally the positions in which the woman's knees are bent allow for deeper penetration, and those where the woman's legs are together give stimulation to the penis and clitoris (see diagram top left).

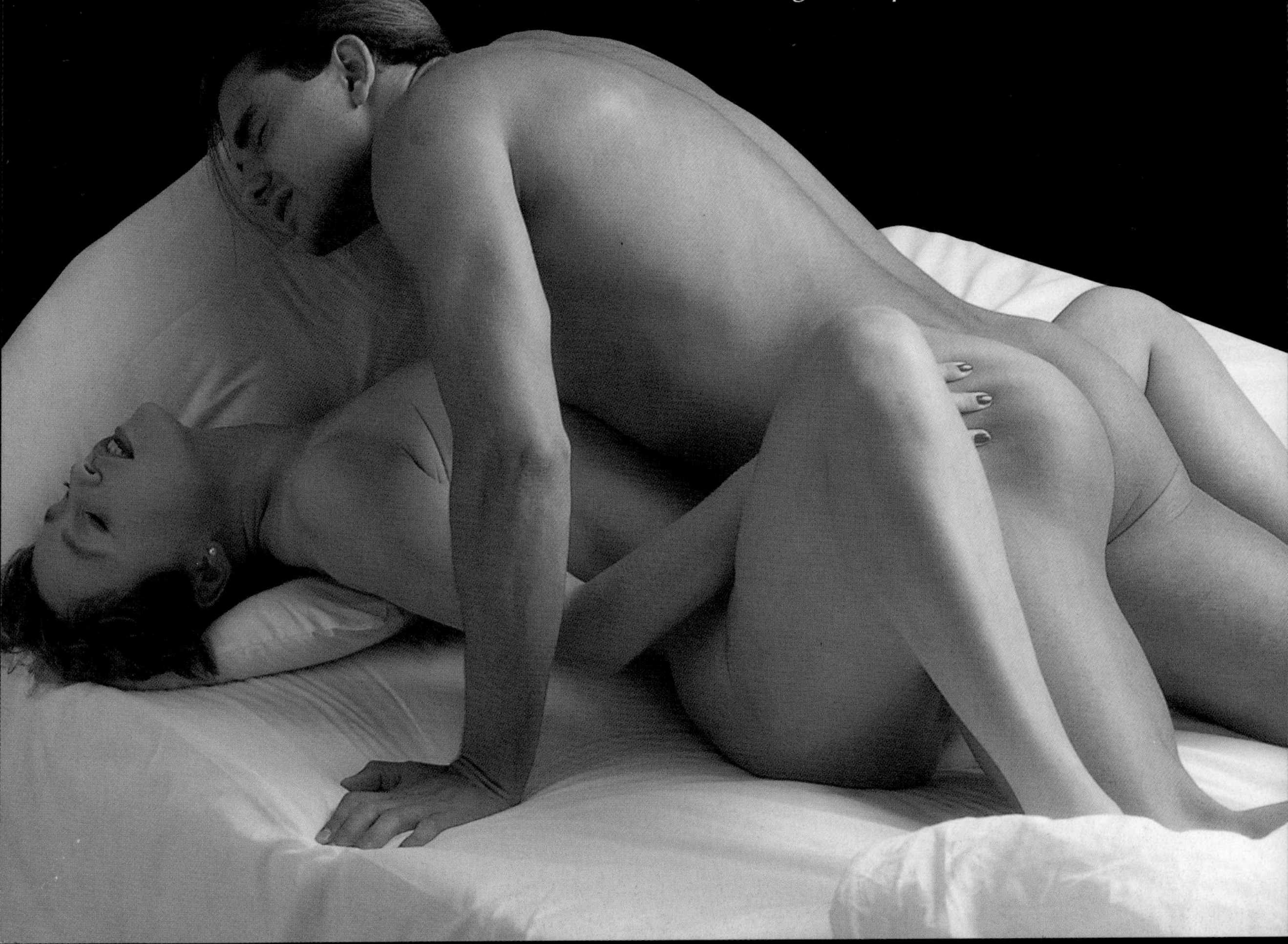

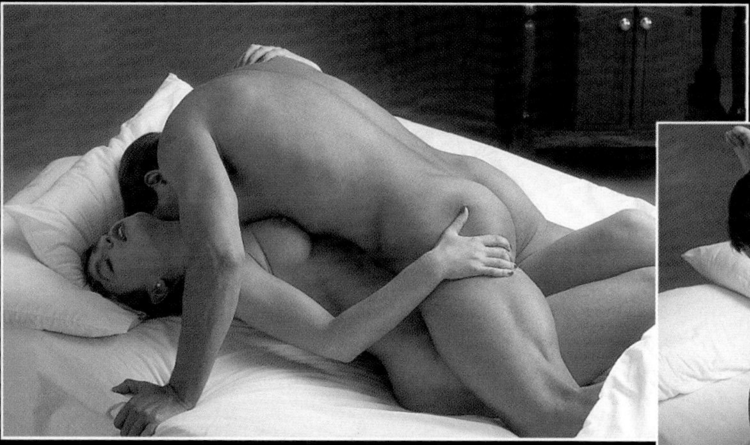

▲ The penis and clitoris receive stimulation in this position. The woman can squeeze the penis with the vaginal lips and muscles. She can exert some control of movement with her hands on her partner's buttocks.

▼ Deep penetration is possible in this position and it is easy for partners to fondle each other's bodies with the hands.

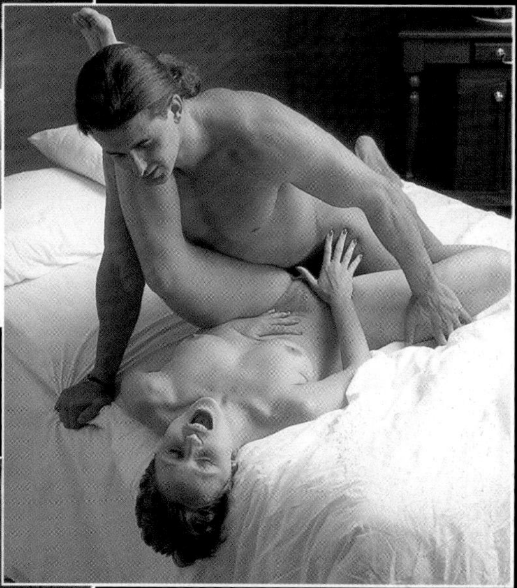

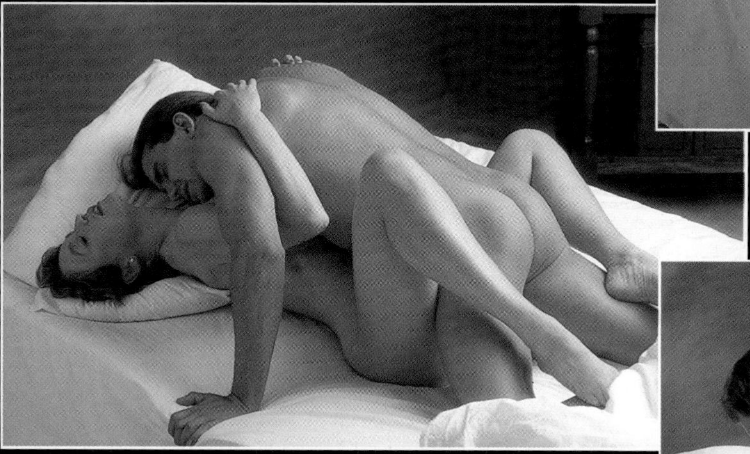

◄ The knees up position allows for deep penetration. The woman's buttocks can be raised slightly to increase depth of penetration.

▼ In this position, the clitoris and G-spot receive intense stimulation. The woman's legs can help control movement.

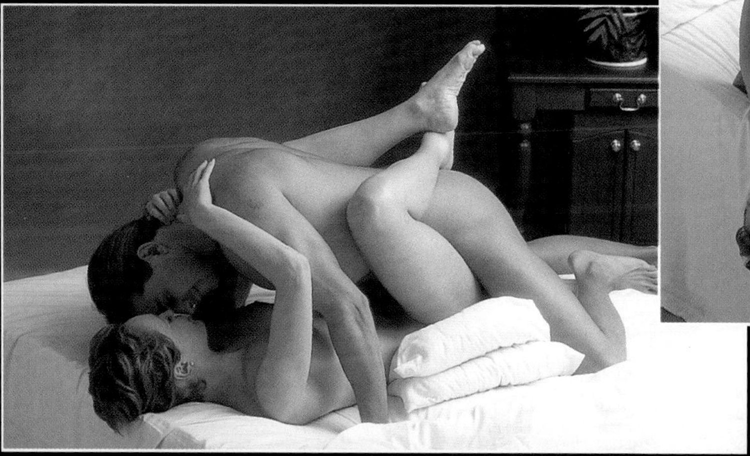

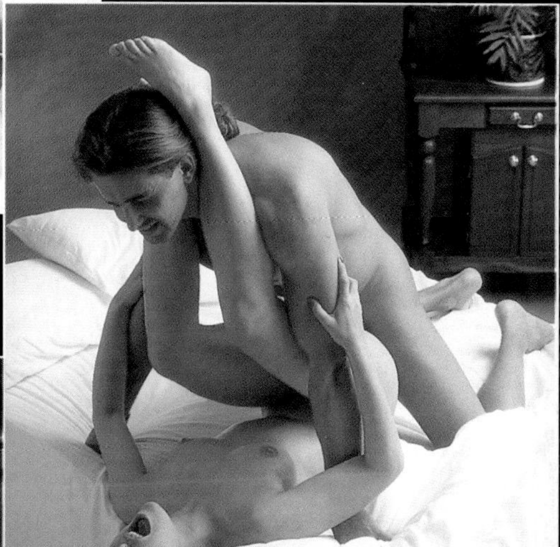

▲ This position allows for deep penetration. The woman's feet around her partner's neck give good balance and control whilst the kneeling position of the man enables him to thrust forcefully if desired.

REAR ENTRY

Rear entry positions can be enjoyed while crouching, kneeling or standing. Either partner can be on top. There is freedom to move and to caress a partner's body with the hands. These positions are also comfortable for the pregnant woman. Penetration and the areas most stimulated are shown below.

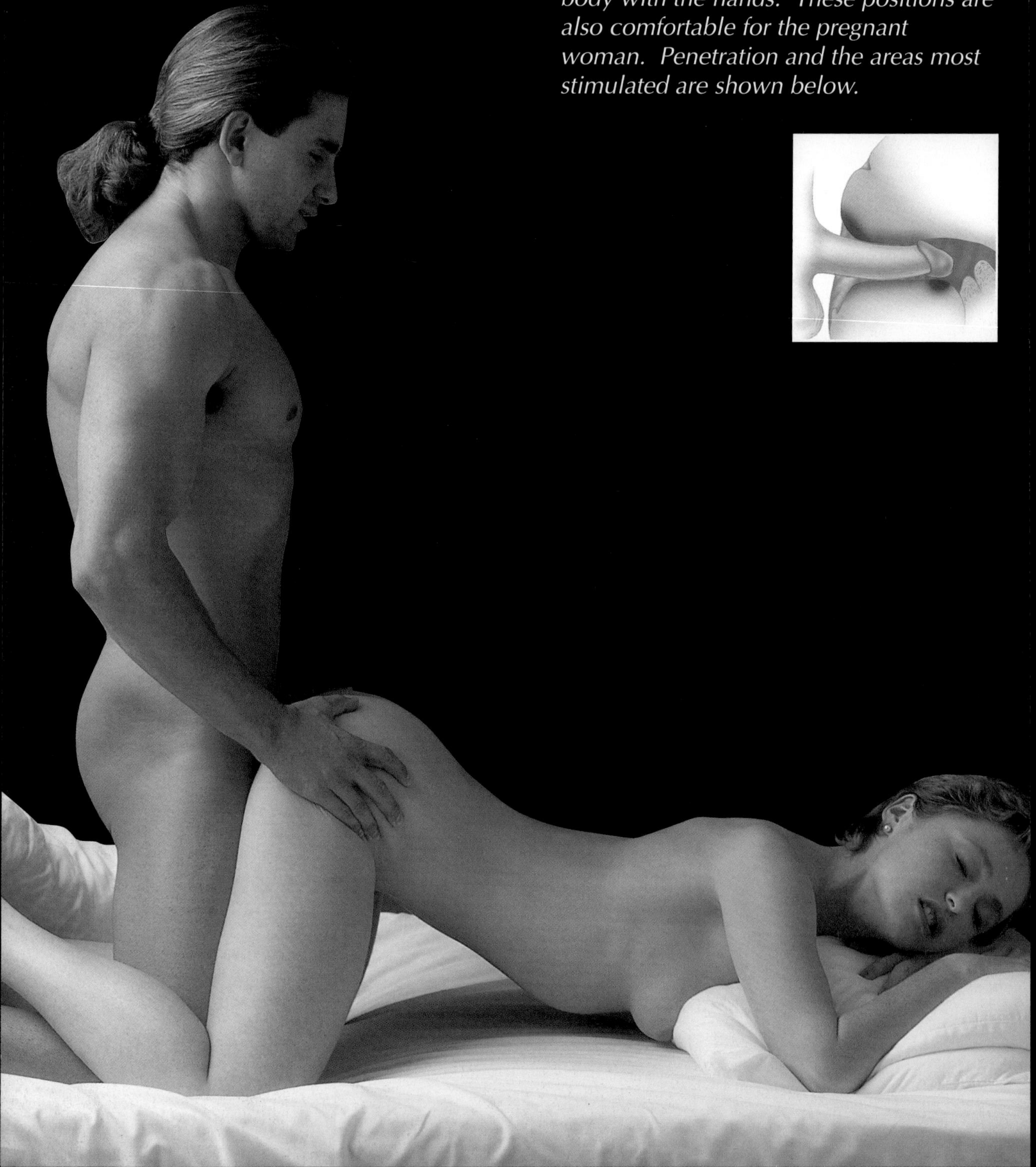

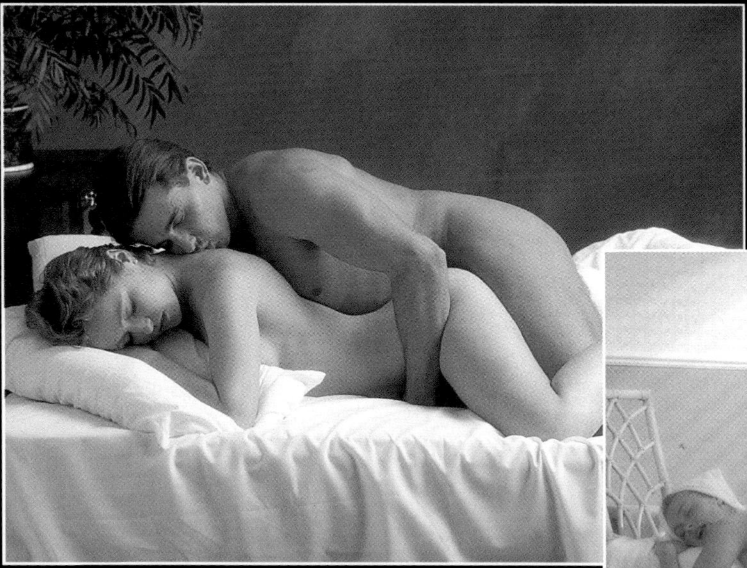

▲ The penis can be squeezed by the woman's buttocks. The man can reach to stimulate the clitoris with his fingers.

▼ The woman's body is well supported by the chair. Deep penetration, friction and thrusting are possible.

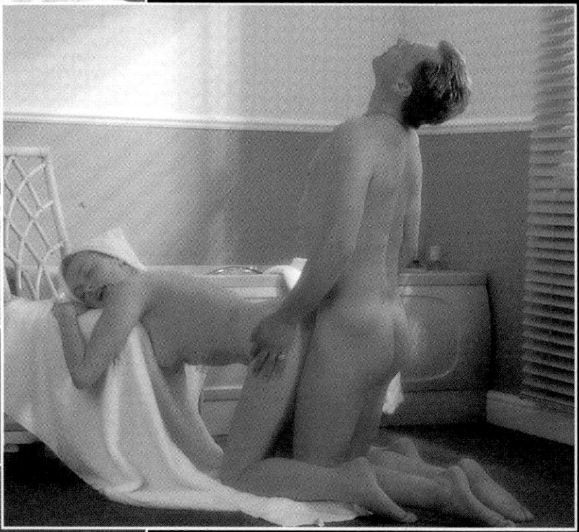

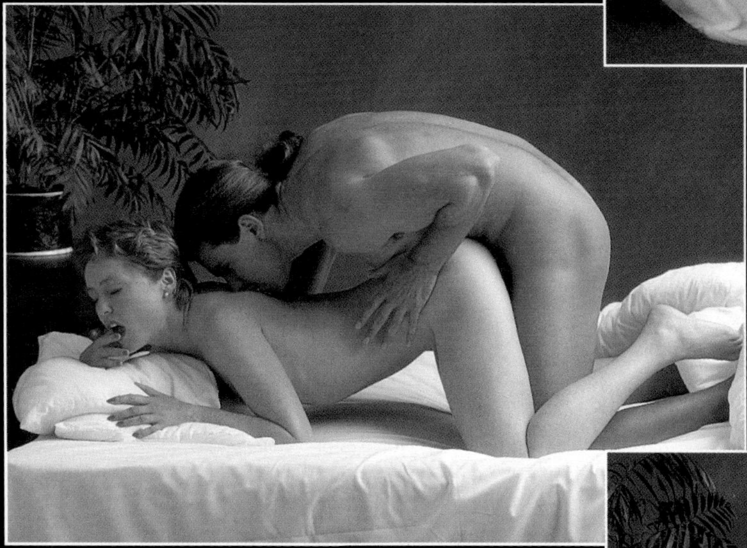

▲ The vagina is tilted upwards slightly which allows for deep penetration. The man's hands are free to caress his partner's body.

▼ The woman can move as she pleases; her leaning back allows for deep penetration. The man can hold his partner's waist or caress her legs.

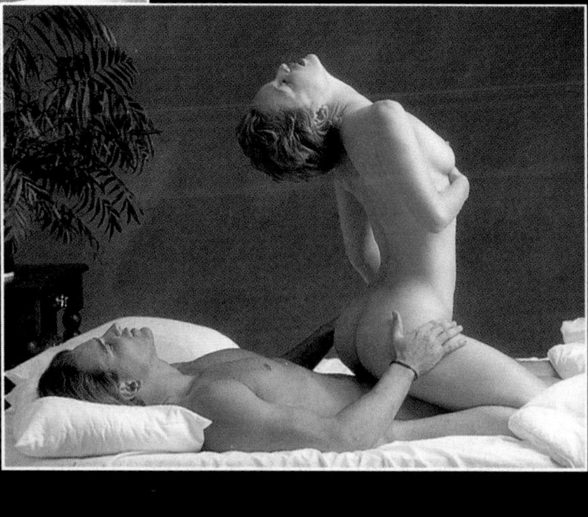

SIDE-BY-SIDE

▼ The woman can open her legs to allow penetration and then grasp her partner with her legs to control the rhythm of movement and increase stimulation.

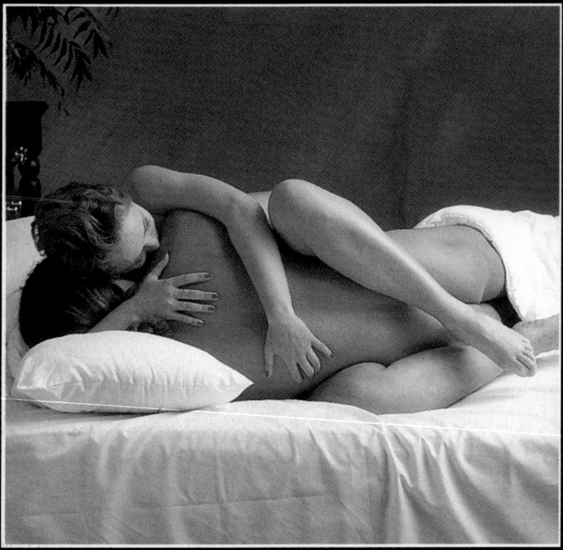

FACE-TO-FACE

The face-to-face positions can be intimate and sensuous. Looking at, kissing and caressing one's partner on the mouth, face and upper body is possible. The hands of both partners can be used to stroke and caress the body of the other. It is a comfortable position if the woman is pregnant or if her partner is heavy. The clitoris can be stimulated by the partner's fingers. The areas stimulated are shown below.

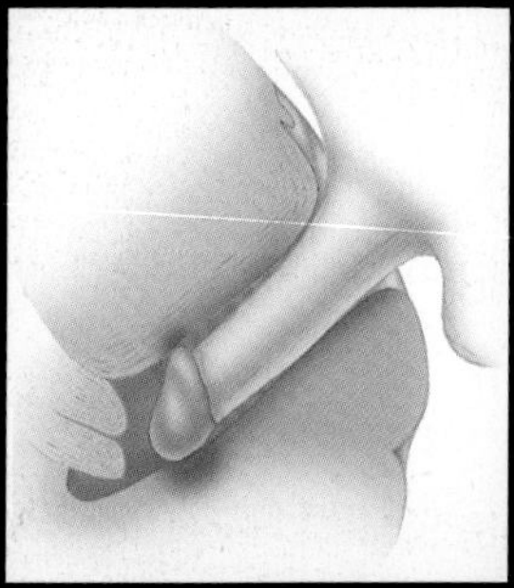

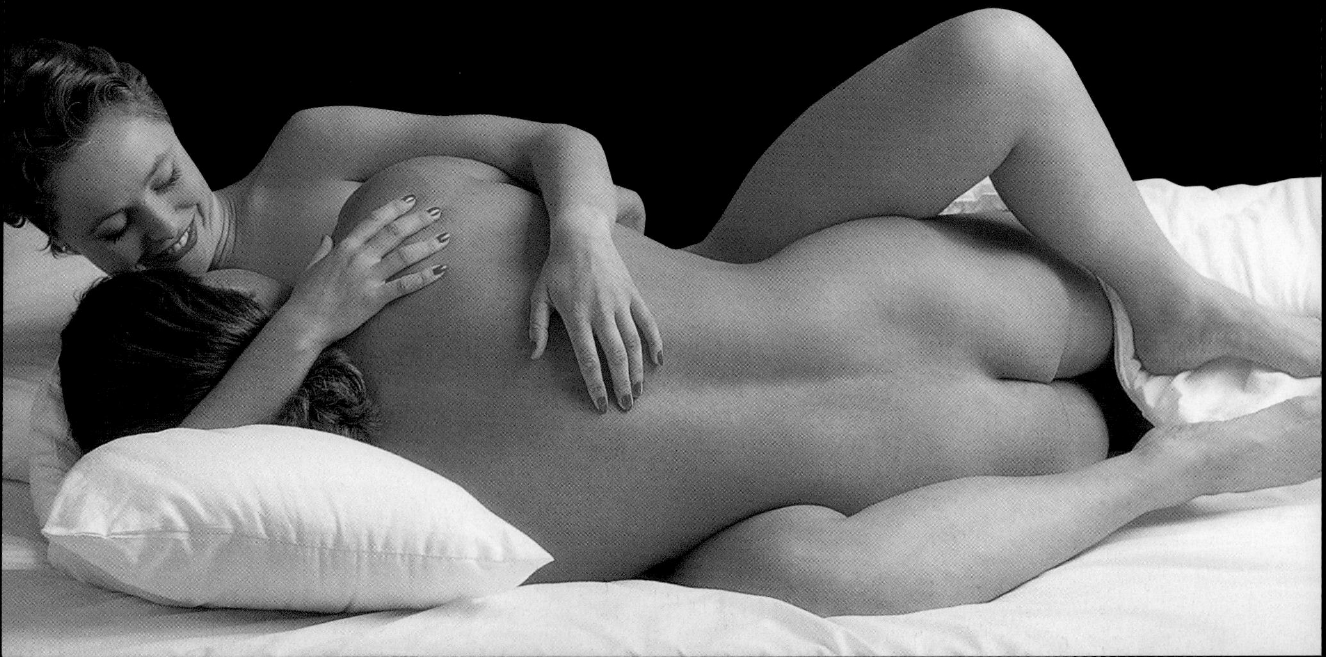

The face-to-back position where the man enters the woman from behind can be relaxed and sensuous. Both partners can move easily. The man can stimulate the woman's clitoris and breasts with his hands and the woman can caress his testicles. If the man leans back, greater penetration is possible. This is sometimes called the 'spoons' position. The areas stimulated are shown below.

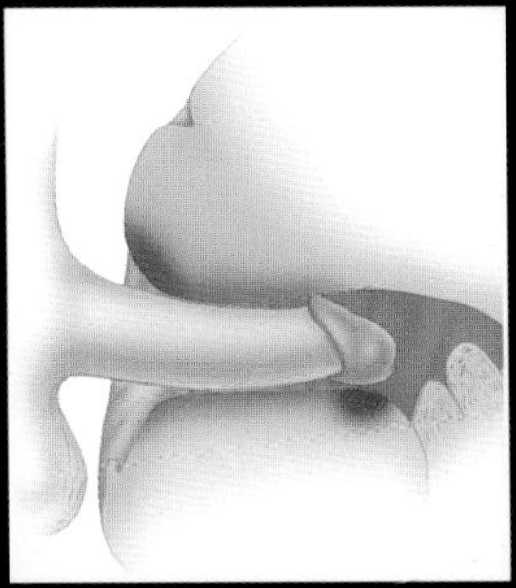

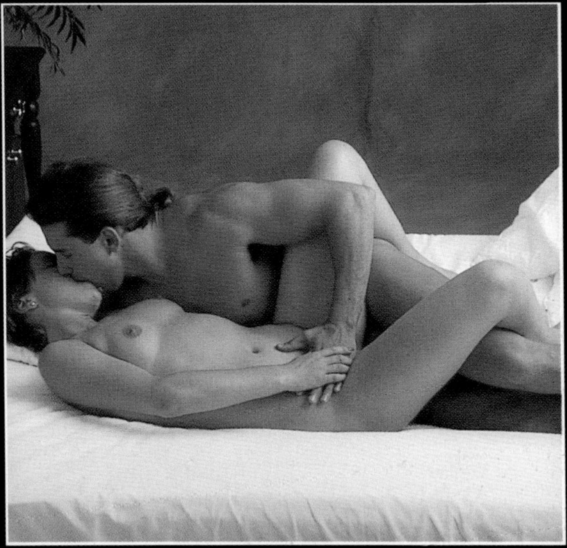

Penetration can be deep.

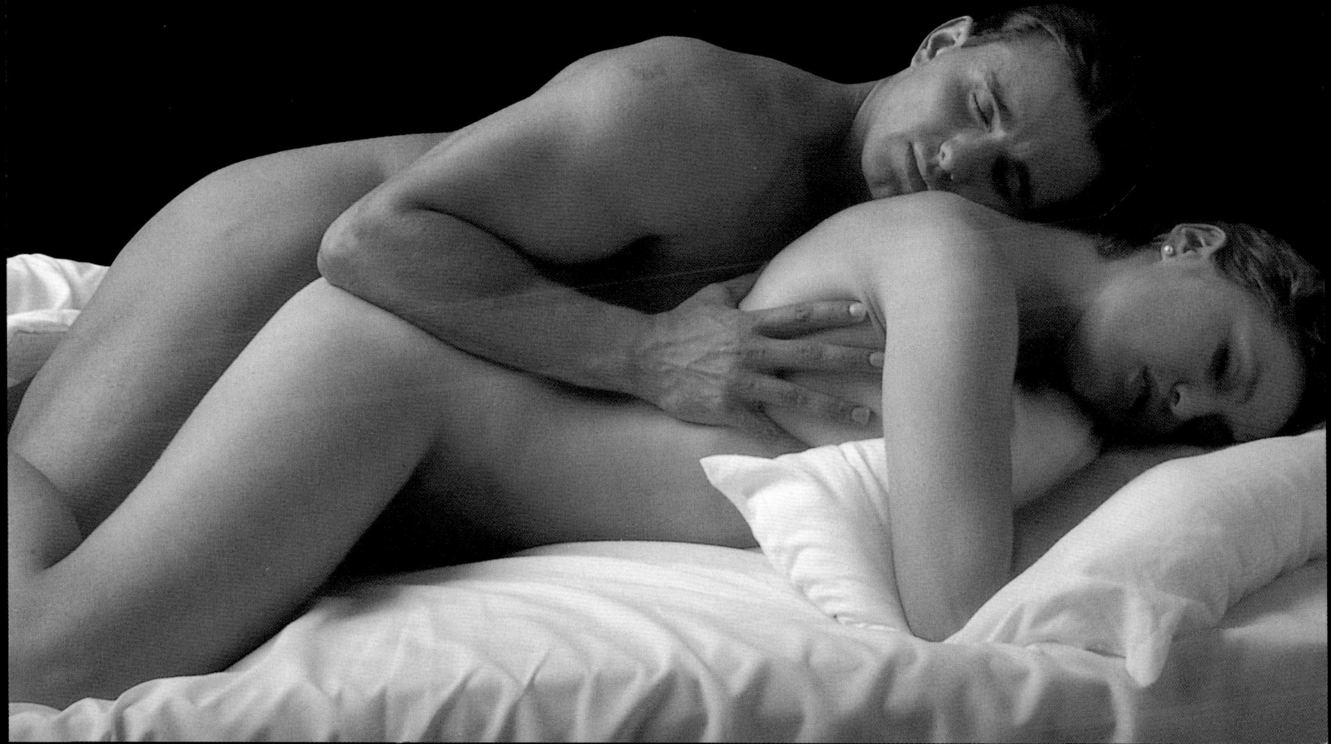

SITTING & KNEELING

The sitting and kneeling positions for sex are close and intimate. Many people find them relaxing. In the face-to-face positions both partners can caress each other's bodies. Some support may be needed to provide freer movement and deeper thrusting. The areas stimulated are shown below.

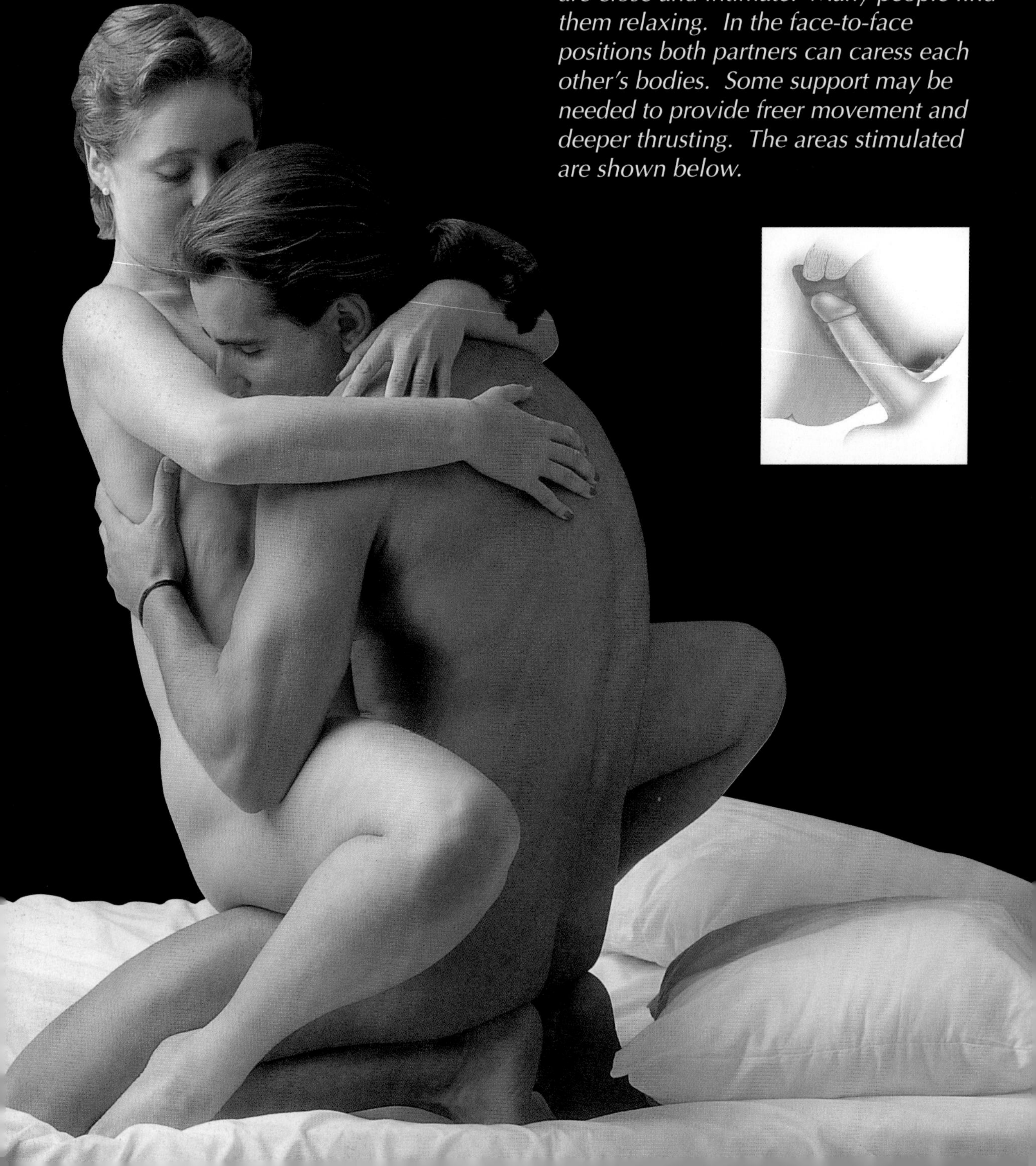

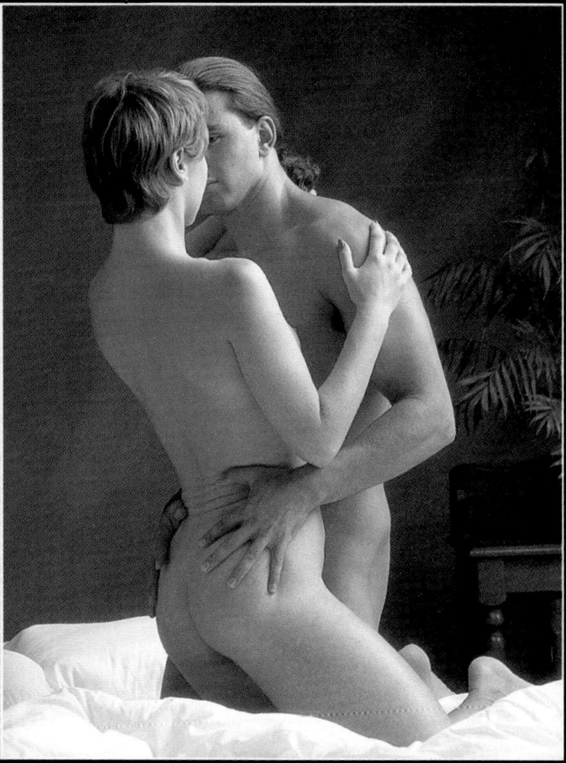

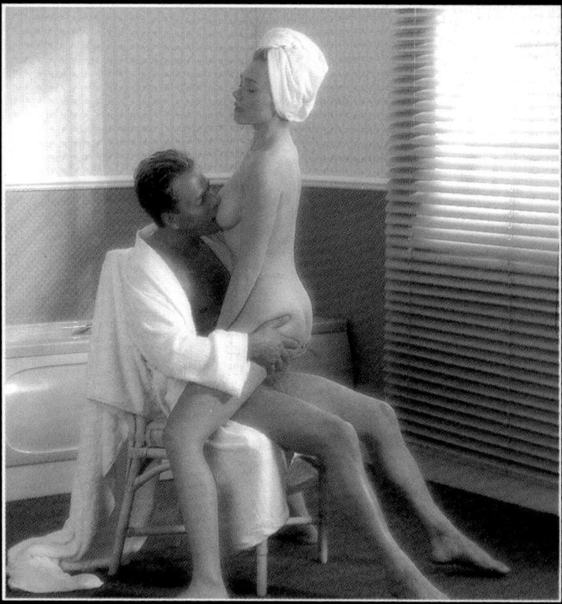

▲ The chair gives support to the man, who can then support his partner. She can control the penetration and thrusting movements.

◀ Both partners are kneeling; they can see, kiss and caress each other's bodies easily.

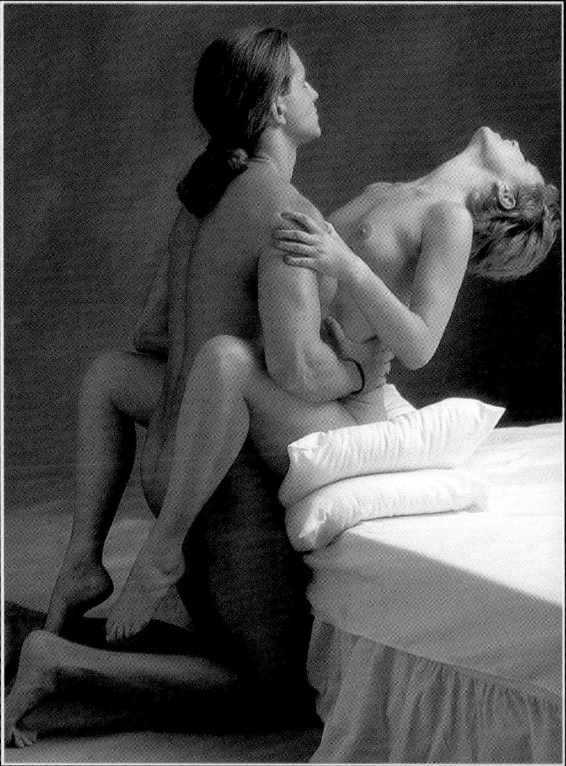

◀ The bed and pillows give good support and alignment for penetration.

▼ In this position, the woman leaning back aligns the vagina with the angle of penetration. The woman's clitoris and breasts can be caressed.

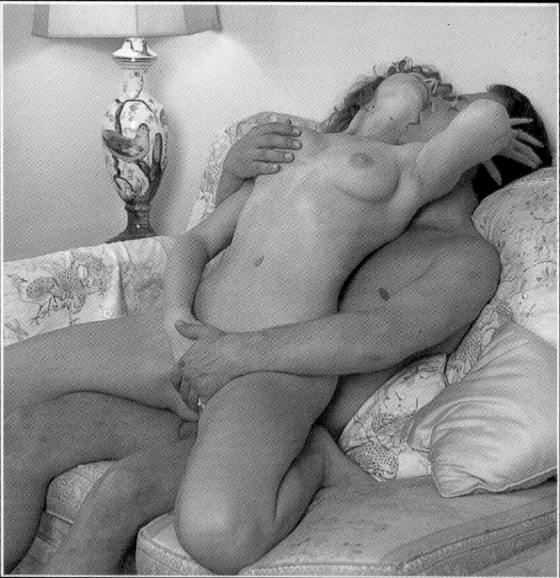

STANDING & ADVANCED

These positions are worth exploring for the sense of challenge and novelty that they provide. They may require a certain amount of agility, and in some cases concern about balance and other factors may affect sexual performance. Some couples find them more athletic than intimate, but others find that they add variety and excitement.

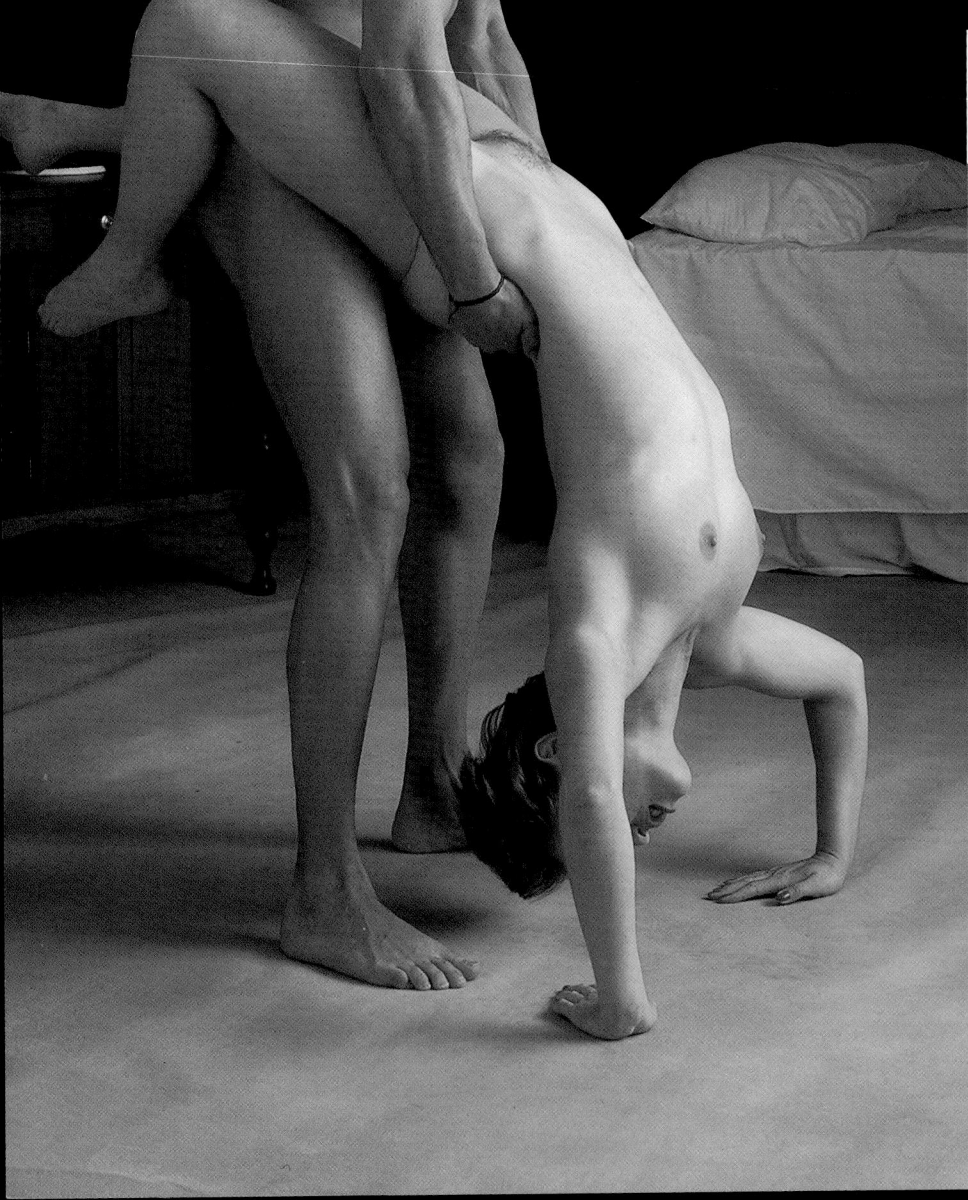

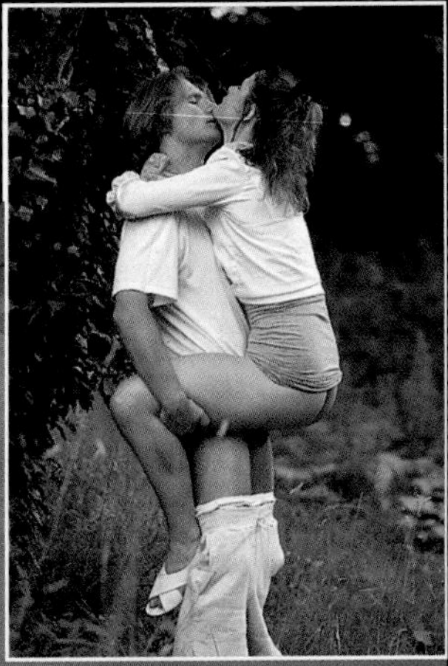

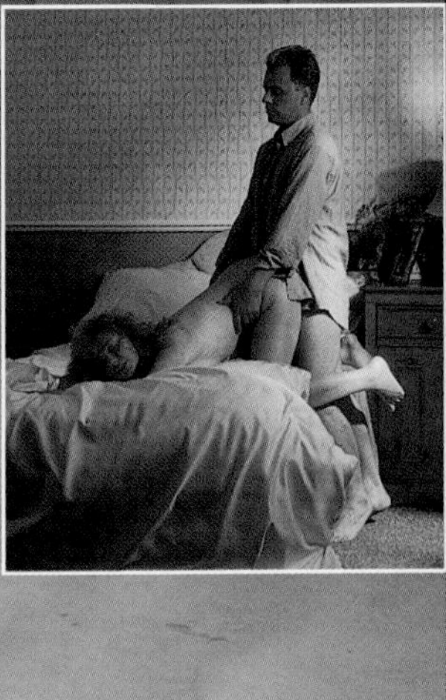

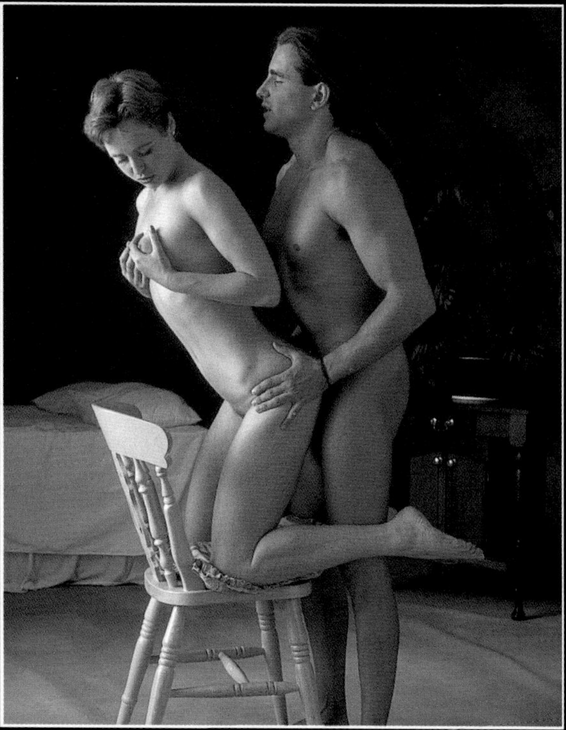

▲ The woman squatting on a chair allows penetration from below. The penis stimulates the G-spot and the man can fondle his partner's breasts and body.

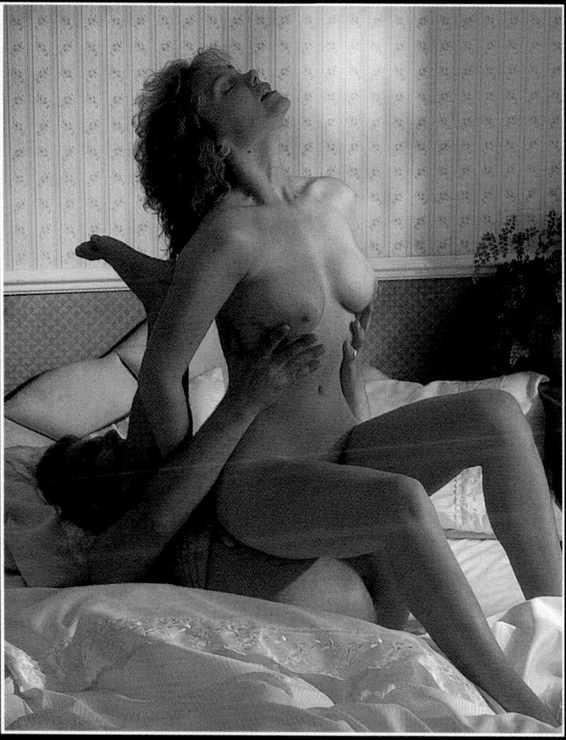

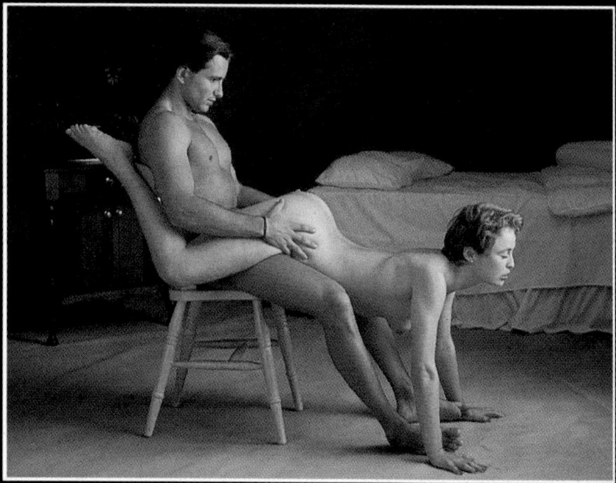

▲ The woman's buttocks and anal area can be stimulated while the man can control movement with his hands on her hips.

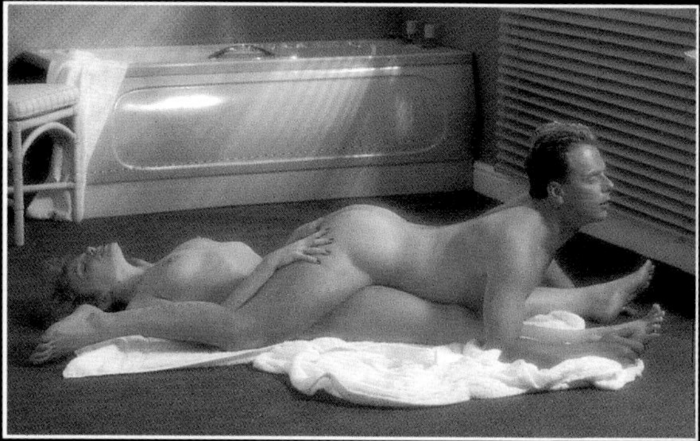

▲ The man's buttocks and anal area are accessible, enabling the woman to stimulate his G-spot. The angle of the penis gives both interesting sensations for him and strong back wall stimulation for her.

◄ ▼ The woman's body is supported by the man's, allowing her to set the pace. She can use her pelvic muscles to stimulate his penis. It may be uncomfortable for the man – and is not for those with bad backs – but the woman can support some of her weight on her feet and by leaning on his legs or ankles.

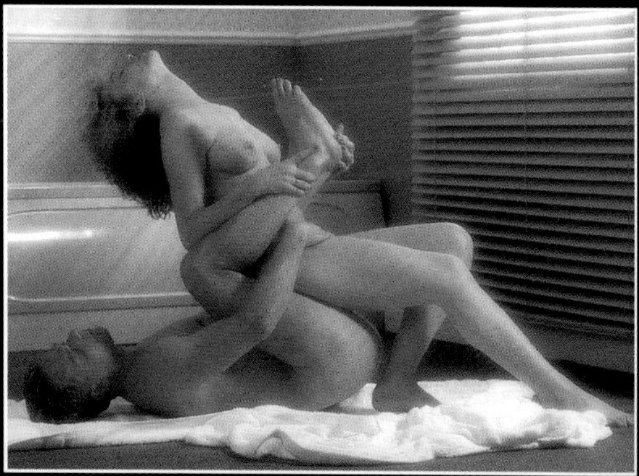

MAN TO MAN

Gay sex is diverse and may be more experimental and adventurous than heterosexual sex. Gay men were the first people seriously to take on board the risks of sexually transmitted HIV and evolve ways of making sex safer but still exciting. Anal sex is not exclusively a male homosexual activity. Gay sex does not always involve anal penetration. Many men feel, however, that penetrative anal sex and orgasm is a way of expressing intimacy and lovingness and of satisfying sexual desires.

Safer sex practices, including using a condom and spermicide, should be used for anal sex. Precautions also apply to oral sex, though the risks are believed to be lower.

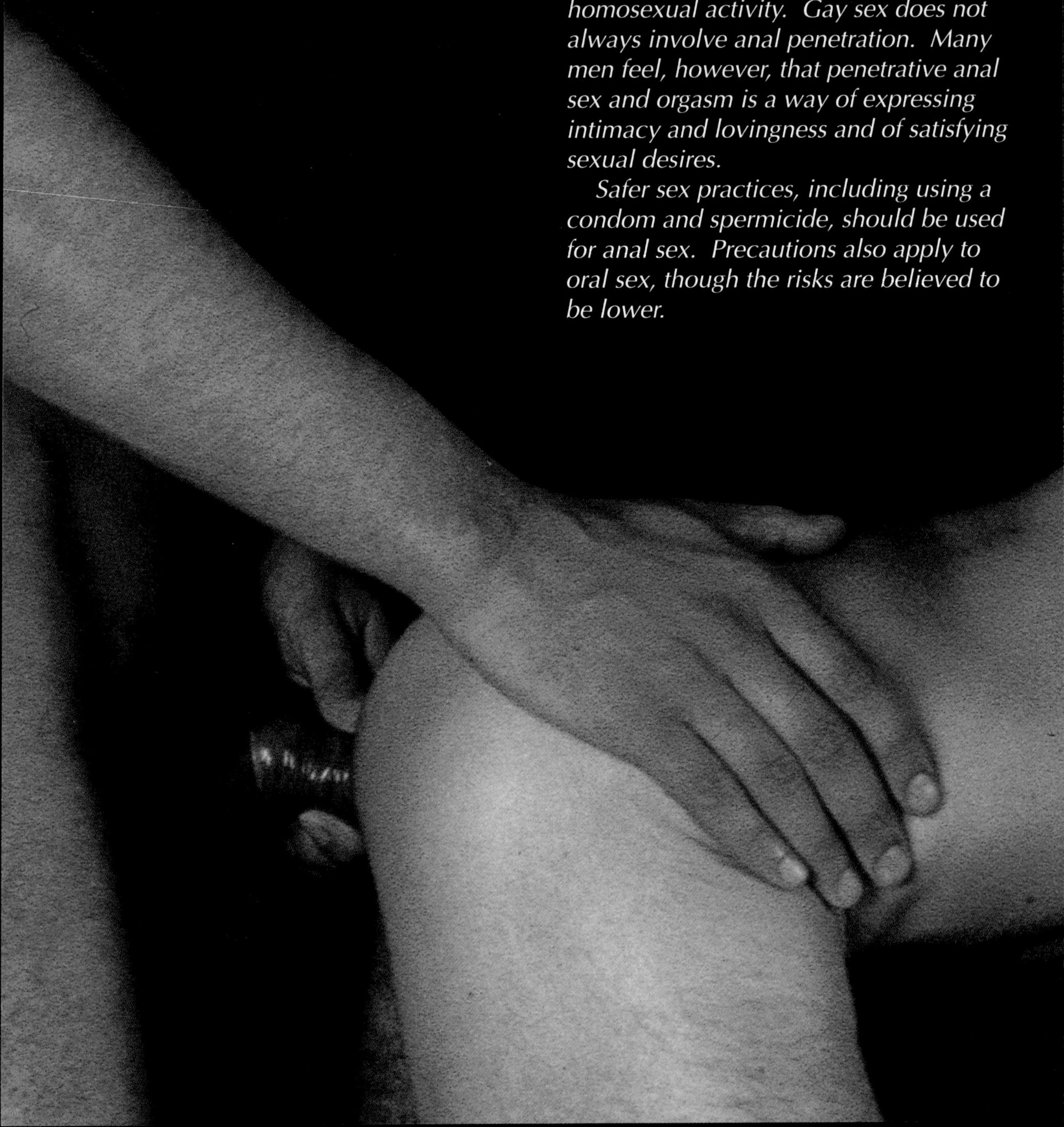

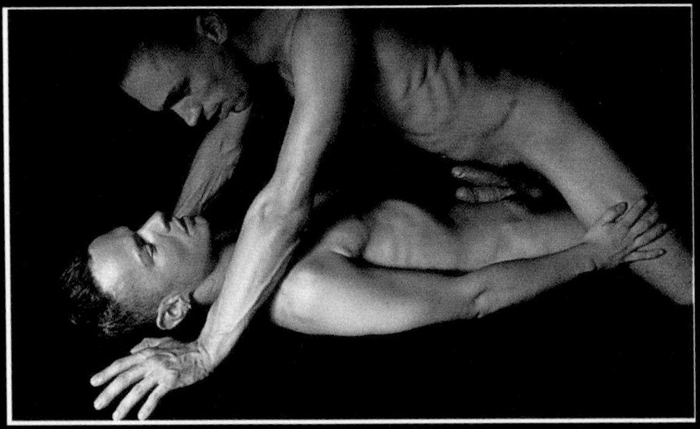

▲ Rubbing penises can bring both partners to orgasm without penetration.

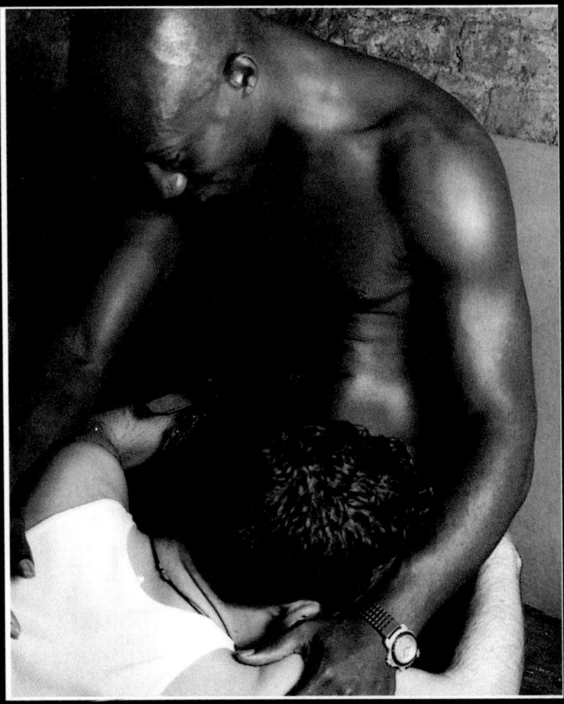

► Gay lovers performing oral sex.

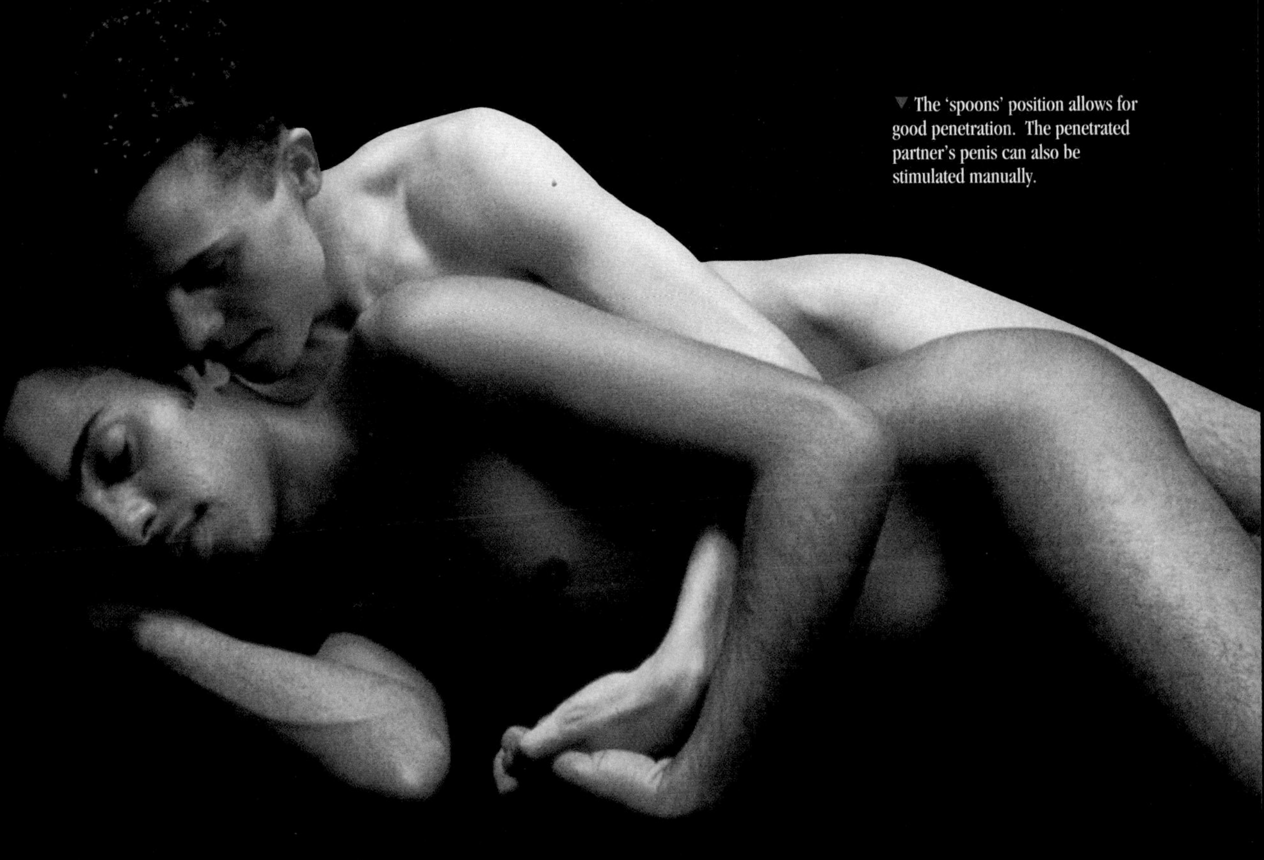

▼ The 'spoons' position allows for good penetration. The penetrated partner's penis can also be stimulated manually.

WOMAN TO WOMAN

Lesbian sex can involve all parts of the body. Vaginal or anal penetration, if desired, can be achieved with the fingers or sex aids, but non-penetrative practices are more common, involving kissing, licking, sucking or stroking the erogenous zones, in particular the lips and mouth, the breasts, vulva and clitoris. Lesbian sex can be as varied as the partners who wish to have it, with scope for great imagination and inventiveness.

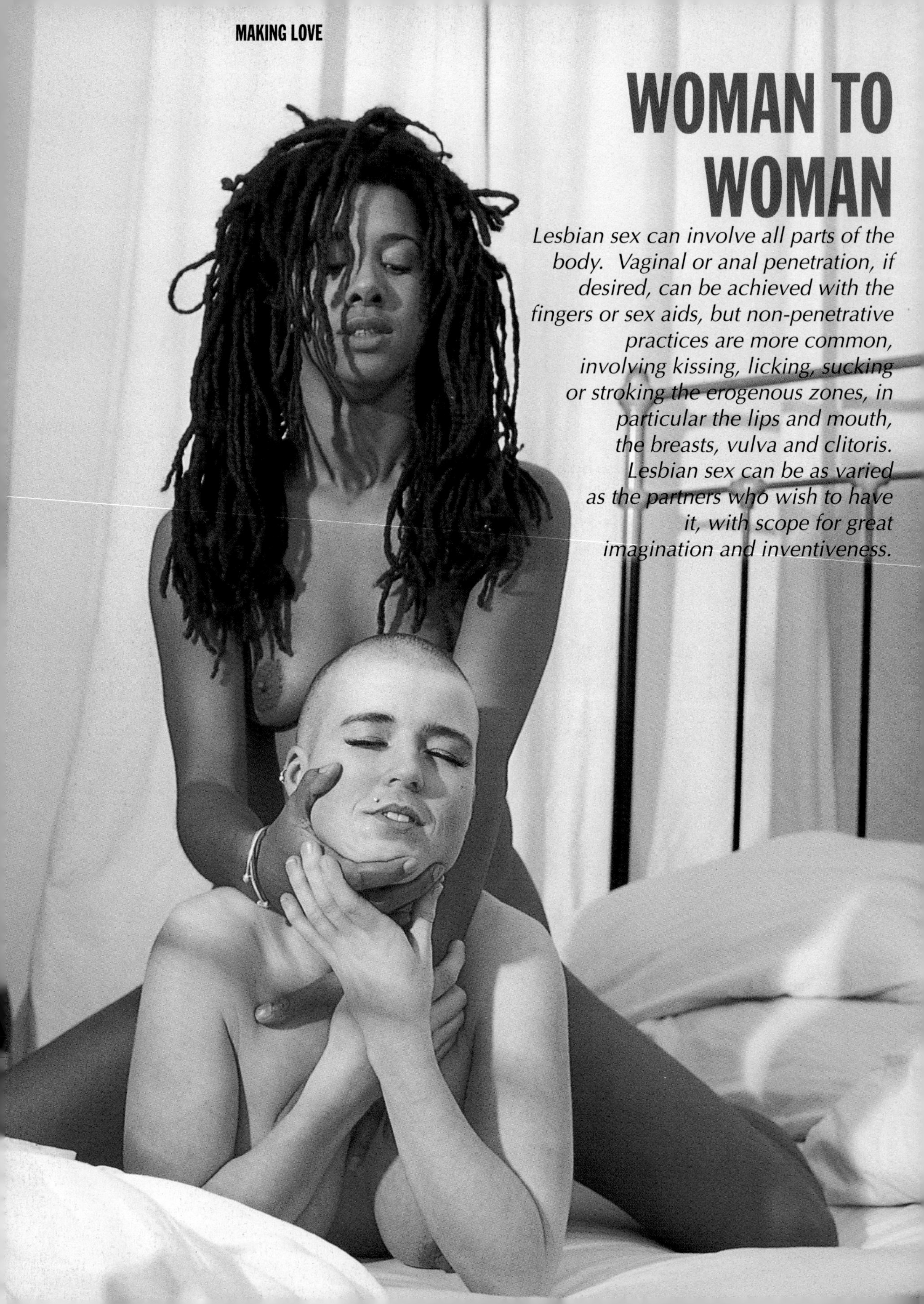

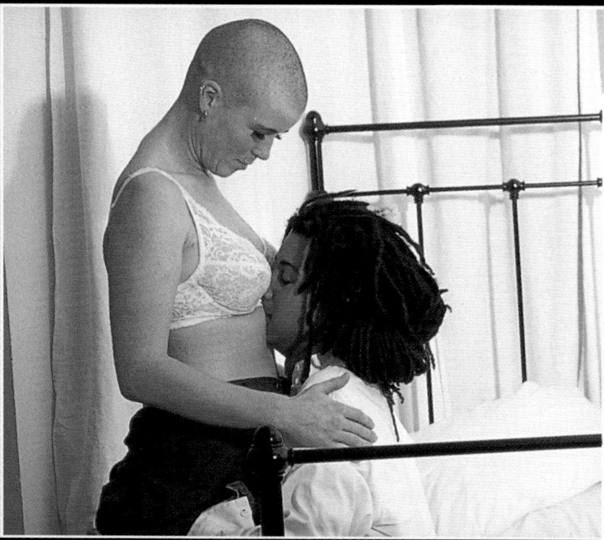

◀ Undressing a partner can be an erotic part of arousal.

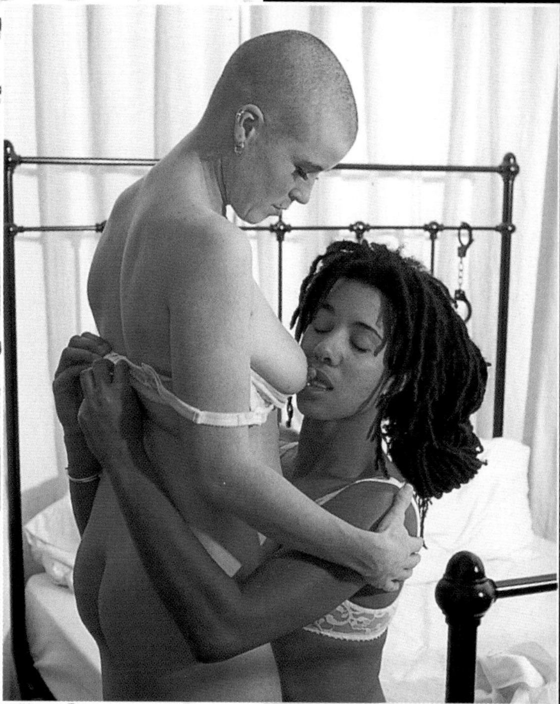

▲ Licking or sucking the breasts can be exciting for both partners.

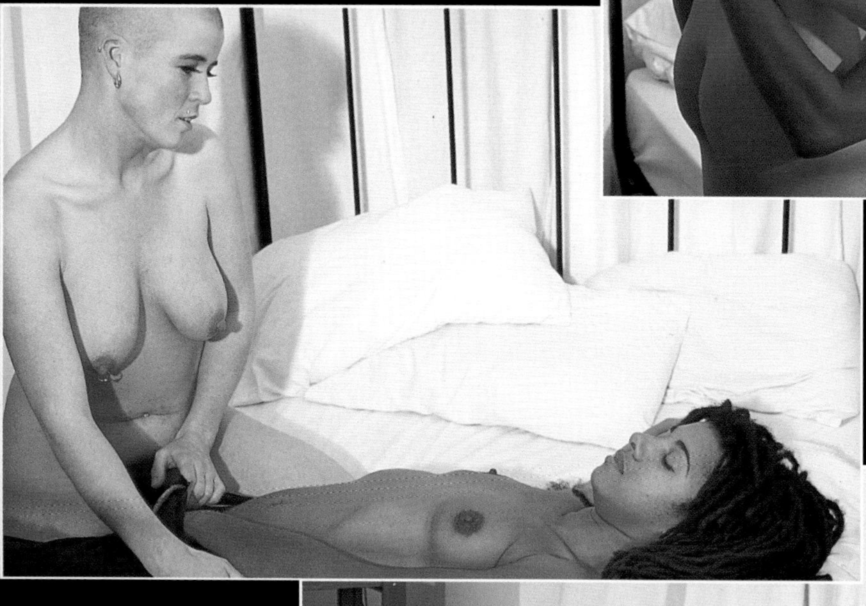

▶ ▲ Stimulating the partner's vulva, especially the clitoris, with the hands or any other part of the body, can be highly arousing.

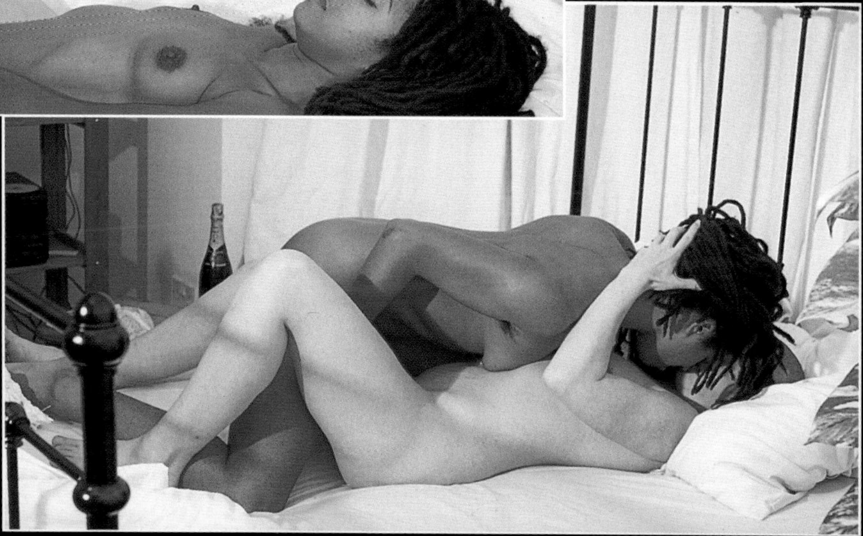

MASTURBATION

More than fifty per cent of women and eighty per cent of men masturbate regularly. Masturbation is a natural, instinctive sexual practice, yet it is also one of the most widely discredited. For centuries the practice of masturbation has been condemned as 'wrong' or 'dirty' in cultures throughout the world. Even now that studies have shown that masturbation is not only common but also generally harmless, people are still trying to free themselves from the legacy of guilt which these attitudes have created.

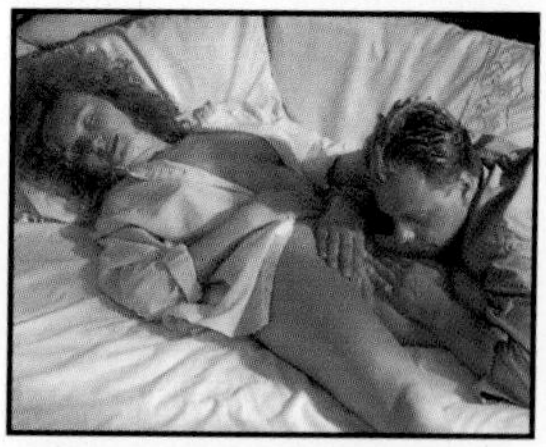

Masturbation can be an intimate way of getting to know your partner and learning what kinds of stimulation arouse them most. It can include stimulating the clitoris – the key to sexual arousal for many women.

Masturbation is taken to mean using the hands, other (non-genital) parts of the body or any object to stimulate the genitals. Most commonly it refers to stimulating oneself, usually to orgasm, but it can also mean arousing a partner in the same way. Mutual masturbation means partners masturbating each other at the same time.

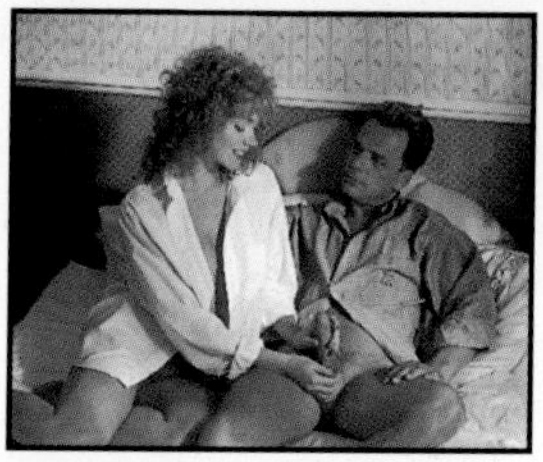

Masturbation can be one of the most exciting forms of stimulation – especially as, for a man, most of the erogenous zones are focused on the genital area.

> *"Don't knock it – it's sex with someone you love."*
> WOODY ALLEN

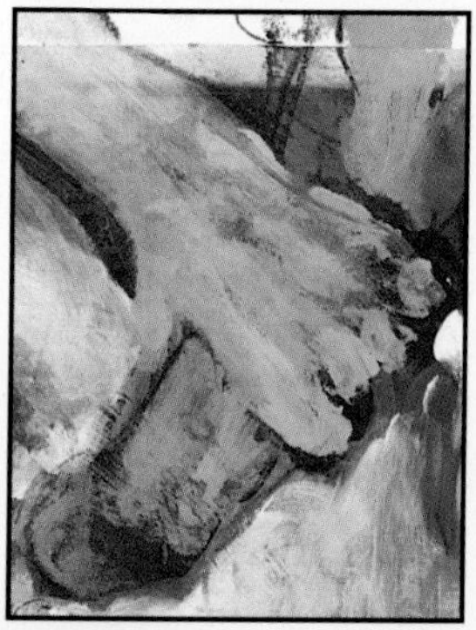

Masturbation is about self-loving and sexual independence. It can be a key part of sexual development as children learn about their bodies and their sexuality from infancy to adolescence.

In adult life masturbation can perform a similar role as people explore their sexuality: it enables people to learn what they find most arousing and what kind of stimulation they need in order to reach orgasm and may be particularly useful for women. Masturbating can be part of fantasizing or using pornography.

It has a part to play both in single life and within a relationship. Many people may, at least occasionally, prefer not to have to make a commitment or deal with another person's needs and emotions.

Slang terms
to wank, to jerk off, to beat off, to toss off, to beat the meat, to choke the chipmunk, to diddle/flog the poodle, to jerk the gherkin, to knock oneself off, to wack off, to bash/beat the bishop, to milk, to jill off, to play solitaire, to pound the pud, to pull the pudding, to do it yourself, to punish Percy in the palm, to have one off the wrist, to touch oneself up, finger job, pocket pool, hand jive, hand shandy, wrist job, Jodrell Bank, J Arthur Rank

See also:
oral sex
sexual feelings
fantasy
pornography

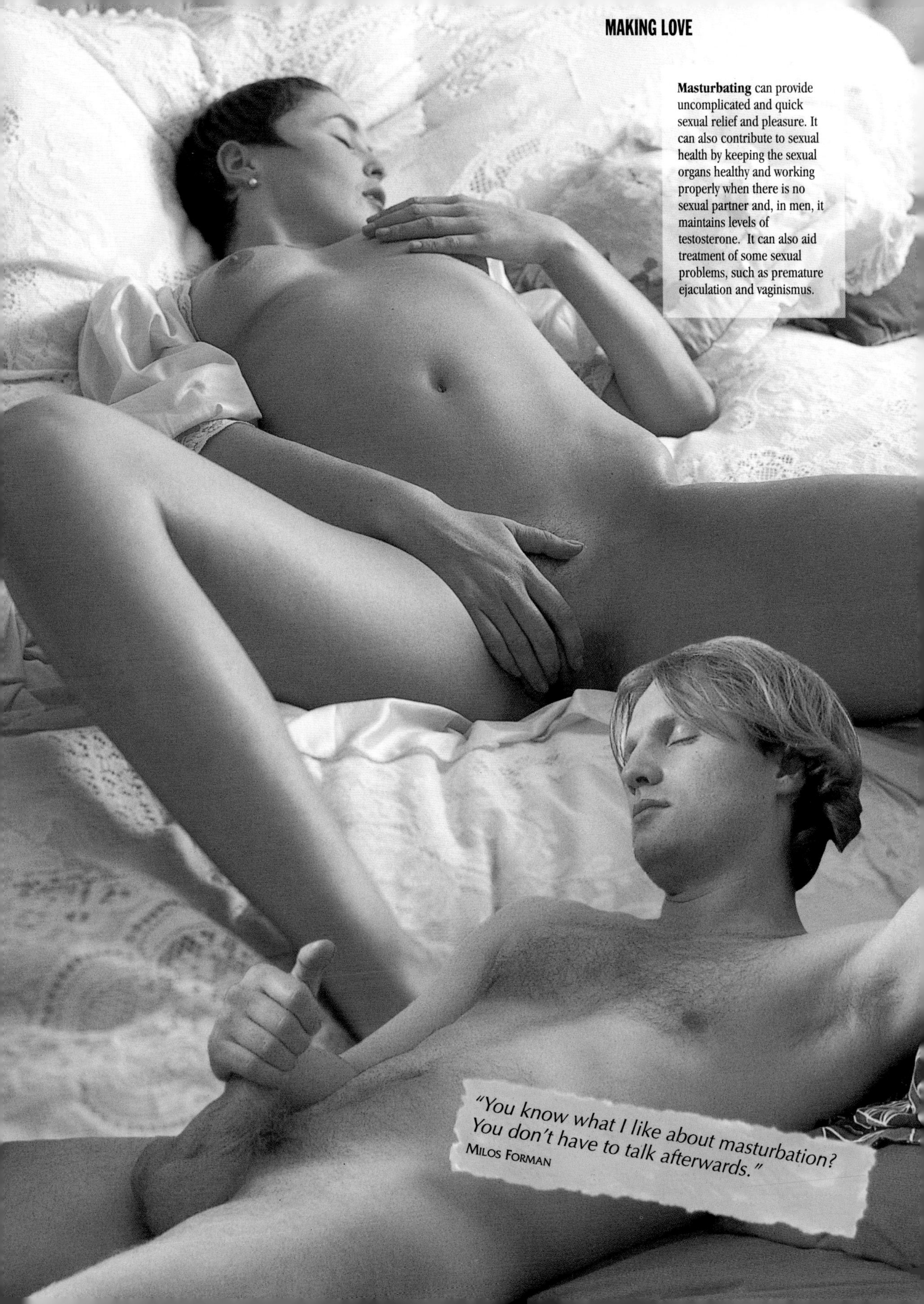

Masturbating can provide uncomplicated and quick sexual relief and pleasure. It can also contribute to sexual health by keeping the sexual organs healthy and working properly when there is no sexual partner and, in men, it maintains levels of testosterone. It can also aid treatment of some sexual problems, such as premature ejaculation and vaginismus.

"You know what I like about masturbation? You don't have to talk afterwards."
MILOS FORMAN

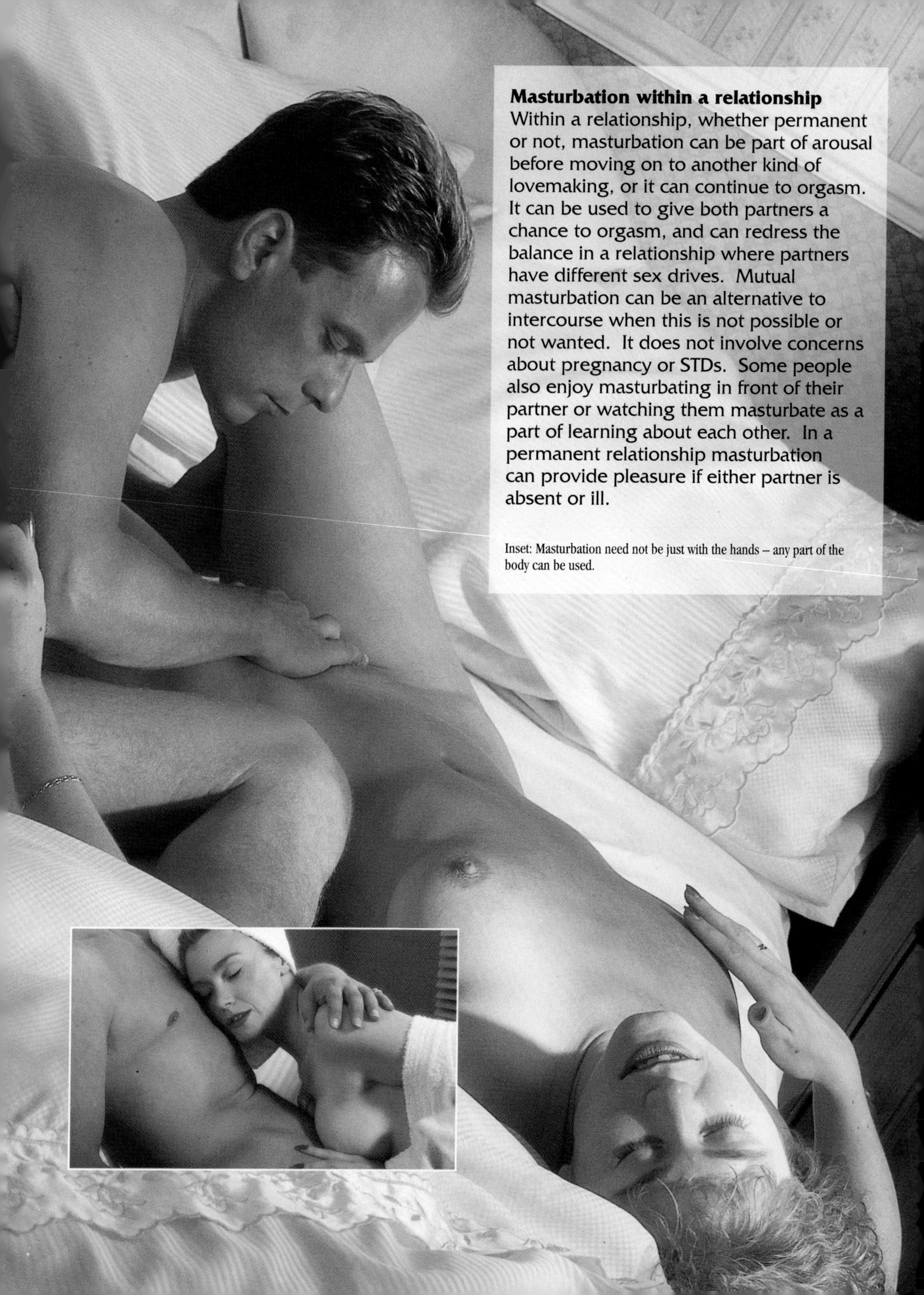

Masturbation within a relationship

Within a relationship, whether permanent or not, masturbation can be part of arousal before moving on to another kind of lovemaking, or it can continue to orgasm. It can be used to give both partners a chance to orgasm, and can redress the balance in a relationship where partners have different sex drives. Mutual masturbation can be an alternative to intercourse when this is not possible or not wanted. It does not involve concerns about pregnancy or STDs. Some people also enjoy masturbating in front of their partner or watching them masturbate as a part of learning about each other. In a permanent relationship masturbation can provide pleasure if either partner is absent or ill.

Inset: Masturbation need not be just with the hands – any part of the body can be used.

Taboos about masturbation: from self-abuse to self-loving

Masturbation was condemned for two reasons: on religious grounds, because sex was supposed to be only for procreation and not for pleasure, and on the basis of a perceived health risk. Eminent and respected physicians and psychologists of the time issued serious health warnings, as every kind of mental or bodily disorder – 'from pimples to insanity' (Kinsey) – was ascribed to masturbation. Cures included castration, various forms of male and female circumcision and restraint. Many children were tied or chained at night to prevent them from touching their genitals in their sleep; bizarre and painful penis harnesses were also used.

Toward the end of the nineteenth century, masturbation among adolescents came to be more accepted, although among adults it was taken as a sign of immaturity, senility, insanity or an inability to form, or maintain, a normal heterosexual relationship.

The major breakthrough came with Kinsey's study of male sexuality. This revealed that ninety-two per cent of men had masturbated at some point in their lives, generally with no adverse effects. (Female masturbation was not investigated until later.) The only substantive negative effect of masturbation was, ironically, the way people had been affected psychologically by its condemnation.

For many people, this legacy of guilt still survives. It is now known that masturbation is not only harmless but can have benefits. It is also probably the most common of all genital sexual practices. But in spite of this, there is still a taboo, people tend to feel guilty and prefer not to discuss masturbation. In relationships it has been seen as a kind of infidelity. Traditional gender roles have not eased the situation: for men masturbation may be interpreted as an inability to form a relationship with a woman and reflect on his 'virility', while women's sexual feelings, fantasies and self-pleasure have not fully acknowledged until relatively recently.

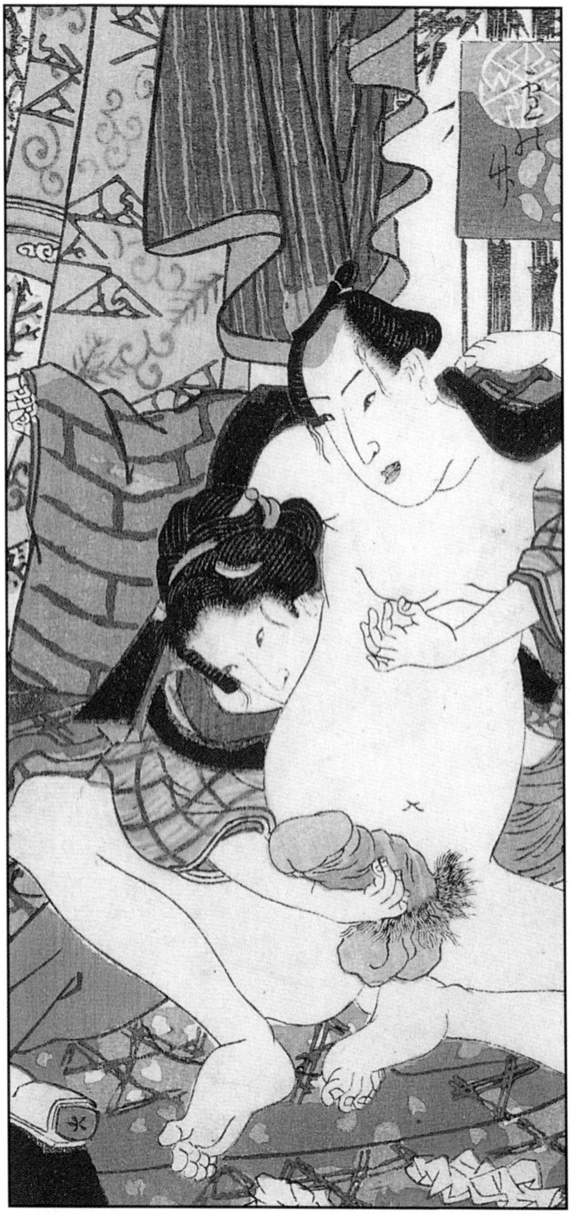

Nineteenth century coloured woodcut (detail) by Kunimori II of Japan. Masturbation has always been part of human sexuality, for both individuals and couples.

"Neither plague, nor war, nor smallpox, nor a crowd of similar evils have resulted more disastrously for humanity than the habit of masturbation: it is destroying the element of civilized society."

NEW ORLEANS MEDICAL AND SURGICAL JOURNAL (1850)

ORAL SEX

Oral sex means using the mouth to stimulate a partner's sexual organs. Oral sex can be one of the most sensuous and erotic forms of lovemaking. Like masturbation, it has been common in many cultures for centuries, and yet remains controversial.

Oral sex can be part or all of a lovemaking experience. It can likewise be used to satisfy either partner before or after the other has reached orgasm. What distinguishes it from other sexual practices is the intense and intimate awareness of the sight, feel and smell of one's partner's genitals which it creates.

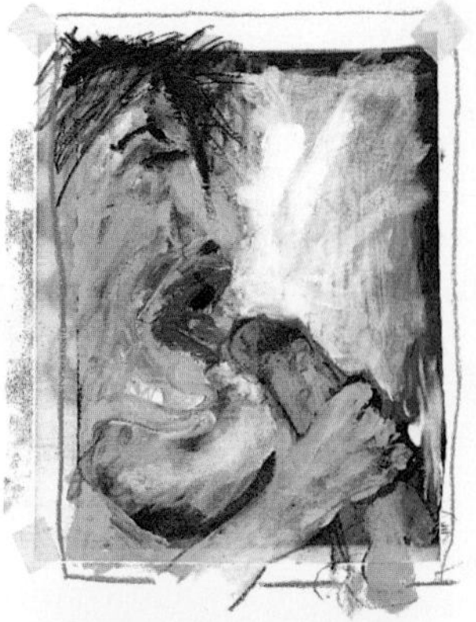

Slang terms

CUNNILINGUS
cunt sucking, Frenching, eating out, going down, eating at the Y, muff diving, clam diving, tonguing, cat lapper, plating, licking, blowing, pussy nibbling, box lunch, head job, breakfast in bed, cake eater.

FELLATIO
cock sucking, blow job, BJ, giving head, deep throat, sucking off, going down on, nob job, Frenching, plating, basket lunch, copping a joint, Derby picnic, Hoover

Cunnilingus

Cunnilingus is stimulating the female genitals with the mouth, in particular the tongue. Kissing and caressing the clitoris and vaginal lips with the tongue can be highly sensuous and arousing – the tongue is soft and can be more mobile and exploratory than the fingers.

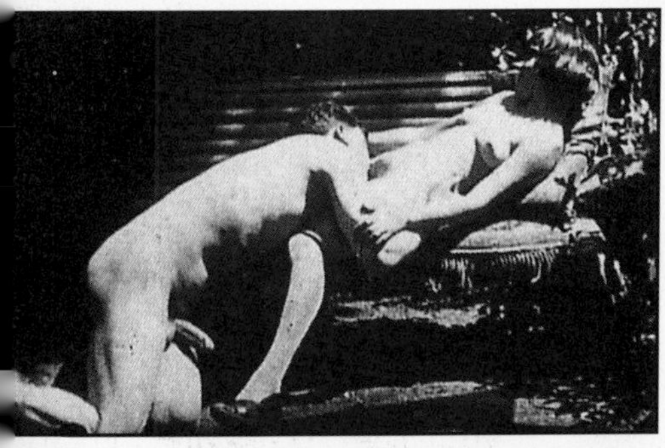

The sensitive inner and outer vaginal lips can be licked and sucked. The vagina itself can be penetrated with the tongue and the G spot can be stimulated, but to bring about greater arousal more attention should be focused on the clitoris.

Cunnilingus may begin with the women's partner caressing the inner thighs and the area around the genitals, moving on to stimulating the clitoris with the tip of the tongue, or to penetrating the vagina with the tongue.

Oral pleasuring of the female can be intensely pleasurable for both partners. However, it is important to discuss and identify what each partner finds most exciting.

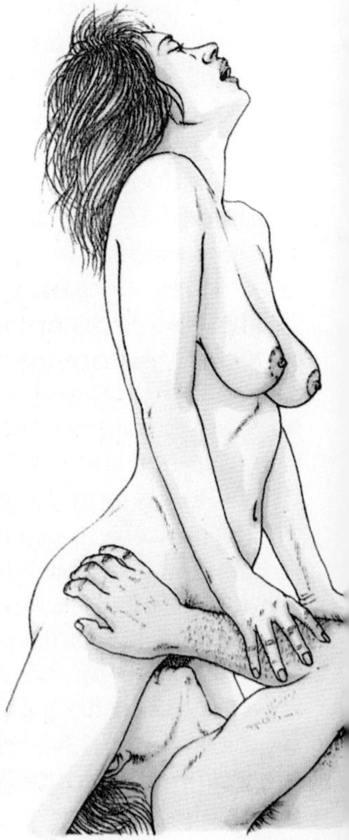

See also:
masturbation
health and hygiene
kissing
safer sex

"You know the worst thing about oral sex? The view."
MAUREEN LIPMAN

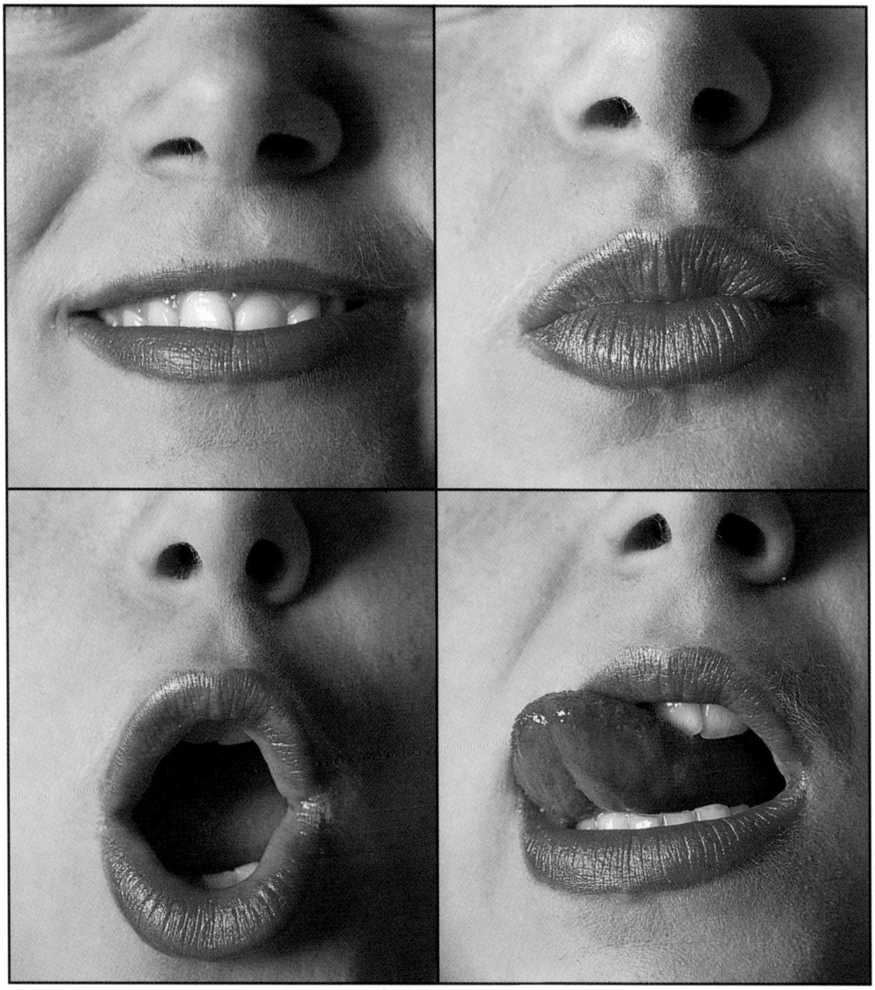

The sexual mouth
The mouth is the only part of the body capable of rivalling and even exceeding the genitals in terms of sensuousness and sensitivity. It is associated with not one but two of life's potentially most sensuous experiences: sex and eating. As well as this, it is mobile and expressive, and can convey anything from doubt or displeasure to excitement, delight and seductiveness. In oral sex, the penis, scrotum and perineum of the male and the vulva of the female – like any other part of the body – can be licked, sucked, kissed, stroked with the lips or lightly nibbled. These factors give the mouth a unique capacity for both giving and receiving oral stimulation.

Fellatio

Fellatio is stimulating the male genitals with the mouth and tongue. It may involve kissing the penis or taking the shaft into the mouth; if this occurs then the penis can be sucked and the tongue used to stimulate the sensitive ridge (the frenulum) on the underside of the penis.

The mouth can be moved to simulate the movements of vaginal or anal intercourse, and the fingers can be used to stimulate the penis further. The partner may wish to thrust simultaneously.

Some people fear gagging or choking, but can avoid this by not allowing the penis to be pushed too far into the mouth. Others, in 'deep throat' fellatio, have learned to repress this reflex.

Fellatio in the nineteenth century
In the superficially prim Victorian era, fellatio (right) and cunnilingus (far left) were as popular as ever.

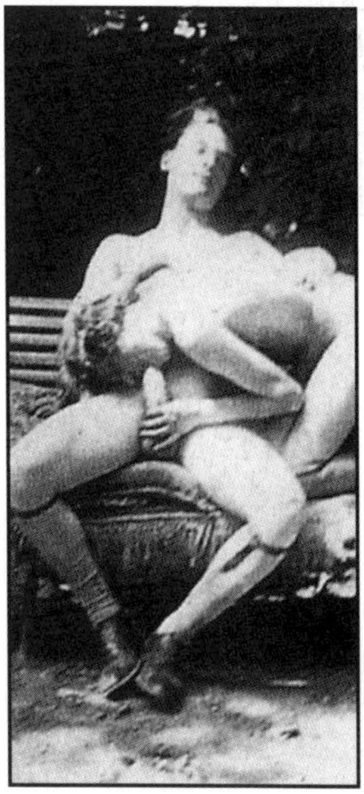

Taboos about oral sex

There are, however, many reasons both personal and cultural why many people prefer to avoid oral sex. A great many will not even talk about it, regardless of whether or not they practise it.

Personal taboos may include any sense of inhibition about this kind of intimacy. Many consider it unhygienic, although if basic personal hygiene is maintained there are generally fewer bacteria on the genitals than there are in the mouth after eating. Many people feel ashamed of their genitals, or conscious of their natural, healthy genital odour, and are for this reason reluctant to let anyone come into such close contact with them. Others have more practical concerns, such as fear of choking or being unable to breathe.

Cultural taboos are not unlike those relating to masturbation in that many are associated with religious beliefs. Certain religions, such as Catholicism and Islam, on the whole only sanction intercourse when it is for reproduction: any other kind of activity – including homosexuality, anal intercourse, prolonged kissing, masturbation and oral sex – may be condemned.

By contrast, a number of cultural groups have celebrated oral sex quite openly. Images of people engaged in oral sex have featured on Chinese perfume bottles and ceramics, Japanese sexual manuals, Hindu temples and Amerindian pottery, as well as, albeit less openly, in Western art and literature.

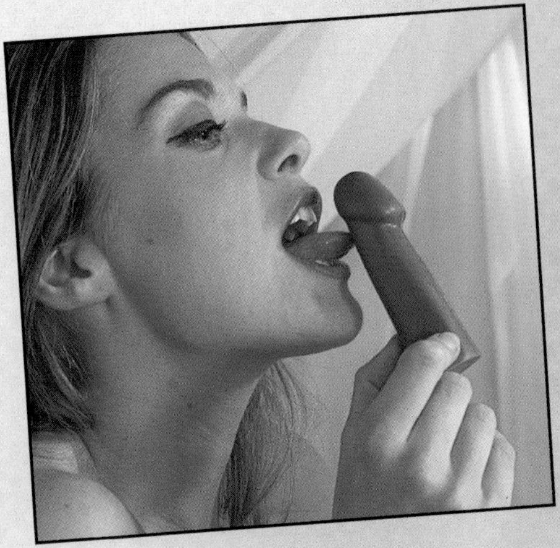

Facts

The amount, consistency and taste of seminal and vaginal fluid produced varies from one person to another. There are, however, some guidelines as to the nature of the taste. Cigarettes and alcohol make bodily fluids taste more bitter; red meats, spinach and foods high in iron give them a sharper flavour; the fluids of vegetarians tend to have a more moderate taste. Only diabetics are likely to taste sweet.

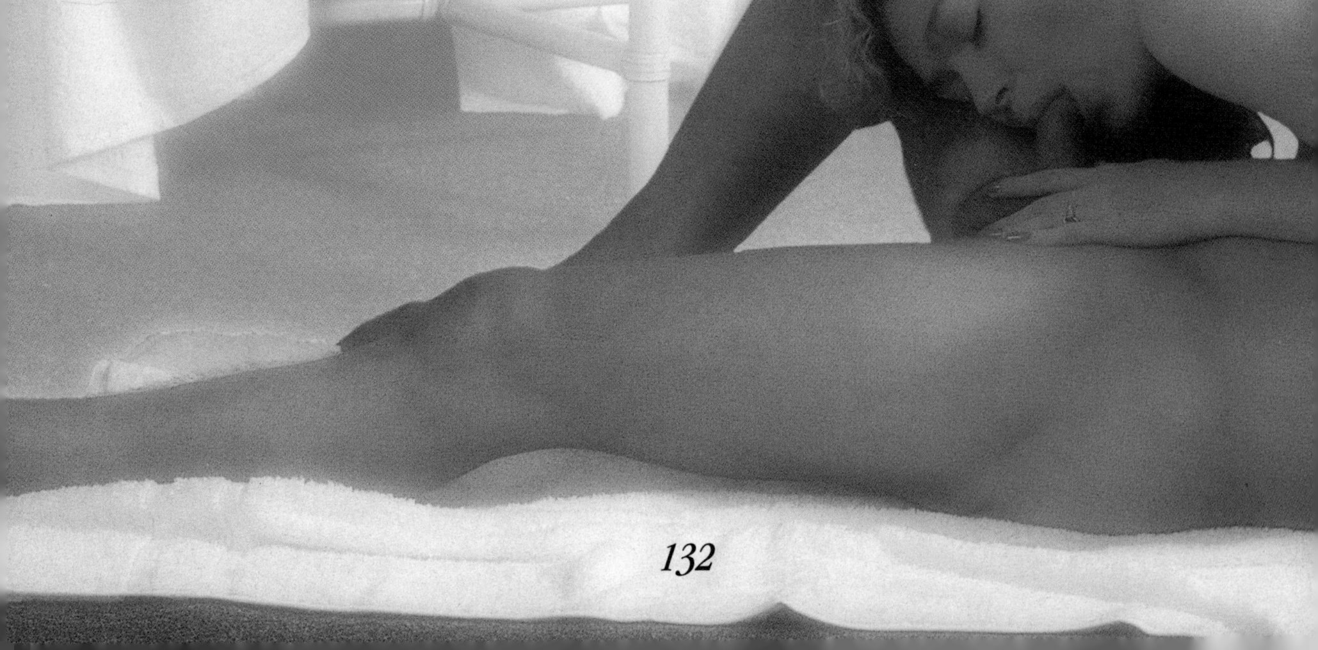

THE '69' OR 'SOIXANTE-NEUF' POSITION

This is called the 69 position (or soixante-neuf *in French) because of the shape of the bodies when they are both positioned mouth to genital area at the same time.*

Reproduction of a Japanese woodcut showing a gymnastic display of the 69 position.

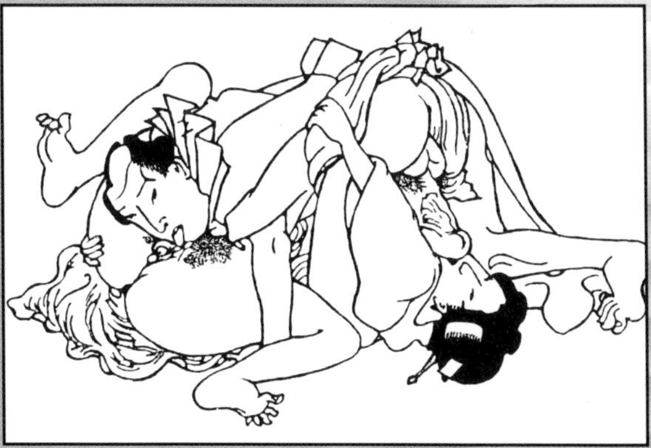

Simultaneously performing cunnilingus and/or fellatio can be highly satisfying and exciting for both partners. A number of positions can be used, with the man on top, the woman on top, side-by-side or even standing; in most of them, the hands can be used to caress the partner's body.

The 69 position may be difficult for partners who are very different from each other in height or physique. Also, some couples prefer to stimulate each other in turn, concentrating on the distinct sensations of giving and receiving oral sex. This may be either as a prelude to penetrative sex or in order to induce orgasm.

"As for that topsy-turvy tangle known as soixante-neuf, personally I have always felt it to be madly confusing, like trying to pat your head and rub your stomach at the same time."
HELEN LAWRENSON

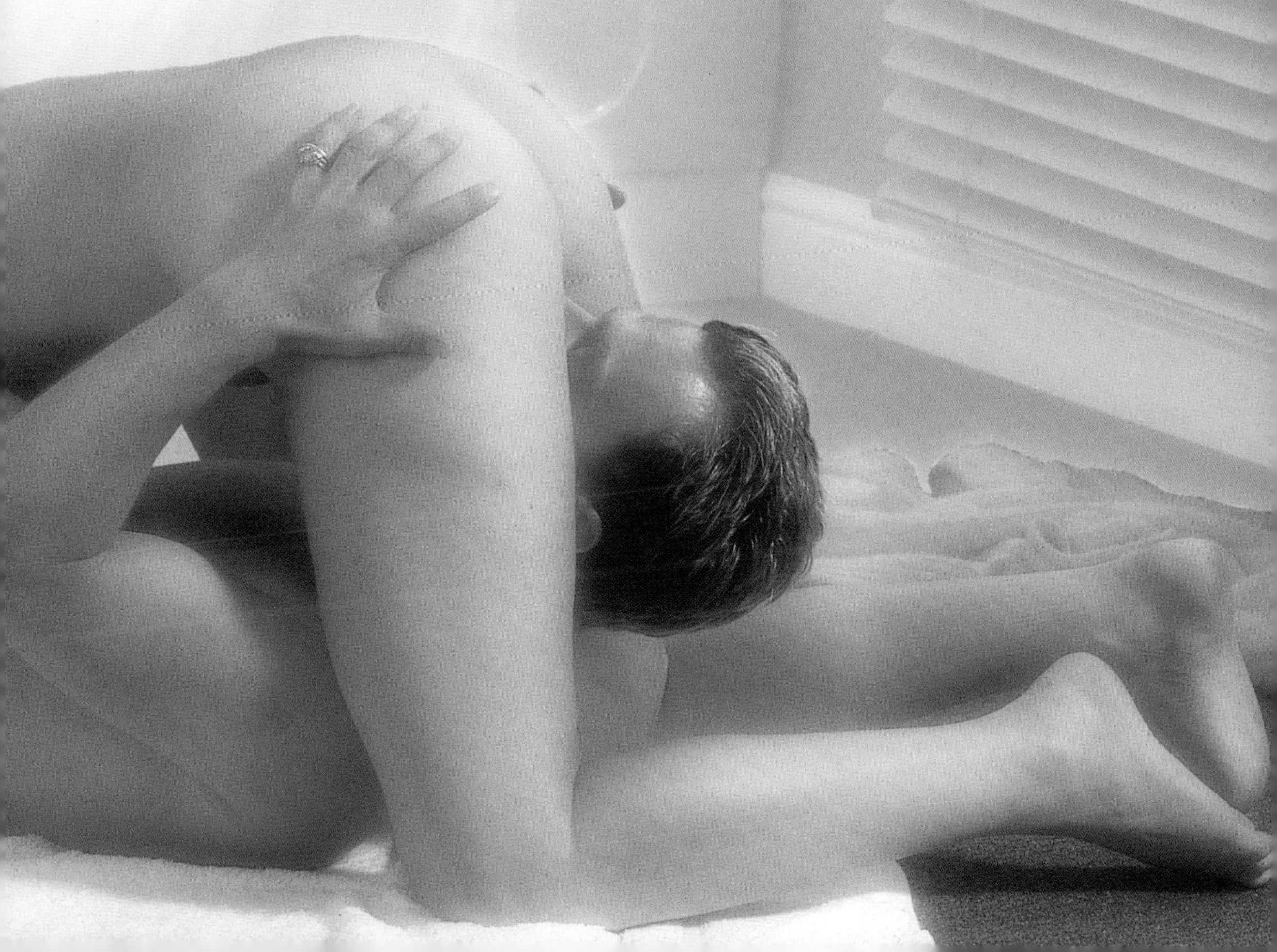

ANAL SEX

Within the range of common sexual practices, anal sex is probably the most controversial of all.

Anal intercourse seems to have been a common sexual activity in all ages and cultures and yet remains a taboo subject, often even between close friends or lovers. For many people it is a highly rewarding sexual experience and fantasy, others find the mere idea repulsive. Amongst some groups, it is used as a method of contraception.

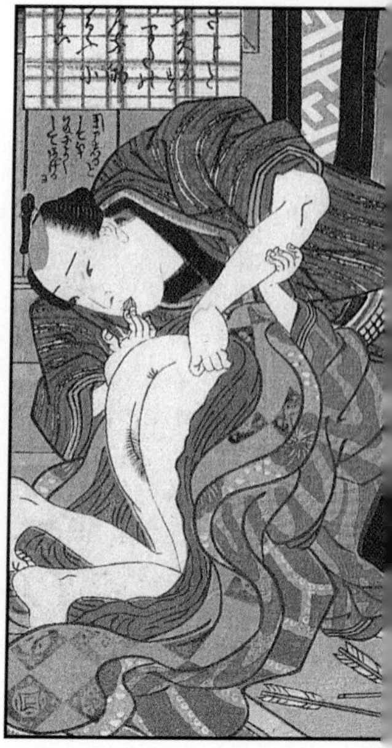

Nineteenth century coloured woodcut (detail) by Kunimori of Japan. The anus is an area of natural curiosity – as well as an erogenous zone of many people.

Attitudes

The notion of anal sex as a taboo may begin in infancy. A child's interest in his or her bodily functions – described by psychologists as the oral, anal and genital fixations – is natural and healthy. The interest in the genitals has been repressed in some cultures, but tolerance is now growing once more. However, the interest in excretion – and hence anything to do with the anus – is often frowned upon and repressed.

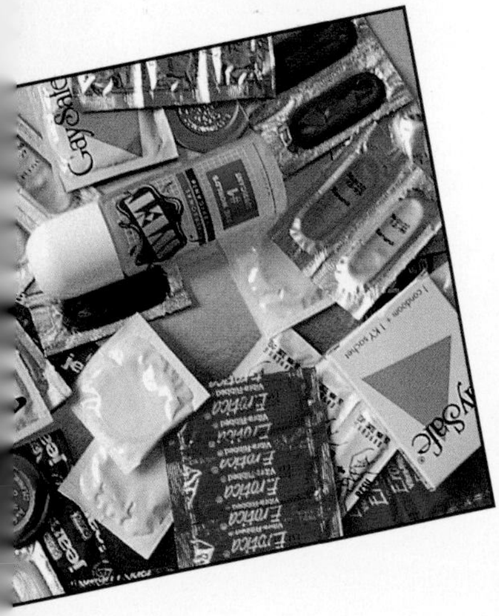

Anal intercourse between heterosexuals is illegal in many countries. It was legalized in the UK at the beginning of 1996.

Pleasure and practicality

It is estimated that at least ten per cent of heterosexual couples and fifty to seventy-five per cent of male homosexual couples have anal sex on a regular basis. In anal sex, the anus is stimulated with fingers or hands, mouth and tongue, the penis, or any other part of the body, with or without penetration. Sex aids and sex toys can also be used, including those which are made specifically for use in or around the anus.

Like the vagina, the tissue of the anus and rectum contains many nerve endings, particularly in the outer parts. Stimulating this area can be highly pleasurable. The anus is also surrounded by the same muscle as surrounds the pelvic bone, that is, the penis and the scrotum in the male and the clitoris and vagina in the female; in women, anal sex can even provide clitoral stimulation. The tightness of the anus can provide great pleasure, especially for the 'giver'.

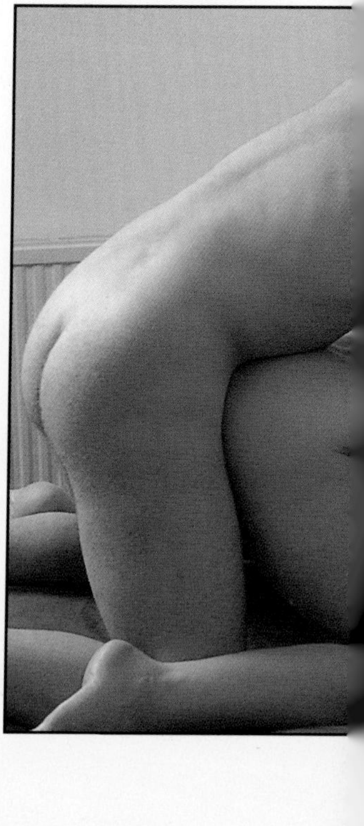

See also:
masturbation
male anatomy
penis
safer sex

Anal stimulation is the only way to stimulate the prostate directly. It also provides homosexual men with a means of having penetrative sex.

Anal sex can also answer certain practical needs. Firstly, as long as the semen does not come into contact with the vagina, it cannot lead to pregnancy. Secondly, having anal sex avoids breaking the hymen, which is taken as all-important proof of virginity in certain cultures, although the hymen can in fact be broken in other ways. People may engage in anal sex for any of these reasons, as well as out of simple sexual curiosity.

FACT: A survey by Cosmopolitan magazine in March 1996 suggested that at least sixteen per cent of British women have tried anal sex, compared to forty-nine per cent of Russian and fifty-two per cent of Italian women.

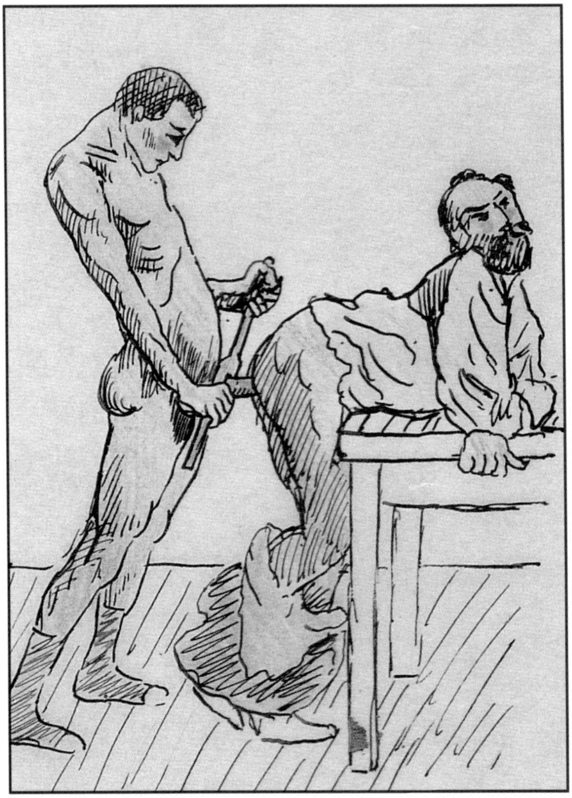

French amateur erotica drawing from the 1890s.

Anal intercourse between homosexuals is also illegal in many countries and often subject to taboos. It is, however, a common form of intercourse between homosexual men.

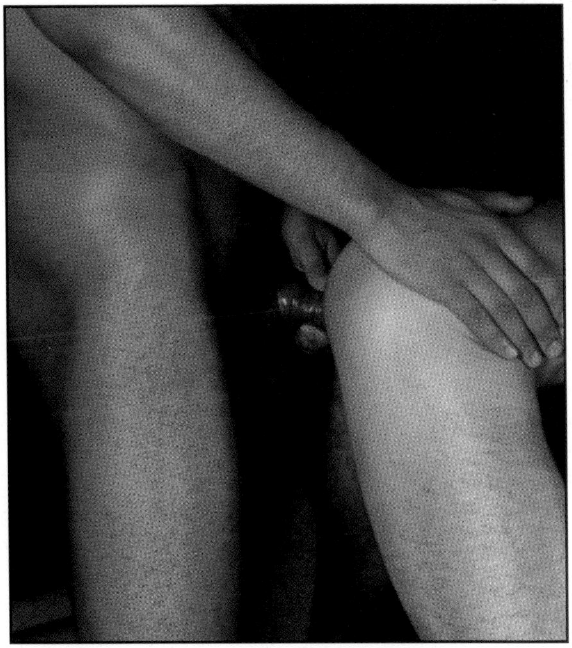

The risks

Practised carefully, in many cases anal sex need cause no problems. However, there are a few risks involved, largely because – unlike the vagina – the anus is not designed for penetration. The walls of the rectum are much thinner and more fragile than those of the vagina and can be damaged comparatively easily. Anal sex can also be painful – receiving anal sex is frequently cited as the sexual practice most disliked by both women and men. However, this can be eased by relaxation, perhaps aided with gentle dilatation with a finger or a small object, and by using sufficient lubrication.

Anal sex carries greater risks of spreading infections and sexually transmissible diseases, principally because of the fragility of the walls of the rectum which makes contact between semen and blood that much more probable. Above all, anal sex seems to be the route by which HIV is transmitted most easily, although the use of a condom with plenty of water-based lubricant substantially reduces this risk. Also, bacteria which exist naturally and healthily in the anus can cause infections when passed to the vagina or mouth.

SEX DRIVE

The term 'sex drive' refers to a person's strength of desire to have sex. It influences the amount and the kind of sex a person needs in order to feel sexually satisfied. It is an innate, instinctive urge common to all animals, but which varies greatly in degree from one person to another. It can also be affected by external influences, causing it to change throughout a person's life and even from one day to the next.

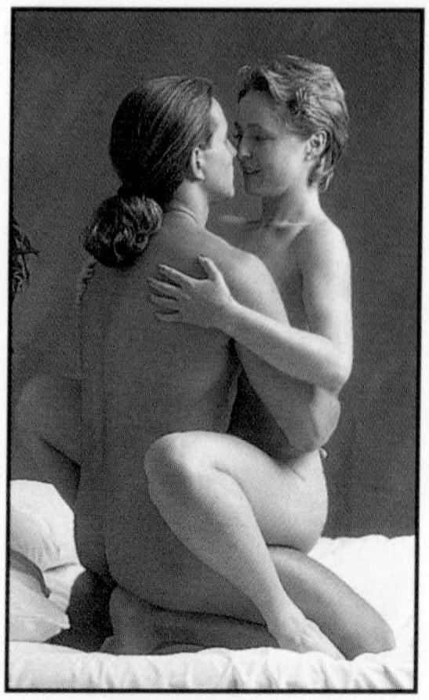

Having the same sex drive can make a couple's sex life highly satisfying. However, most people find that their sex drives can be a problem, but mutual understanding and flexibility can often resolve it.

What determines a person's sex drive?
Sex drive is instinctive: it is not a conscious force. It can be enhanced or controlled consciously, but the strength of the urge itself is more deeply rooted.

At one level, sex drive is about reproduction: it is the instinct that ensures the continuation of the species. It has been suggested that the human enjoyment of sex evolved as a means of ensuring reproduction. Biologically, sex drive is caused by androgenic hormones, in particular testosterone. This is produced in the adrenal glands and the testes in men, and the adrenal glands and the ovaries in women. In men testosterone is produced in greater quantities and is responsible for the male secondary sexual characteristics such as greater body and facial hair, and the occurrence of more muscle and less body fat than females. Anything that affects the production of testosterone – such as castration and use of synthetic hormones, as well as psychological factors – affects the sex drive in men and women.

FACT: Freud was the first person to use the term 'libido', the Latin word for desire, in a sexual sense. He was the first to point to sex drive as a fundamental source of human motivation.

Incompatible sex drives can be a problem for some couples, but mutual understanding and flexibility can often resolve it.

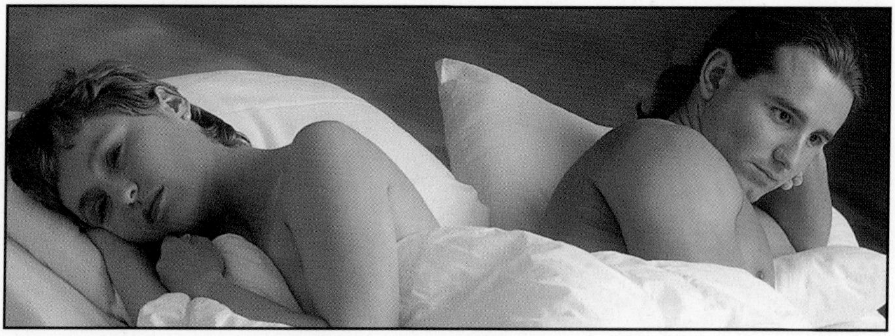

See also:
sexual feelings – male
sexual feelings – female
sexual attraction
fantasy
aphrodisiacs
growth and change

The links between state of mind and hormone production are still not fully understood. However, the two are connected and can affect sex drive. Stress and anxiety are known to reduce sexual desire, just as happiness and a sense of security can boost it. Negative influences may be specifically to do with sex or apparently quite unconnected, but they can be very powerful. Many are rooted in sexually repressive attitudes during childhood, in cultural background or upbringing.

Throughout history, people have been searching for effective aphrodisiacs, that is, substances or products which increase sexual desire. A fail-safe aphrodisiac has yet to be found, although many people swear by certain substances. In spite of this, a balanced diet, regular exercise and good general health have all been shown to boost sexual appetite, capacity and enjoyment.

Differences in sex drive

Attitudes to female sexuality have always been somewhat ambivalent. While men have almost always been expected to have strong sexual desires, some cultures have recognized and even worshiped female sexuality but others have completely denied it. In the West in the nineteenth century, women were seen as divided into two types: those who had sexual desires and were 'loose' or immoral, and those who were chaste and suitable for marriage. Sex drive was not part of the ideal of femininity.

It is now acknowledged that both sexes have a sex drive, although some stigma remains for women: a man with many partners may still be seen as a 'stud' while a woman is more likely to be seen as a 'slut' or a 'slag'. Statistically, women are more likely than men to have low sexual desire, although among men it is not uncommon. A study carried out in the USA estimated that of the twenty per cent of the population suffering from Inhibited Sexual Desire (ISD), a third were men.

Biological differences may have some influence here, in that a man is constantly fertile while a woman is only fertile for a few days each month and so has less biological need of a high sex drive. However, sex drive and fertility do not seem to be related. A man's sex drive declines steadily from his late teens or early twenties even though he can remain fertile until late in life; a woman's sex drive tends to build until her early forties when it may gradually start to decline, while she loses her fertility around the age of fifty.

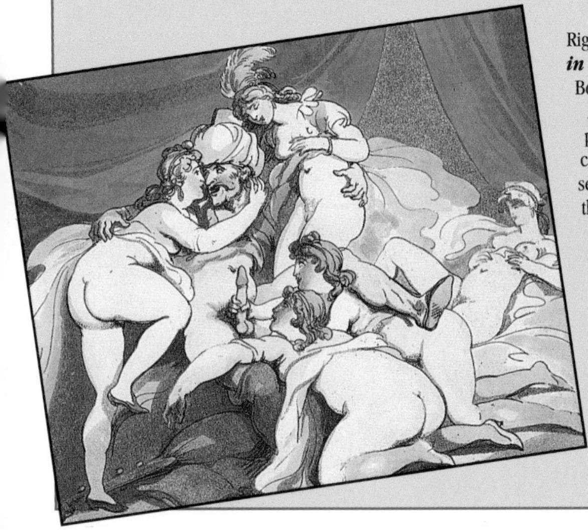

Right: ***Two Athenian Women in Distress*** (detail), by Aubrey Beardsley, 1896 illustration for Aristophanes' *Lysistrata*. The picture depicts women of fifth century Athens, who went on a sex strike when annoyed about their men always being at war. They ended up as sexually frustrated as the men – if not more so.

Left: ***The Sultan*** (detail), by Thomas Rowlandson, from a nineteenth century sequence of caricatures of the English aristocracy.

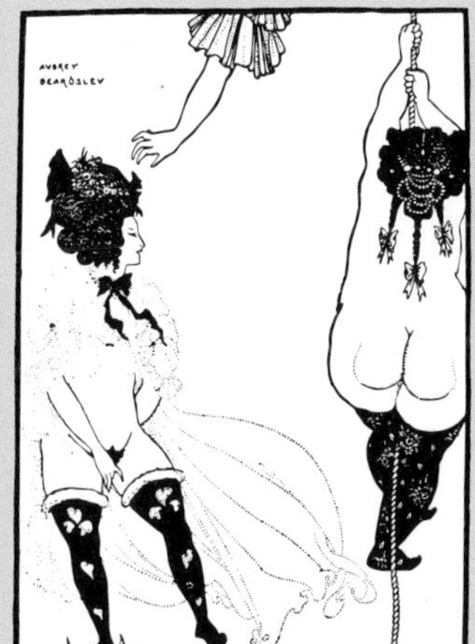

ORGASM

Orgasm, for most people, is the highest point of sexual excitement, the release of sexual tension built up in the course of arousal. It is also arguably the most complex part of sexual excitement, both in its nature and in the way it is perceived.

Orgasm can be anything from purely physical sensations experienced in the genital area to a psychic experience in which immediate, physical consciousness of the body is lost. Many attempts have been made to classify orgasm, but the reality is that it varies enormously from one person to another and from one sexual act to the next.

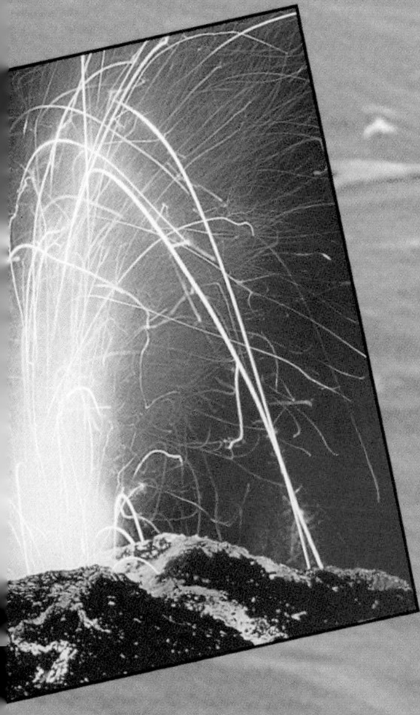

The importance of orgasm

The main difference between male and female orgasms is that men's are more reliable and happen faster. This does not mean that women are condemned to sexual dissatisfaction, but it does mean that a woman's partner may need to learn what she needs to achieve orgasm so that he or she can give her that stimulation. This may involve a partner learning to delay their own orgasm or using other – non-penile – kinds of stimulation.

At the same time, placing undue emphasis on orgasm as the sole indication of successful sex can detract from sexual pleasure. The media in general – and films in particular – frequently portray orgasm as the primary objective in sex: the message is that orgasms should be frequent, simultaneous and preferably multiple. For many, orgasm is the ultimate sexual experience, but often it is not possible and pursuing it single-mindedly can prevent people from enjoying many of the other satisfying aspects of sex. Some Eastern sexual practices are even based on delaying orgasm or preventing it completely.

This same media pressure may have given rise to the phenomenon of the faked orgasm. The notion is that if the man or woman does not reach orgasm there is something wrong. In reality, only if a person is unable to reach orgasm – a condition known as anorgasmia – may there be cause for concern, and the condition is often curable.

See also:
clitoris
penis
sexual intercourse
sex drive

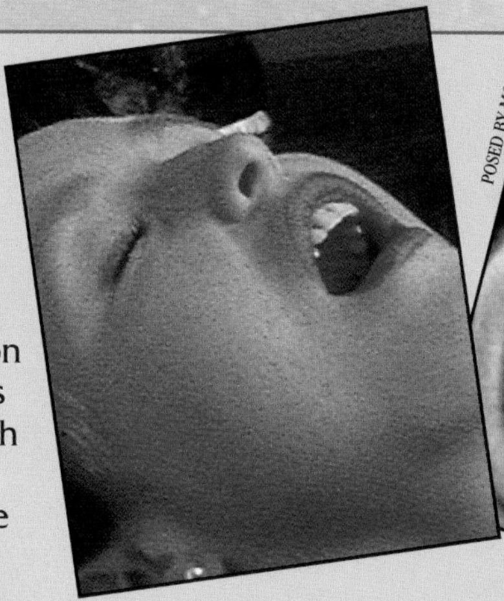

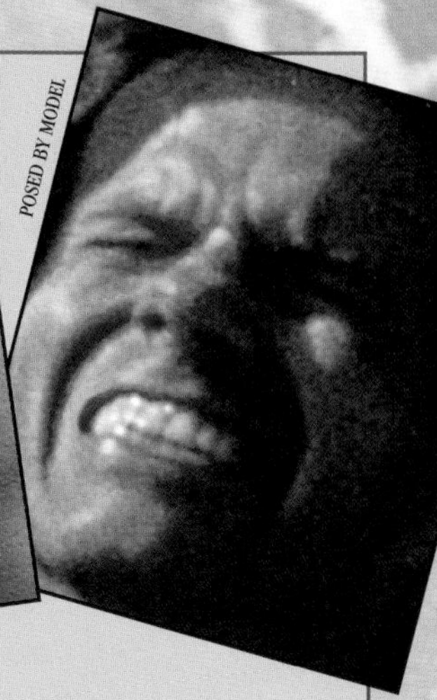

Female orgasm

Orgasm in females is much more complex, mainly because women can reach orgasm through more varied kinds of stimulation. The female orgasm does not depend on vaginal penetration. For most women, sexual arousal is focused on the clitoris rather than the vagina and it is direct or indirect clitoral stimulation which produces orgasm.

The debate about any differences there may be between clitoral and vaginal orgasms has yet to be resolved. Biologically there is no difference between the two as they involve the same muscles. Nor has the existence of a female G-spot been proven conclusively. However, women's reports of their own experiences reveal that many have an area of highly sensitive tissue or 'G-spot' located on the front wall of the vagina and that this can create an orgasm which is more intense and powerful than that which is focused solely on the clitoris. For most women the clitoris is more important, but for others it is the G-spot. Orgasm may focus on one or the other or both.

Most women do not reach orgasm with every sexual act; only about fifty per cent have regular orgasms. The reason for this may be evolutionary in that female orgasm, unlike male, is not necessary for reproduction. However, it is thought that women tend to have orgasms which are more intense and which last longer. Women are also much more likely to be able to achieve multiple or prolonged orgasms, possibly because they do not have to maintain an erection and have no refractory period like that experienced by men. A woman's ability to have an orgasm can also vary, as can the nature of the orgasm itself: both can be affected by the menstrual cycle, by emotional stress and by innumerable other factors, both physical and psychological.

Male orgasm

Sexual activity will – if uninterrupted – usually lead to orgasm, which is generally accompanied by ejaculation. The pleasure experienced tends to be focused on the genitals and is closely linked to ejaculation. A refractory period during which re-arousal is not possible usually follows ejaculation. The duration of this period is variable, but generally increases with age.

It was long thought that there was only one kind of male orgasm. However, research has revealed considerable variation, including the incidence of male orgasms without ejaculation. Some men are able to delay orgasm, either by halting stimulation for a few moments when orgasm is felt to be approaching, by mental exercises or by using conscious muscle control to prevent ejaculation. Either technique can make it possible for a man to experience more than one orgasmic peak, similar to the multiple orgasms experienced by some women, or the so-called status orgasmus or prolonged orgasm in which the sensations of orgasm can last for as long as a minute. Delaying ejaculation can also help a man to maintain his erection long enough to ensure that his partner reaches orgasm, or to enable the couple to achieve simultaneous orgasm if desired.

LOCATIONS

The bedroom is regarded as the most suitable place for sex by sixty-eight per cent of women and men. In the West, most people, most of the time, make love in the bedroom, and usually at night. There are many potential reasons for this, not the least of which are comfort, privacy and convenience. However, this is another area in which cultural norms vary enormously.

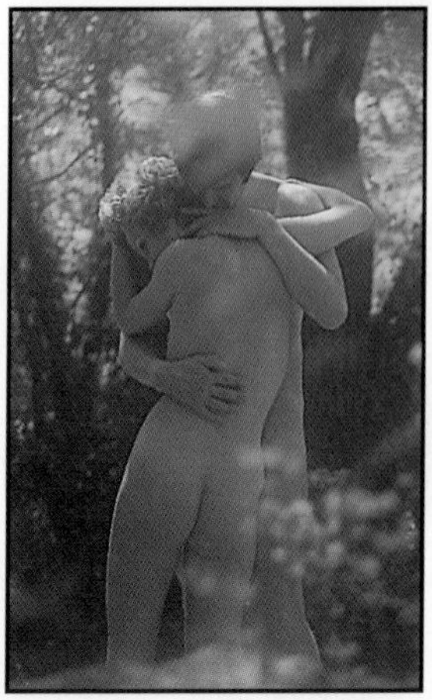

Cultural differences
In certain West African and Latin American cultures sex outdoors is forbidden and strictly punished. At the other extreme are the tribes of Papua New Guinea among whom sex indoors is taboo. Between the two come certain parts of Africa and Oceania where both are considered normal and acceptable. Sexual activity in these cultures tends to be less repressed and treated as much more normal than it is in many Western societies.

Similarly, in the West it is widely believed that night-time is the most appropriate time of day for sex. This custom is more widespread, probably for practical reasons since, regardless of the culture, the daylight hours tend to be taken up by work. However other groups have more deeply rooted reasons, such as certain African tribes who believe that breaking the taboo against daytime sex will cause sickness among their people and animals, and the one tribe who believe that it will produce albino offspring.

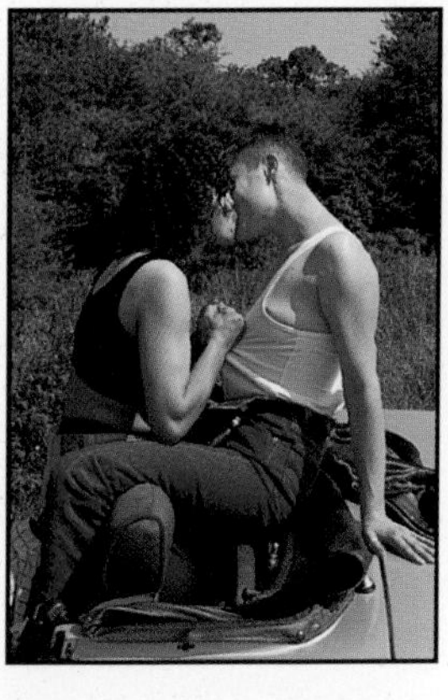

In the West
Even though the norm in the West is to have sex at night, indoors and probably in the bedroom, people have always experimented with other options. This may be out of necessity (to avoid those with whom accommodation is shared) or simply to add excitement.

For many, a sense of the forbidden or the taboo can be highly arousing. In the right circumstances and with due forethought, great variety in terms of location can be brought into lovemaking.

See also:
food and sex
fantasy

Outdoors and public places
Making love in the open air is the wish of many and, hence, a common sexual fantasy. While those who have an enclosed garden can be assured of privacy, sexual activity in any other place outside the home or hotel carries its risks – of discovery and of prosecution. Most countries have some laws against sexual activity in public. For many people these risks, and a sense of doing something forbidden, are part of the excitement (although it is important not to cause offense).

Making love in a field, wood or park can provide a romantic sense of returning to nature and can also rekindle memories of courtship. Camping creates an environment which is slightly more private and very intimate, if potentially uncomfortable. It may be for the same reason – the memories of courtship – that parked cars enjoy such enduring popularity for lovemaking, although for some the possibility of being watched is a major source of excitement. In the USA, more than sixty per cent of women and men with their own homes still like making love in a car.

In terms of other public places, it seems that every possibility has been at least attempted. People have made love on trains and buses, on aeroplanes (becoming members of the 'Mile High Club'), at the cinema, theatre and opera, in lifts, libraries, restaurants and fairground rides. Some have suffered the consequences of getting caught, but most have had uniquely thrilling and memorable experiences.

Indoors

Any kind of accommodation can offer a variety of alternative locations for lovemaking. If sex is confined to a single room different pieces of furniture can provide variation, and other rooms may be available, as long as other residents or family members are absent and there is privacy from neighbours and passers-by.

While the bedroom is the most common choice of location, people can have sex in any number of different places, at home or elsewhere.

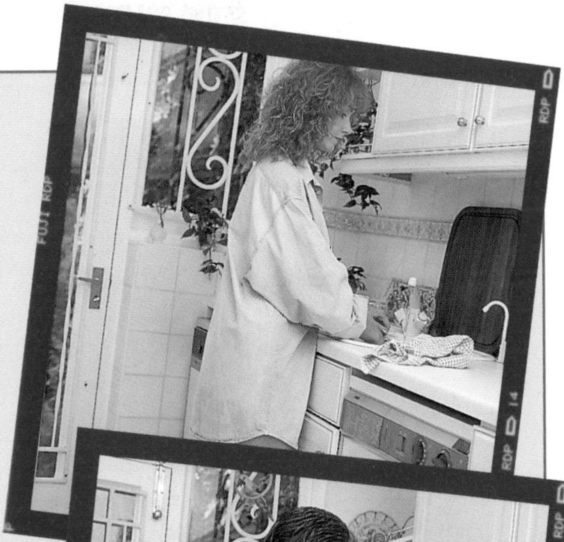

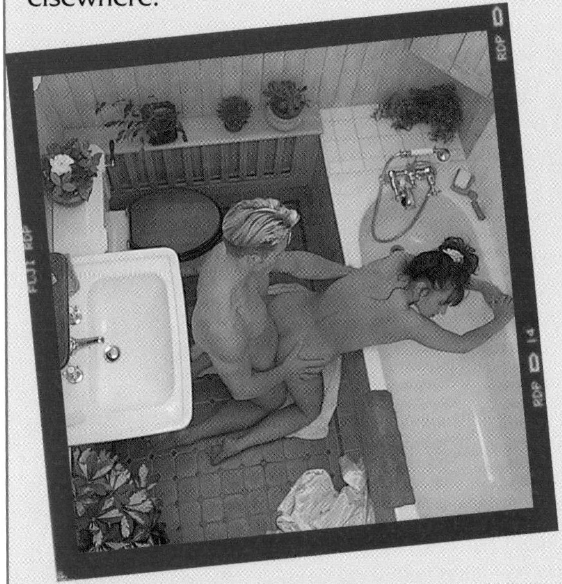

The bathroom often has the added advantage of having a lockable door. Making love in a shower or bath may be highly sensuous, and candlelit baths very romantic!

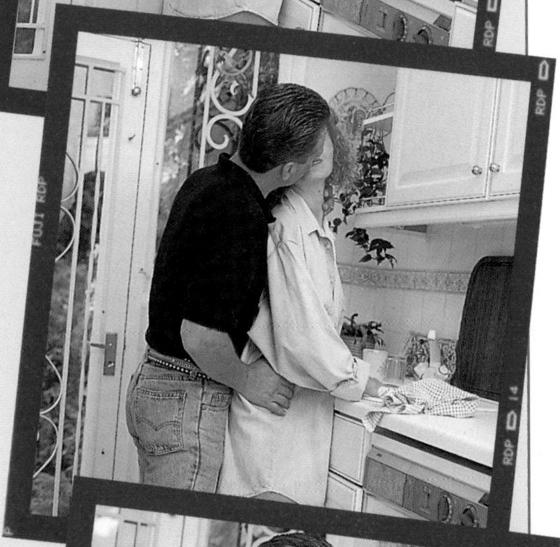

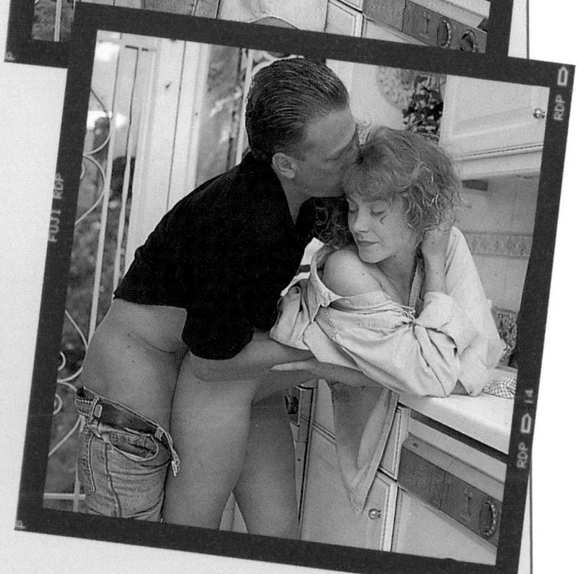

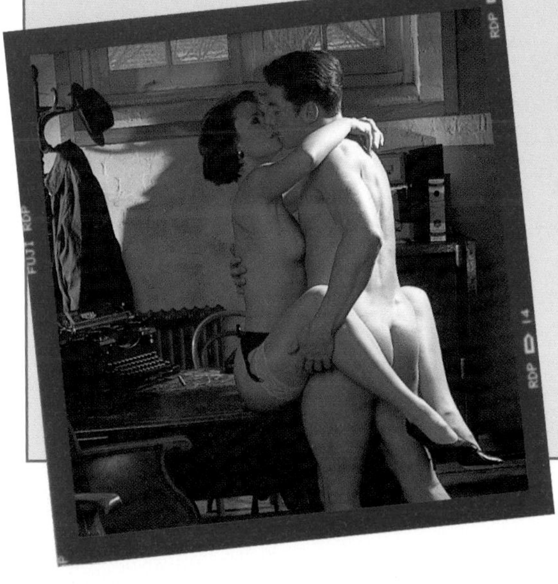

Spontaneous lovemaking in the kitchen, study or elsewhere is possible. The living room is one of the most popular choices. Over ninety per cent of women and men have made love in the living room at least once.

DRESSING & UNDRESSING

Throughout history clothes have been used to express sexuality. From codpieces to crinolines, changing fashions have drawn attention to different parts of the body as sources of sexual attraction. However, we rarely have the opportunity to make the most of the sexual potential our clothing offers. Very often, the place to do this is within the context of a sexual relationship.

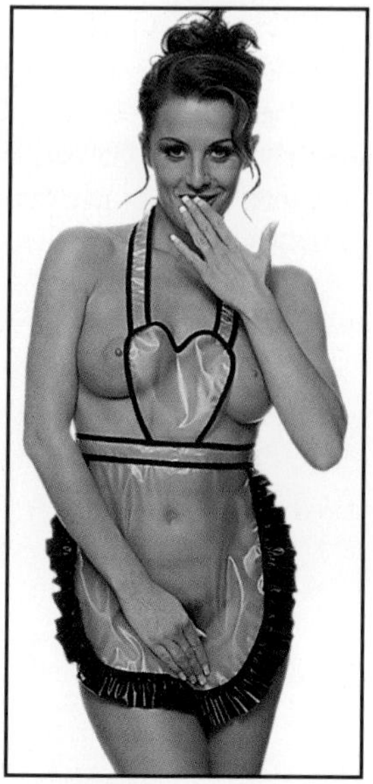

Dressing for sex can be an opportunity for expressing fantasies or experimenting with role-playing games.

Dressing for sex

Surveys suggest that while most people make love naked, many men and women find certain ways of dressing arousing. They may be aroused by the image of the clothing or by the teasing element of not being able to see the whole body straight away. Some like the idea of dressing up as a prelude to naked lovemaking while others like certain types of clothing to be worn throughout. In particular, many men find women more attractive partly dressed than completely naked.

The clothing most commonly worn for making love is underwear. The clichéd example of stockings and suspenders for women seems to enjoy an enduring popularity, and underwear designed specifically for sex – such as crotchless knickers and nipple-less bras – is still widely sold in sex boutiques. Even edible substances, from liquorice to flavoured gelatine, have been used to make underwear.

"Brevity is the soul of lingerie"
DOROTHY PARKER

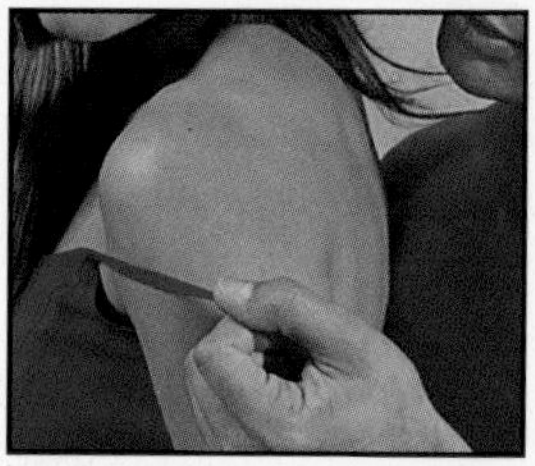

Dressing for sex can also mean indulging fetishes. Materials such as leather and rubber have long been seen as slightly risqué, even though many people are aroused by the feeling of these and/or other materials against the skin.

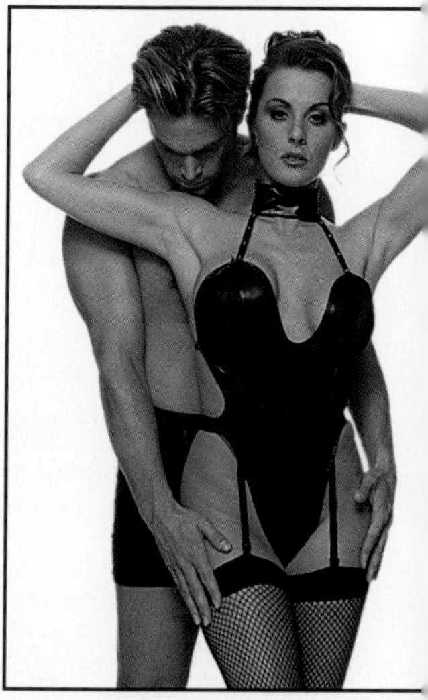

Special materials, such as leather, rubber and fake fur, have become increasingly popular and widely available – including for underwear. Specialist shops continue to produce leather and rubber goods to individual specifications.

Costumes are also popular, and many people enjoy using these in role-playing games. These may involve one partner dressing as an authority figure such as a doctor or nurse, a police or army officer, or a nun or a priest. Alternatively they may be more fanciful, with exotic costumes or period dress. This can be one way of fulfiling sexual fantasies within a relationship.

See also:
fantasy
sex aids and toys
exhibitionism and voyeurism
bondage
touching
attitudes and values
sexual feelings

Undressing in style

The actual process of removing clothing can also be an exciting part of lovemaking, and one that is too often hurried, rather than enjoyed and explored. Various aspects can be considered.

● WHO UNDRESSES WHOM? People either undress themselves or each other, both together or one at a time. One person may watch the other undress; one may 'strip' for the other. Some people like to undress together in front of a mirror. One can remain partly or fully dressed while the other is naked.

● WHAT DO YOU TAKE OFF? Rather than removing all your clothes at once, they can be removed gradually as lovemaking develops. Some articles can be left on throughout.

● QUICKLY OR SLOWLY? Hurried, frenzied stripping suggests eagerness and passion, but slow undressing, continuing to touch each other in the process, can be seductive and sensuous.

● LIGHTS ON OR OFF? Seeing a partner's face or genitals during lovemaking is important for many people. However, seeing each other's bodies as more is revealed can be highly arousing, especially the first time; on the other hand, when lovers see each other less clearly or not at all, the focus is more on the feel of the clothing and skin which can also be very erotic.

● WHAT ABOUT UNDERWEAR? The variety of styles and fabrics available for underwear provides choice: in the end it is a question of working out what the wearer finds comfortable and what both people find arousing. It has been said that many people feel socks should not be left until last, although high-heeled shoes may be kept on!

"The Duke returned from the wars today and did pleasure me in his top-boots."
SARAH, 1ST DUCHESS OF MARLBOROUGH (1769)

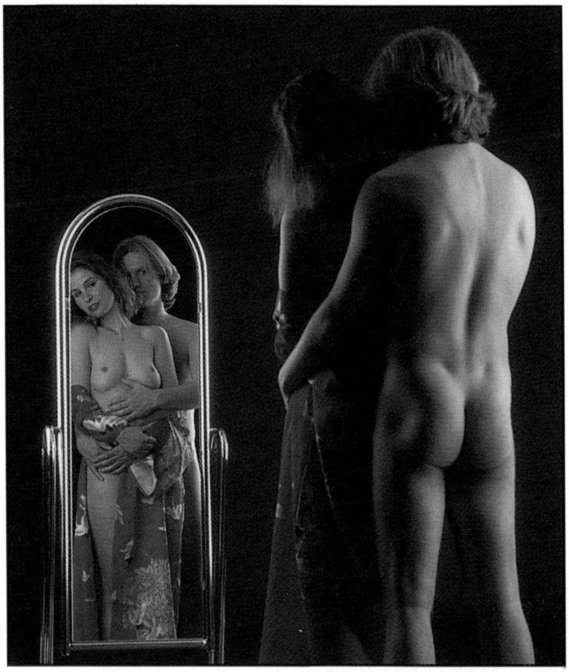

"No woman so naked as the one you can see to be naked underneath her clothes"
MICHAEL FRAYN, CITED IN THE OBSERVER, 15.10.95

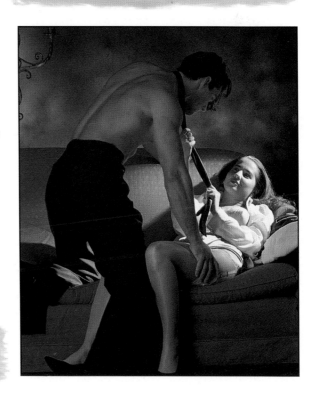

SEX & FOOD

Making love and eating are among life's greatest pleasures. They are natural, instinctive activities, but as humans we can also enjoy them as highly sensuous experiences. The two come close in oral sex, but it is also possible to combine them, experimenting with different kinds of food and different ways of eating.

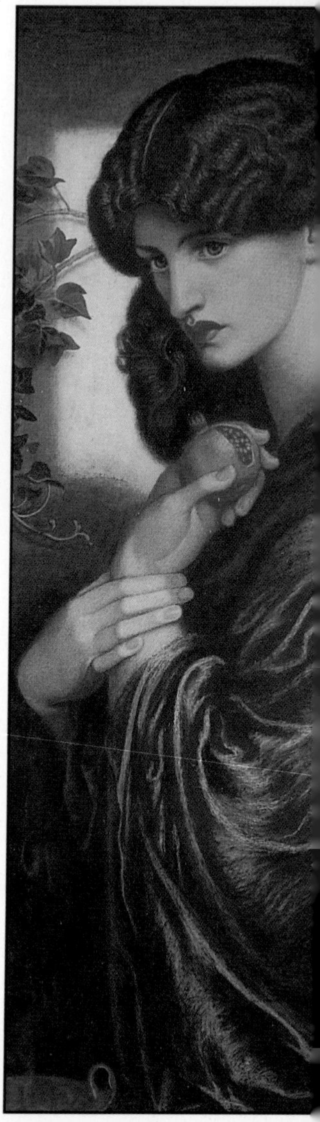

Proserpine (detail), by Dante Gabriel Ros

Food before sex, and during, and after...
Food has long been seen as a traditional preamble to sex. A dinner date can create an opportunity to get to know a person as a part of developing intimacy and can add romance at any stage of a relationship. However, sex and food can be mixed in any number of ways; whether in a formal dinner in a restaurant or a take-away on the back seat of a bus, a naked picnic in the bedroom or strawberries and cream in the bath, eating together or on each other can be both erotic and intimate.

Types of food
The kinds of food eaten can add to the enjoyment. While large amounts of rich or heavy foods may not be a good idea, foods with a variety of different flavours, textures and smells can stimulate the senses. Some foods may be seen as more explicitly sexual, such as asparagus (traditionally eaten with the fingers) or oysters. Many foods are reputed to have aphrodisiac qualities. While none has been conclusively proven to be effective, many people do claim certain foods to be so – experimenting with them can be exciting.

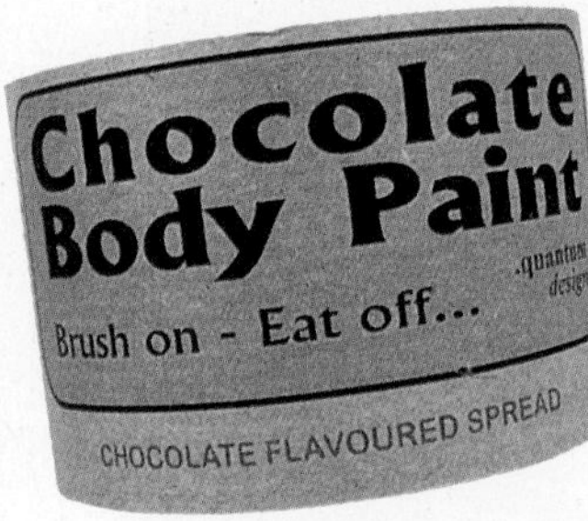

Edible sex aids are now widely available, openly acknowledging the implicit link between sex and food. This chocolate-flavoured body paint is sold in department stores throughout the UK.

Feeding each other
Feeding each other can be almost instinctive in a close, loving relationship. It is a natural gesture of affection and intimacy – mouth-to mouth kissing originates from primates feeding their young from their own mouths. Many people feel a strong urge to nurture their loved ones: to feed one another can be seen as an extension of preparing food together or for each other. With carefully chosen foods, this can be sensuous as well as affectionate.

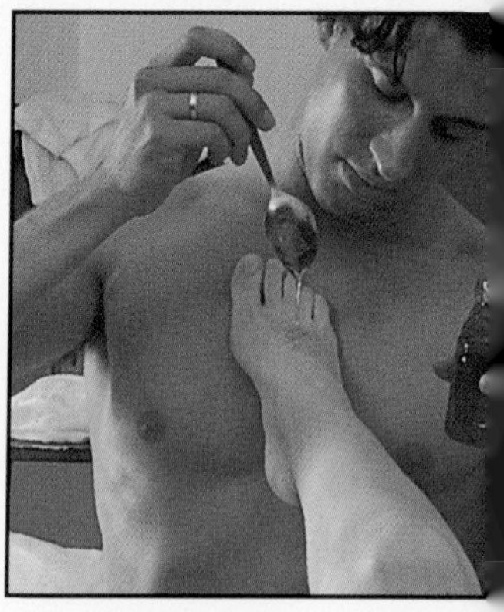

See also:
oral sex
aphrodisiacs
kissing
locations

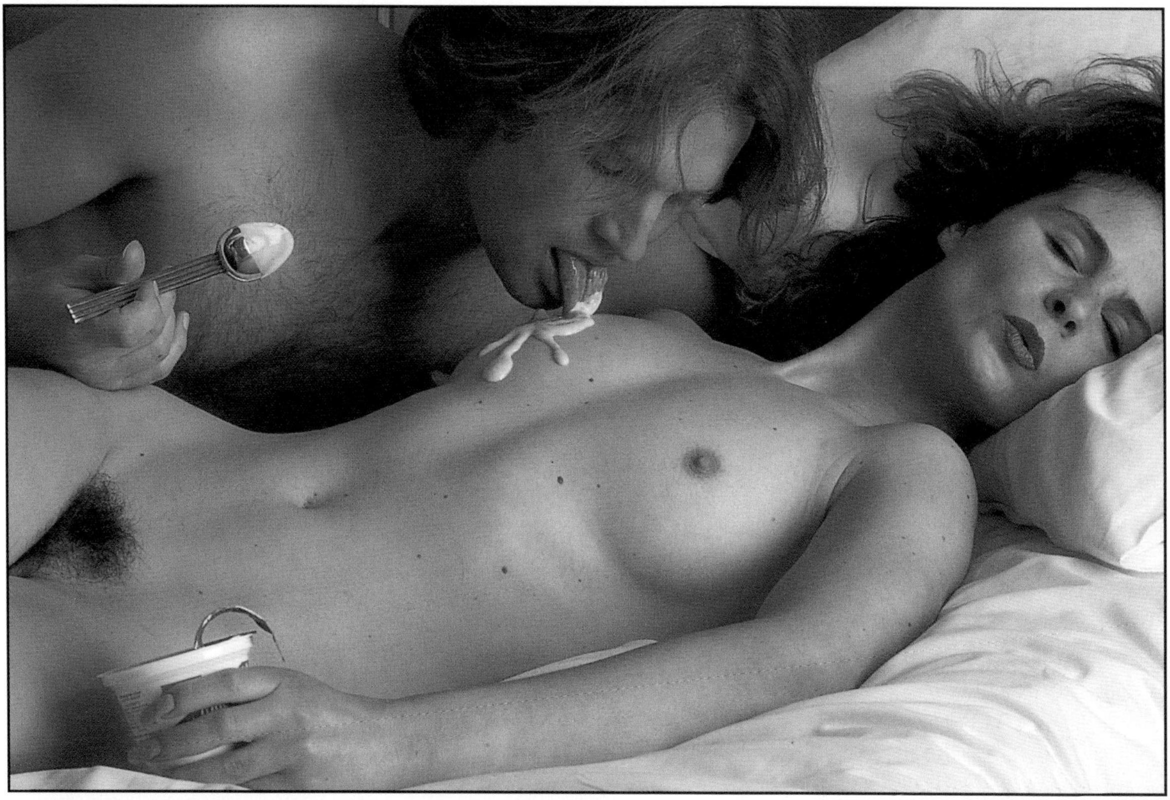

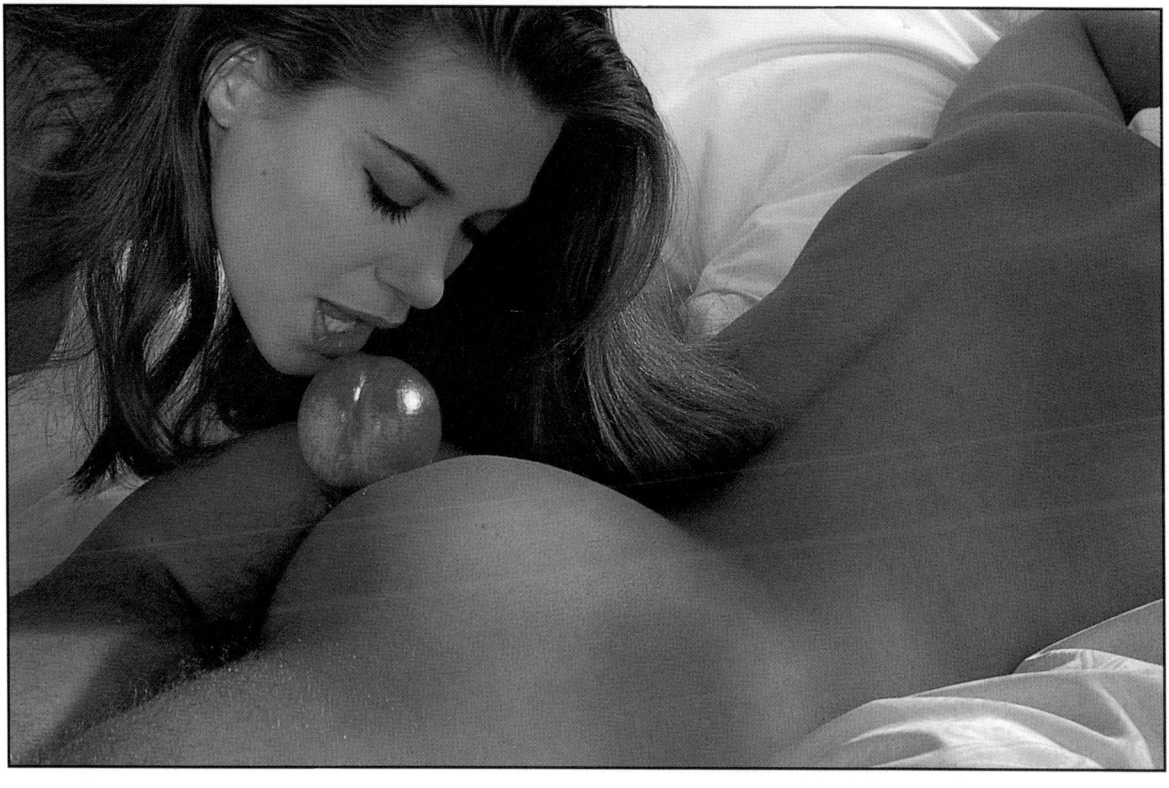

APHRODISIACS

The term aphrodisiac is used to describe anything said to increase sexual desire or performance.

The search for effective aphrodisiacs has been going on for centuries. People have experimented with everything from books and pictures, to all kinds of magic and ritual, but probably most common of all are foods, drinks, plants and chemical substances.

Many of the substances that have been long used as aphrodisiacs have never been scientifically proven to be effective. In spite of this, they remain popular. This may be due to a certain novelty value, or a sense of adventure associated with reputed aphrodisiacs.

The placebo effect -- where the substances seem to work for no other reason than that people believe they will – can also be very powerful. Similarly, taking a supposed aphrodisiac can give people an excuse to lose their inhibitions and express their sexual nature more openly.

The dangers associated with losing inhibitions lie in regretting actions after the event, forgetting to follow safer sex guidelines or becoming involved in bondage or similar practices without taking the necessary precautions. Some sexual practices require considerable care and attention.

FACT: The word aphrodisiac is derived from the name of the goddess of love in ancient Greek mythology, Aphrodite. Aphrodite is said to have been born from the sea, which may be why aphrodisiac qualities are so often attributed to sea food.

APHRODISIAC FOODS

Food has always been associated with sex, not least for the reputed aphrodisiac qualities of some foods. The types of food linked with sex vary, for reasons ranging from those with some scientific basis to those which can only be described as superstitious or anecdotal.

Foods with symbolic value

Certain foods may have been linked to sexuality by visual association, on account of their similarity to the sexual organs of either gender. Asparagus and the roots of ginseng and mandrake can be seen as phallic while oysters, mussels and bearded clams have been likened to the female genitalia, for example. These associations may even have influenced the shapes in which some chocolate bars are designed.

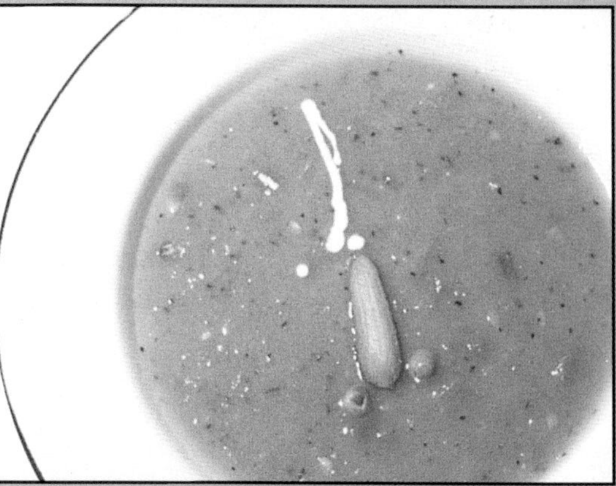

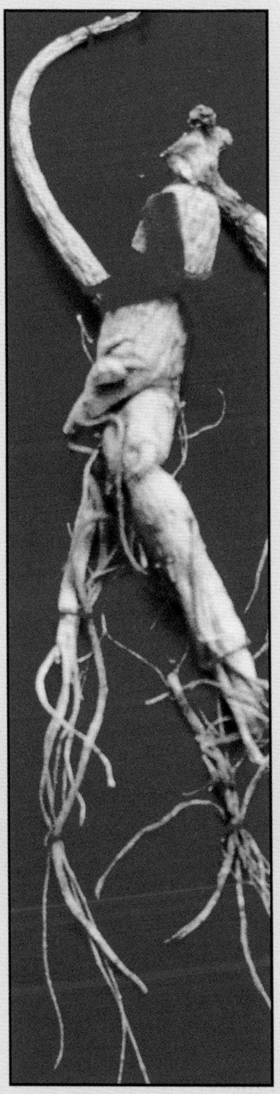

Edible plants

Chillies, onions, fennel, garlic and other spicy and strongly flavoured foods are often connected to sexual passion and with machismo.

A number of plants generally used as tonics are also perceived as sexual stimulants. Several of these have been shown to contain hormones or chemical stimulants, including hops, pollen and honey, cocoa, liquorice water, and parts of plants such as sarsaparilla in South America and hydrocotyle asiatica in the east. Ginseng in particular can stimulate the flow of hormones and many people report aphrodisiac effects soon after having taken a dose. Guarana is made from the ground seeds of a plant from the Amazon basin and is sold as a stimulant in the form of powders, tablets, chewing gum and fizzy drinks. 'Love bombs' contain herbs and spices from Brazil, combined with ginseng and royal jelly (from queen bees). Chocolate, one of the traditional gifts from lovers or people courting, is thought to contain stimulants similar to those produced in the brain by people who describe themselves as being 'in love'. Liquorice, fennel and ginger have all been used in commercial preparations sold as aphrodisiacs.

Plants rich in certain vitamins, including B6, C, D and E, are also eaten as sexual stimulants and to maintain potency and fertility.

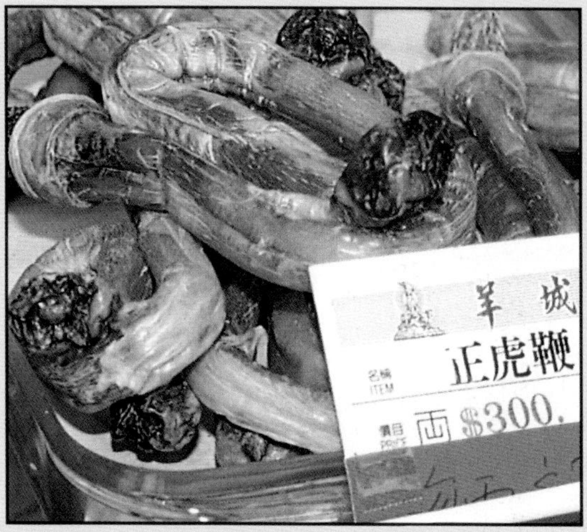

Animal products

The life-sustaining properties of blood have long been recognised and linked to sexual potency. Various sexual practices involving blood may have contributed to this connection, as well as the sexual connotations of blood-thirsty myths related to vampires.

The sexual organs of animals have also been eaten as aphrodisiacs, in particular those of the males of various large species. Bull's testes or 'prairie oysters' and sheep's testes known as 'mountain oysters' are considered delicacies and are often believed to have aphrodisiac properties. While they do contain male hormones, these would probably be destroyed by cooking or by digestive fluids. Extracts from the testes and penises of other animals have also been used. Tiger and deer penises may be bought dried for use as aphrodisiacs in many parts of China. As a general rule, the more rare and difficult to catch the species is, the more highly its aphrodisiac properties tend to be asserted.

The use of powdered horns and tusks of various animals are probably considered to be male aphrodisiacs on account of their phallic appearance.

Seafoods of all kinds have also been associated with sexuality, perhaps because of their sensuous textures and their links to sexual aromas. The fact that oysters are generally eaten alive may have led to their being attributed with life-giving properties. This may also be true of the custom of eating fish eggs – literally a source of life – as caviar. Again, the relative rarity of both adds to the excitement.

SEX & DRUGS

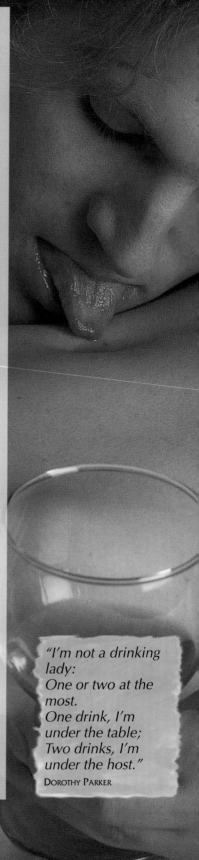

Substances which produce altered states of mind have been part of sexual experimentation throughout the ages. Many reputed aphrodisiacs are drugs occurring naturally or prepared synthetically. However, these drugs can be extremely dangerous to health. In some countries, many are illegal and others may only be available on medical prescription. There is rarely any control over the purity and strength of such drugs if they are obtained illegally, also increasing the risks of side effects, addiction and overdose. However aware of the consequent risks people may be, they continue to use them in the hope of altering or enhancing sexual experience.

Alcohol

In the past, some of the traditional 'love potions' were in fact alcoholic drinks. Many of these are now made commercially as Advocaat, Chartreuse, Drambuie, Sloe Gin, Vermouth and other brands. Today, the West favours wine and champagne, while in China men may drink ginseng brandy, for example.

Alcohol can help to ease shyness and lessen inhibitions. It can also heighten sensations of warmth and affection, making people more open to advances. There is, however, a negative side. Alcohol can act as a depressant; large quantities can make people tiresome, aggressive or violent and reduce physical and mental dexterity. Alcohol can also affect a man's ability to have an erection. It can be addictive and expensive. Prolonged and heavy use affects the central nervous system and testosterone production, and can cause impotence in later life.

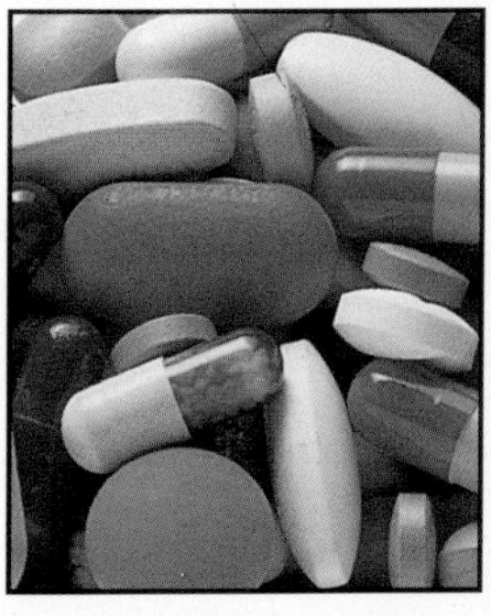

"I'm not a drinking lady:
One or two at the most.
One drink, I'm under the table;
Two drinks, I'm under the host."
DOROTHY PARKER

NATURALLY OCCURRING DRUGS

Cannabis (marijuana)
The plants from which cannabis – and opium – are extracted have probably been cultivated for longer than any other. Cannabis can be taken from either the Cannabis sativa or Cannabis indica plants. Like alcohol, cannabis may be used to overcome inhibitions and for relaxation. It can also increase awareness and sensitivity of the skin and organs. In women, it can increase the likelihood of orgasm. It can make sex more lethargic and leisurely, or make it seem to last longer through its effects on the perception of time. The effects vary greatly from one strain of the drug to another.

Cocaine
Originally used as a local anaesthetic, cocaine is derived from the leaves of the coca plant Erythroxylon coca. It has been a popular recreational drug for centuries, although it peaked in popularity during the 1920s and again after the 1960s. It also has a reputation as an aphrodisiac: the feelings of exhilaration which it creates may increase people's sense of desirability. For some people it reduces inhibitions and increases libido, and may produce enhanced feelings of empathy and eroticism. Whilst promoting these feelings, it can either boost a man's ability to have an erection or severely reduce it and has similarly varied effects on women's sexual capacity. Crack is a refined form of cocaine whose effects are more intense but do not last as long; it is also dangerously addictive.

Spanish fly and yohimbine
Yohimbine is derived from the bark of the tree Corynanthe yohimbe. Spanish fly is available as a powder made from dried, ground cantharis, mylabris or lytta beetles. They function by causing dilation of the blood vessels which can result in prolonged erections as well as irritation of the skin and mucous membranes (when taken orally, this effect is focused on the bladder, the urethra and the genital area). Both have been described as aphrodisiacs, but their effects can be painful as well as dangerous. The amount which is sufficient to create sexual arousal can also be fatal.

GHB
GHB (gamma-hydroxy-butyrate) can be found in over-ripe guava fruit but also occurs naturally in humans as a neurotransmitter. It has been linked with the production of androgenic hormones, which can boost the development of body muscle and enhance the sex drive. It is available in many sex shops.

Mescaline
Mescaline is derived from the peyote cactus, Lophophora williamsii and the San Pedro cactus Trichocereus pachanoi. It is a psychedelic drug with similar effects to LSD and psilocybe mushrooms. American indians have used it for centuries in rituals and to add a new level to sexual experience. Mescaline is rarely available in its pure form.

Opium
Opium is derived from the Opium poppy, Papaver somniferum. Its active ingredient is morphine, from which heroin (diamorphine) is refined. Opium is probably best known for its use in Chinese opium dens which provided opium and prostitutes; they were known as 'Fume and Flower dens' where the fumes were the opium smoke and the flowers were the prostitutes' vaginas. Opium, and heroin in particular, can be extremely dangerous and highly addictive. Accidental overdoses are not uncommon.

'Magic' (psilocybe) mushrooms
Mushrooms of the genus Psilocybe grow wild in some countries but can sometimes be cultivated. They are similar in appearance to some poisonous mushrooms but contain the hallucinogenic chemical psilocybin. Their effects are similar to those of mescaline and LSD but less intense.

SYNTHETIC DRUGS

Amyl nitrite
Amyl nitrite, also known as 'poppers' or 'amyl', speeds up the cardiovascular system and may intensify sexual experience when sniffed just before orgasm, although this does involve interrupting sex play at the height of arousal.

Amphetamines
Amphetamines, also known as 'speed', are sometimes taken to boost stamina for sex, although they can make it difficult to achieve and maintain an erection.

Ecstasy
Ecstasy, or 'E', is methylene dioxymethamphetamine (MDMA) a chemical originally used as a diet pill. It was later rediscovered as a recreational drug, potentially enhancing sexual sensation and desire, with feelings of intense happiness and affection. The drug can also be highly dangerous, especially in impure forms. 2CB is a drug in the Ecstasy group of psychedelics, which has been developed to have a stronger aphrodisiac effect.

LSD
LSD, also known as 'acid', is lysergic acid diethylamide, a psychedelic compound which produces hallucinations (either blissful or horrific), enhances sensory perception and intensifies moods. It can make sex seem more pleasurable and experimental and increase feelings of closeness. Acid is physically – but not psychologically – harmless and non-addictive. It may be dangerous for people with certain mental illnesses.

Barbiturates and other anti-depressants
These drugs can lower inhibitions, but they reduce sensory perception. Despite having been commonly available on prescription, barbiturates in particular are now recognised as dangerously addictive. Newer 'designer' drugs, such as Prozac, are increasingly being offered.

Medical research
Drugs are increasingly available on prescription and illegally for recreational use. Scientific research on their effects on sexual activity may be limited, but sex-enhancing or -inhibiting side-effects are often noted in prescribed use.
Trazodone hydrochloride, a drug prescribed for depression, has been known to cause priapism in men and increased libido in women. On the other hand, thiazide diuretics which may be prescribed for hypertension can destroy a man's ability to achieve or maintain an erection. The treatment for cancer, chemotherapy, has been found to destroy sexual drive, although testosterone can counteract this in women.

Natural health and fitness
One of the best and safest ways to boost or maintain sexual potency and libido in the long term is through good basic health. Regular exercise can help to increase sexual desire and enjoyment.

Yoga, Tai Chi Chuan, Chi-Kung, martial arts and dancing are particularly thought to enhance sexuality. A balanced diet and sufficient sleep are also important, while stress and anxiety often have negative effects. Reliance on any drug, including even those which are in common daily use such as caffeine, nicotine and alcohol, may have a detrimental effect on sexual potency.

PORNOGRAPHY

Pornography *originally meant writing about prostitutes: the word is derived from the Greek words* porne, *a prostitute and* graphos, *to write. The term later came to refer to any form of image or text designed to be sexually stimulating. The way this kind of material has developed has led to strong negative connotations with the term pornographic, and to the increasing use of the word erotica when referring to sexually stimulating material which is considered neither obscene nor offensive.*

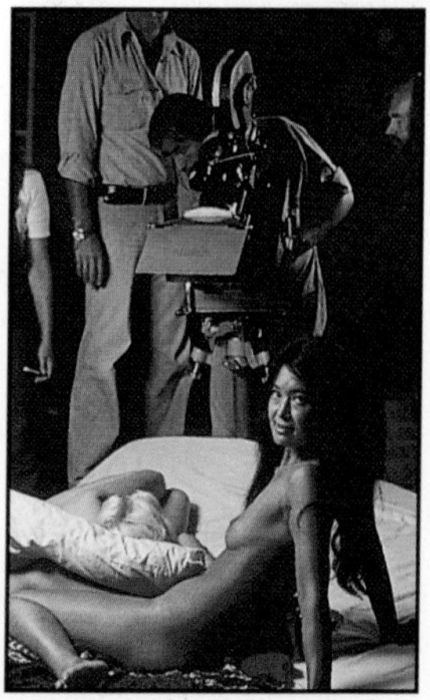

Is this woman being exploited? – or is she making a living and supplying a market?

Use of pornography

Pornography, in the sense of sexually stimulating material, does, however, play a role in many people's sex lives. It can function as a substitute for those people who have a fear of, or difficulty with, forming relationships, for example, or who find the idea of physical intimacy with another person unpleasant. Those who are not in a relationship can find sexual relief with the aid of pornography; it can also add excitement to an established relationship and aid seduction in a new relationship. It can function in a number of ways:

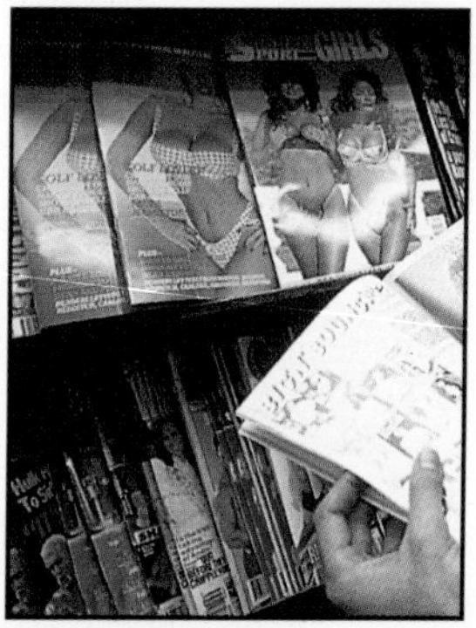

● **Pornography as an aphrodisiac**

Erotic images are widely used as sexual stimuli, either alone or with another person. An enormous range of films, books, audio tapes, paintings and photographs are available, whose intention is to describe sexual interests or simply to arouse. These belong to an ancient tradition. *The Bridal Roll* in Japan, pillow books in China, Vatsyayana's *Kama Sutra* in the Hindu world and many other such books were designed to arouse, inform and provide ideas for love-making. Many are poetic and beautifully illustrated. Far from being considered offensive, they were taken as an important part of the art of loving.

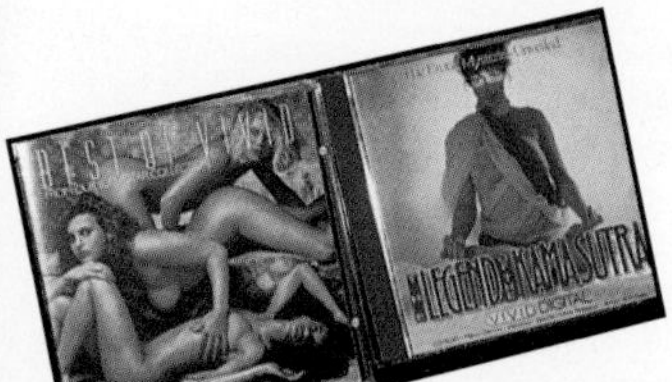

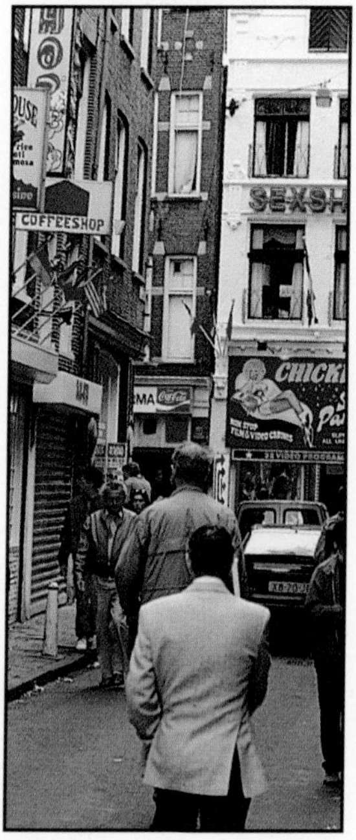

● **Pornography and fantasy**

Pornography and sexual fantasy are implicitly linked, and can fulfil several of the same roles. Both can function as

See also:
sexual feelings
masturbation
cybersex
fantasy
body decoration – make-up

aphrodisiacs and are associated with the unobtainable or unusual. There is a great demand in pornography for that which is not considered acceptable in a given society or within the context of a relationship. Whether it is extra-marital sex, oral sex, painful sex or the sight of pubic hair, fantasy and pornography can provide it. The same patterns are followed in prostitution, where the activities most commonly requested by individuals in a given society are culturally taboo. Similarly, the countries where sexual repression is greatest tend to be those who have the highest consumption of pornography.

● **Pornography for educational and group interest**
A number of sex publications deal with specific sexual tastes, enabling people to discover different forms of sexual activity and to exchange ideas. Some titles are more for interest and information, while others are more for titillation. Some are even used as vehicles for campaigns for greater sexual freedom under the law.

Pornography and society
While it is clear that pornography has a valid place in many people's sex lives, it has been a contentious issue in many societies for centuries. There is widespread legislation against pornography on the basis that it is 'obscene' or 'seditious'. People have long reacted against pornography, believing that it has some capacity to 'deprave or corrupt', as it is written in British law. This fear may be founded on a fear of sexuality as an innate and powerful part of human nature. It may also be caused by the teachings of certain religious faiths. The result of it is a rejection of anything that represents the enjoyment of sex for its own sake, pornography being a prime example: in American law erotic material must have 'serious literary, artistic, political or scientific value' in order to be considered acceptable.

The problem is reaching a definition of what should be considered obscene, and therefore unacceptable. While explicit sexual scenes involving children are almost universally condemned, many others will be the subject of argument: while for one person seeing a woman's breasts will be obscene, for another an image of group sex will be perfectly acceptable. Notions of obscenity are as varied as notions of attractiveness: neither can be generalised.

The main criticisms of modern pornography are that many see it as sexist, exploitative and degrading, although women who work in the sex industry tend to deny this. In many cases this is true. Certainly the film and magazine markets continue to be dominated by men and oriented to a primarily male market. It was long thought that women did not respond to pornography, but studies have since shown that some women respond as strongly as some men, but to different kinds of stimulus. The demand for pornography for women is growing fast. Many men and women equally have no interest at all in pornography.

The strongest criticisms are provoked when unwilling subjects are involved, such as children or animals. The advocates of this kind of material are few and very little of this kind of material is produced. There is also a widespread belief that pornography can incite sexual crimes.

There is, however, no substantial evidence to support this. If anything, repressing pornography can have a negative effect. Studies carried out in Germany, Denmark and Sweden show that after the legalisation of pornography, incidence of sexual assault either increased less than non-sexual assault or did not increase at all.

With the advent of the Internet, pornography is becoming more widespread. This makes it more commonplace and hard to control. It is possible that the taboos about using pornography as an aphrodisiac make it more widely acceptable and popular. Alternatively it has been suggested that the greater sexual liberation which it promotes will reduce the need for it. Either way, sexually explicit writing and images are an important part of human sexuality and will remain a part of popular culture for the foreseeable future.

SEX AIDS & TOYS

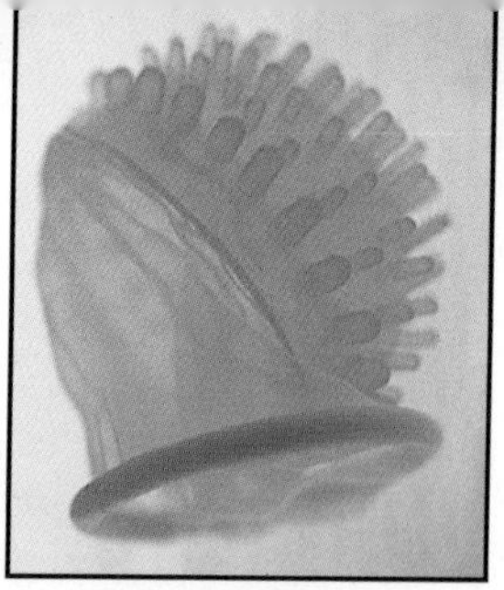

In many countries sex aids are achieving a major change of image. No longer only to be found in sex shops, and now sold to increasing numbers of women as well as men, they are being used more and more widely to increase pleasure, add excitement and combat sexual problems.

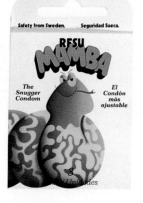

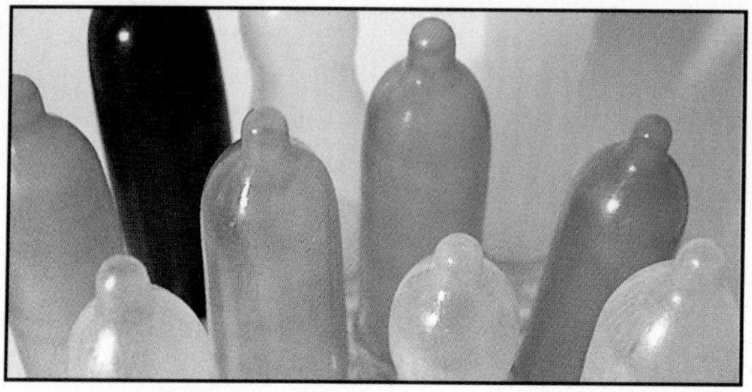

Condoms

While condoms are most commonly used as contraceptives and as part of safer sex practices, they can also be used as sex aids.

One of the most common fears about condoms is of reduced sensitivity. The outer ring of the female condom may also provide some clitoral stimulation. Male condoms are available in a wide range of colours and flavours: flavoured ones are sometimes used by people who find the idea of oral sex disagreeable, although the taste is rarely very pleasant.

Few condoms are produced for pleasure. There are, however, condoms made with padding, ribbing or extensions, to make the penis seem larger or to create stronger or different sensations in the vagina. Padded condoms can help to boost a man's confidence if he is concerned about penis size, but in reality the difference will barely be felt - or may not be felt at all - by his partner. 'Ticklers' – textured condoms or ones with shapes at the tip – can provide some extra stimulation to the nerve endings at the mouth of the vagina, the vulva and perhaps the cervix, although this is unlikely. More ornate and attractively packaged condoms are produced in Japan.

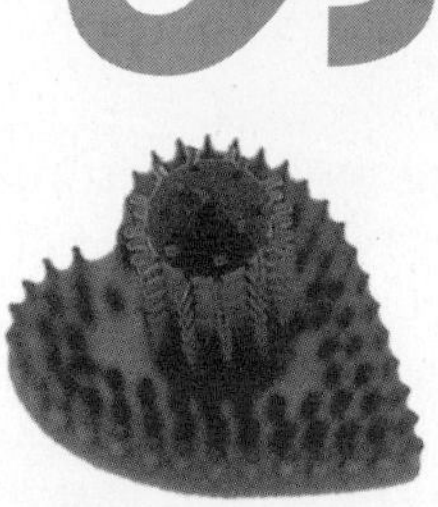

See also:
masturbation
aphrodisiacs
contraception
health and hygiene

Precautions

- Sex aids should not be shared without thorough cleaning. Sexually transmitted infections and diseases can be transmitted on sex aids just as they can be passed through genital contact. Condoms can be used on vibrators and dildos.
- Any kind of sex aid which i used in or around the anus should be thoroughly cleaned before coming into contact with the mouth, urethra or vagina. Bacteria which exist normally and healthily in the rectum can cause infections in other parts of the body.
- Dildos and other objects used in the same way must be used with caution as objects can be drawn into the vagina or anus and become lodged inside, requiring medical attention for removal.
- Most padded, textured and 'tickler' condoms are not safe to use as contraceptives or for safer sex. Only condoms specifically labelled as contraceptives should be considered reliable. Many manufacturers of condoms now make ribbed as well as flavoured varieties.
- Any oil-based lubricant can damage the latex rubber of a condom or diaphragm.

Vibrators

Vibrators are probably the most common sex aid. Whether powered by batteries or mains electricity, they vibrate rhythmically to give sensual pleasure. There are several basic forms.

Most vibrators are like battery-powered dildos. Mains-powered vibrators are also available. Again they come in various shapes, sizes and textures. Some are smooth with a hard plastic or metallic finish while others are covered with latex and are made to look like a penis. Those which are covered in latex are less cold to the touch and tend to be less noisy.

Other shapes include those which are not unlike electric toothbrushes, and the 'butterfly' which is an oblong pad which fits against the vulva. Massage devices, which can also be used as vibrators, can be bought in some pharmacies.

Vibrators can be used by women or men, together or alone, on any part of the body. They can produce exciting sensations when pressed to earlobes, nipples, the lower back, the thighs and above all to the genital area. They are most commonly used by women around the inner and outer labia and on the clitoral hood and clitoris. Some women place a piece of soft fabric between the vibrator and their skin to improve sensation. For a man a vibrator may be pressed against the shaft of the penis, or the tip of the vibrator may be used on the glans of the penis or around the scrotum and anus. They should not be used in the bath or shower unless they are clearly labelled as waterproof.

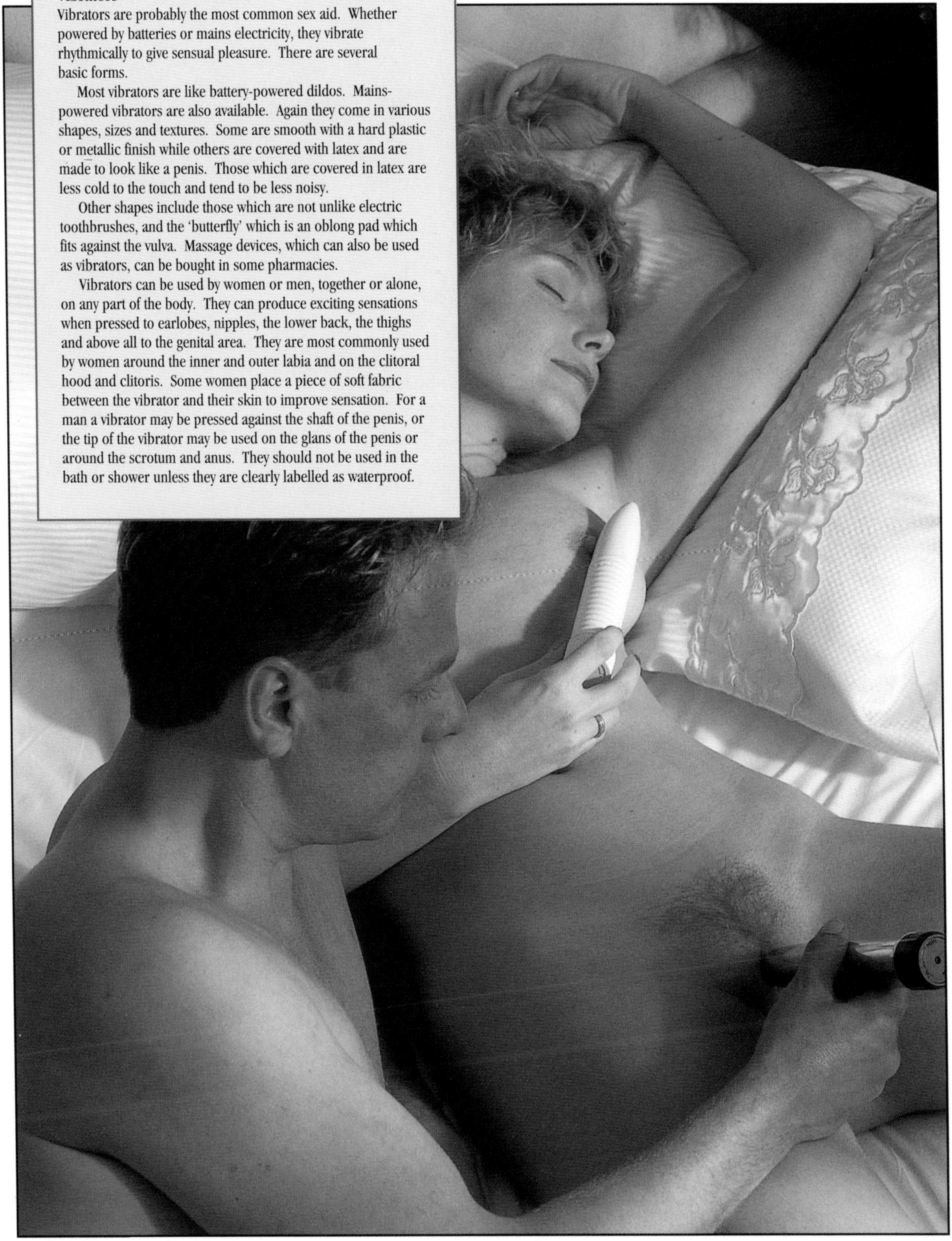

Dildos
Dildos are objects that can be used as penis substitutes. They are probably the oldest form of sex aid, featuring in ancient Greek and Babylonian art and in the Bible.

They are usually realistic in design, and are made in many shapes, sizes, materials and colours. Some are curved to stimulate the G-spot. Some have a bulb on the end, sometimes in the form of testicles, which can be filled with liquid and squeezed to imitate ejaculation. Most are slightly exaggerated in size but much larger ones are also available. Double-headed dildos are also made.

If desired, dildos can provide a means of having penetrative sex for lesbians and for some disabled people. They can add fun to love-making and prolong it, and may be used as a form of safer sex.

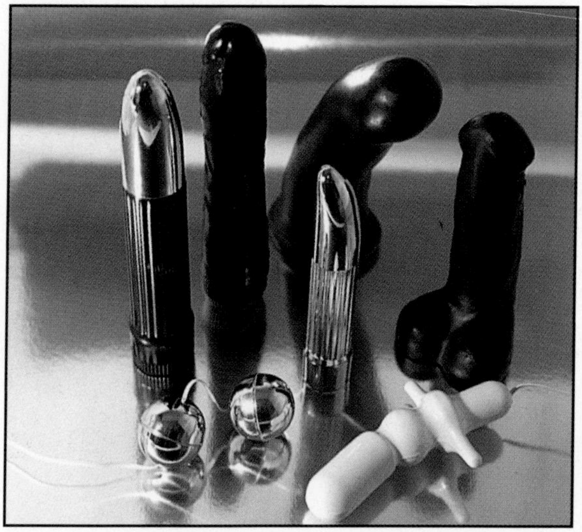

Butt-plugs and anal vibrators
Latex attachments for anal stimulation are available for ordinary vibrators, but there are also dildos and vibrators designed specifically for this purpose. They are not usually made to look like a penis and often have a longer or bigger hand grip than vaginal vibrators to prevent them from becoming lodged or drawn up inside the rectum. They should not be used too roughly or without lubrication as the anus and the walls of the rectum are very delicate.

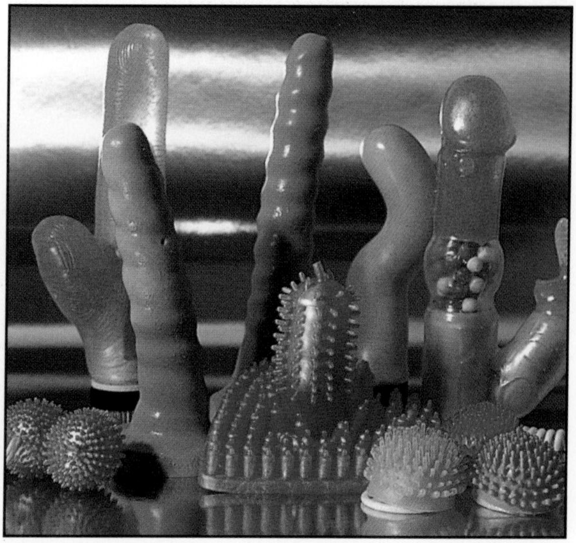

Love balls
Love balls, also known as love eggs or *Ben-wa-balls*, consist of two hollow balls connected by a cord. They contain smaller balls or weights which can move around inside them. They are put into the vagina, the weights inside cause them to move around as the woman moves. They can be used during love-making or for keeping the woman in a state of arousal at other times.

Some women find them highly arousing while for others they may have no effect at all other than causing mild discomfort. They can make a slight noise. They can be good for exercising the pelvic floor muscles. They should not be used in the rectum.

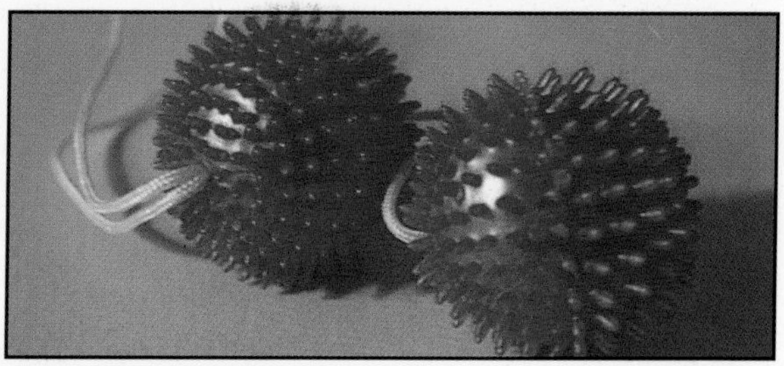

Thai beads
Thai beads consist of a number of plastic beads either on a string or a flexible rod. They are inserted into the rectum and moved in and out during intercourse or pulled out quickly or slowly at orgasm.

Penis vibrators
There are two types of vibrator made specifically for use on the penis. One is in the form of a ring which fits around the base of the penis with an attachment which vibrates against the shaft. Others are substitute vaginas, made as latex or rubber tubes with or without a vibrating mechanism. Some can be 'pumped up' to grip the penis more firmly. They may be plain or decorated. Sometimes they are fitted into a model of a woman's head to simulate oral sex; sometimes they are part of an entire plastic torso.

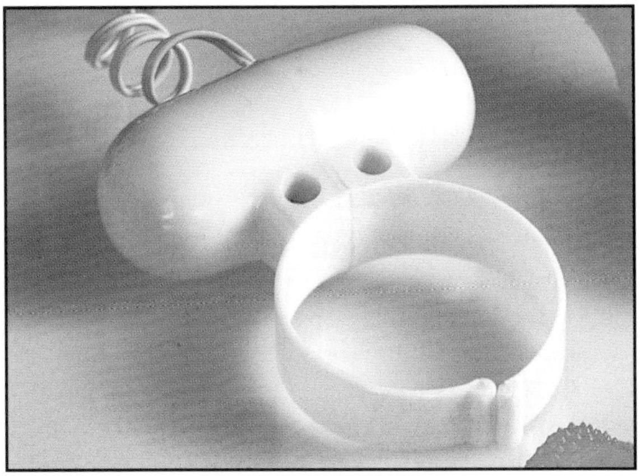

'Stay longer' creams and sprays
These products contain a small amount of local anaesthetic, the idea is to reduce penile sensitivity and delay orgasm and ejaculation. In some men they are successful, but with the inevitable loss of some sensation. Ejaculatory control can be developed more effectively by increasing awareness of sensations in the penis.

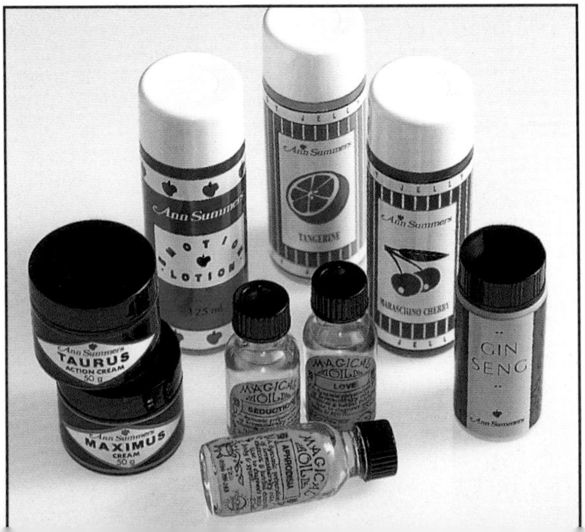

Breast developers
Like the majority of penis developers, these are usually used more as a toy than as a serious sex aid. They function by stimulating the breasts by massage, water jets or with the use of a vacuum. While the sensations created can be arousing, there will be no permanent change to breast size.

Arab straps, cock and ball straps, cock rings, gates of hell
These are all devices used to help maintain a man's erection. They are made up of rings of metal, leather or rubber, which may be held together with leather straps or rubber bands. Tightly fastened to the penis in the course of arousal they constrict the blood flow out of the penile tissue, maintaining the erection. They can be stimulating both for the wearer and their partner, providing extra friction against the sides of the vagina or rectum. Some people also find their appearance arousing. Some men just use an elastic band.

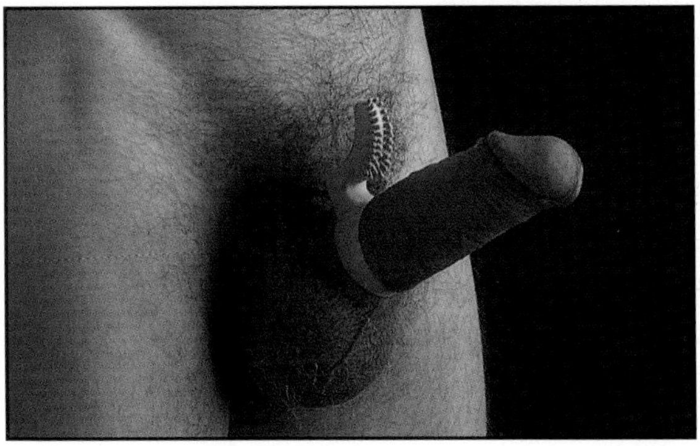

Clitoral stimulators
These are rings made of latex, rubber or plastic which fit around the base of the penis, with some form of projection which is designed to stimulate the clitoris during vaginal intercourse. There are many different designs.

Controlling the amount of pressure on the clitoris can be difficult, as can keeping the projection from twisting around to face the wrong direction. However, many people enjoy using them and they can also help maintain the man's erection by functioning like a cock ring.

BODY DECORATION

Humans have always adorned their bodies, for purposes ranging from tribal identification to ritual celebration. Body decoration has many links with the expression of sexuality, where it can function as a specific sexual signal, a means of boosting attractiveness or a way of enhancing sexual pleasure.

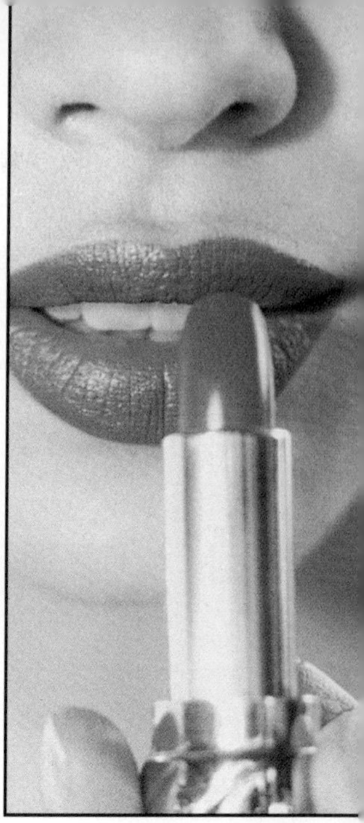

Women's magazines are full of advice on the most common form of body decoration – make-up.

Make-up

Make-up has been used for centuries by members of both sexes but particularly by women. It is mainly used on the face, to draw attention to particular features or to present the face in a more attractive or alluring way, as well as to conceal whatever might be considered a defect. It can be used on the body in the same way.

There are many psychological interpretations of why people use make-up. It is sometimes thought that, however subconsciously, we may be imitating the open, unthreatening and even needy appearance of a baby's face: we do this by drawing attention to the eyes and mouth and making other 'adult' features, such as the nose, less prominent. However, it is more widely believed that make-up was originally used to simulate the effects of sexual arousal, making the eyes look larger and darker, the lips redder, and the skin more flushed.

Body make-up can create the same effect. In India henna has been used for centuries to redden nostrils, earlobes, fingertips and toes, all of which darken due to the increased blood flow during arousal. Rouge has been used on the nipples in some cultures. Nowadays red nail varnish for finger and toe nails is quite common, and rouge or blusher can be used lightly over the breasts, shoulders or any other part of the body.

FACT: Among the Ila Bantu people of Zambia a bride is expected to pluck out all the facial and pubic hair of her new husband the morning after the consummation of their marriage.

FACT: In ancient Rome prostitutes painted their lips bright red as an explicit signal that they would perform oral sex.

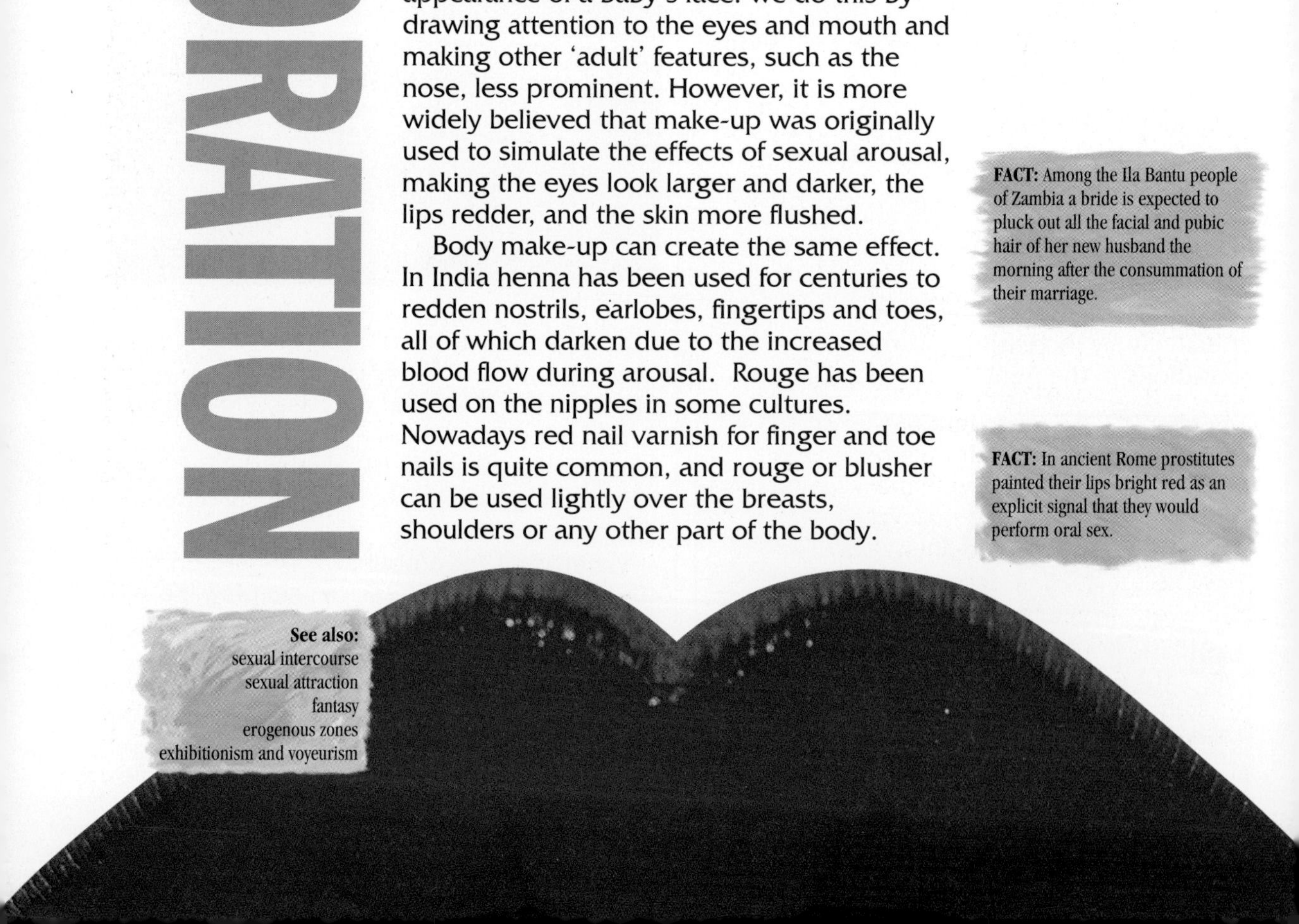

See also:
sexual intercourse
sexual attraction
fantasy
erogenous zones
exhibitionism and voyeurism

Body painting

Used for tribal identification and ritualistic purposes, body painting probably began in prehistoric times. It survives as a cultural practice primarily among tribal peoples in Africa, America and Australia. In other cultures it is enjoyed by many for sexual stimulation.

As well as conventional make-up, theatrical make-up and special non-toxic body paints are available. The paint can be used to decorate the body and to emphasize its contours. Particular attention is usually paid to the most sensitive or expressive areas, such as the hands, feet, face, ears, nipples and genitals. Actually applying the paint, whether with a brush or with fingertips or hands, can be a sensuous experience for both partners. Only non-toxic substances should be applied to the skin, and care should be taken to allow the skin to breathe by not covering the entire body.

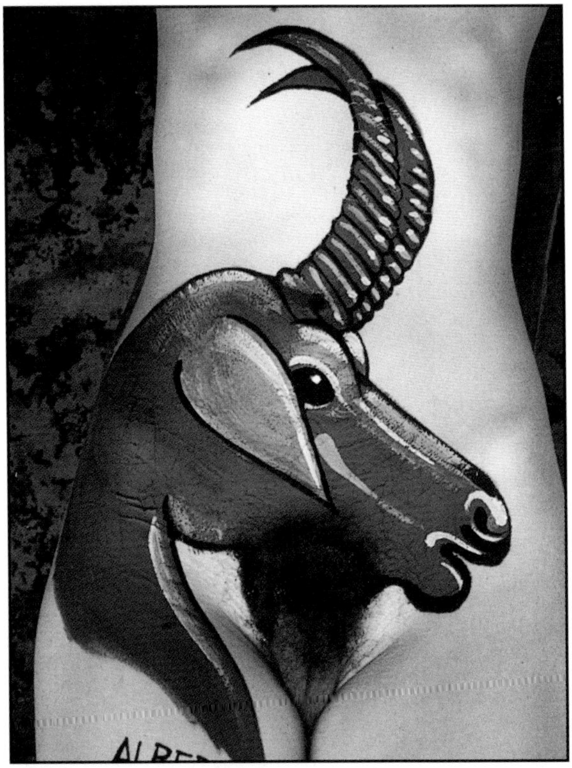

Body hair dressing

Attitudes to body hair vary enormously from one cultural group to another. In some groups from southern Africa, India and Pakistan, both men and women are expected to remove all body hair. In others, the sight of pubic hair is considered so explicitly erotic that it features prominently in pornography, as in Japan. In many Western cultures, male body hair has long been seen as acceptable while women have been expected to remove it: some see hairy men as more masculine and hairless women as more feminine. This is echoed in images of men and women in Western art. More recently, with greater liberation among both women and men, people have begun to ignore society's dictates and follow their own preferences.

The appearance or the feel of skin and body hair can be arousing, as can any change in the way body hair is looked after. It can be bleached, dyed, trimmed, shaped or removed completely to reveal areas of skin which are never normally seen. Many people enjoy the actual process of shaving their own or their partner's body hair. Shaving can enhance the sensitivity of the skin.

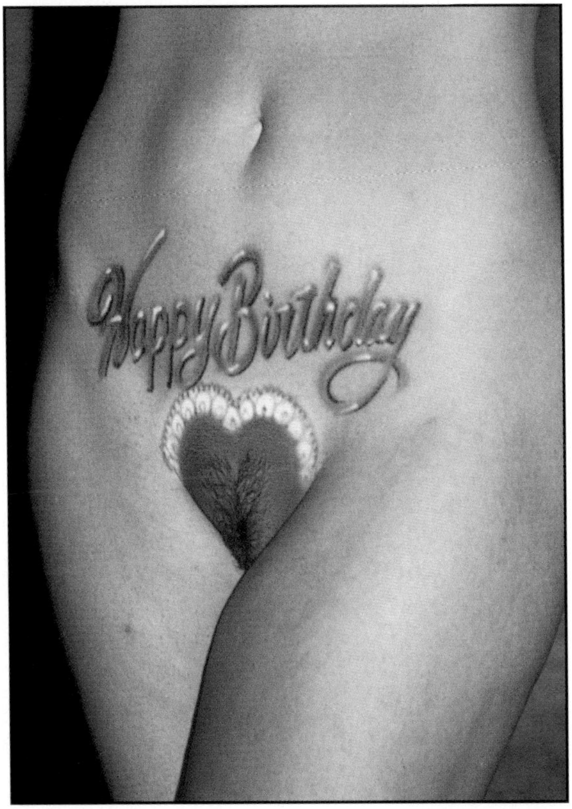

Tattooing and body piercing

Many people choose to decorate their bodies more permanently. While for some the mere idea of marking or piercing the body may be unacceptable, practices such as tattooing and piercing are becoming increasingly popular. The motivation behind these practices may or may not be sexual. They create a more positive body image and a sense of personal empowerment in some people, and many find the appearance or the experience of tattooing or piercing arousing. In recent years these practices have also become increasingly fashionable.

Both tattooing and body piercing can be enjoyed simply as adornment or specifically for sexual pleasure. They can be sexually arousing in various ways. Many people are aroused simply by the fact that they or their partner has a part of their body pierced or tattooed, particularly if this is on an intimate part not seen by anyone else. For others the enjoyment is more symbolic, to do with the choice of the image or words tattooed or if the ring used for piercing is taken as a sign of commitment. Both practices can involve a certain amount of pain and this can also be seen as symbolic, harking back to the origins of such practices as initiation rites and proof of adulthood or social status. Body piercing adds another dimension in that manipulating or gently pulling on the rings or rods used can be highly arousing.

Neither practice need be dangerous if carried out hygienically by a reliable professional, although in some countries both are illegal, particularly if carried out for sexual purposes.

Designs may consist of words, pictures or both and tend to be intensely personal. The areas considered most obvious are the arms, chest and back. However, designs in 'secret' places, where only lovers will find them, are also popular, and tattoos on the genital area are not uncommon. The shaft of the penis is easy and not too painful to tattoo, as is the skin of the thighs and abdomen surrounding the pubic area. The glans of the penis and female labia are more difficult to tattoo, requiring simpler designs. Most tattoo artists will not put designs on the face or palms of clients.

FACT: The oldest verified colour tattoos were found on a 5,300-year-old Stone Age man in Italy and a 4,200-year-old Egyptian priestess.

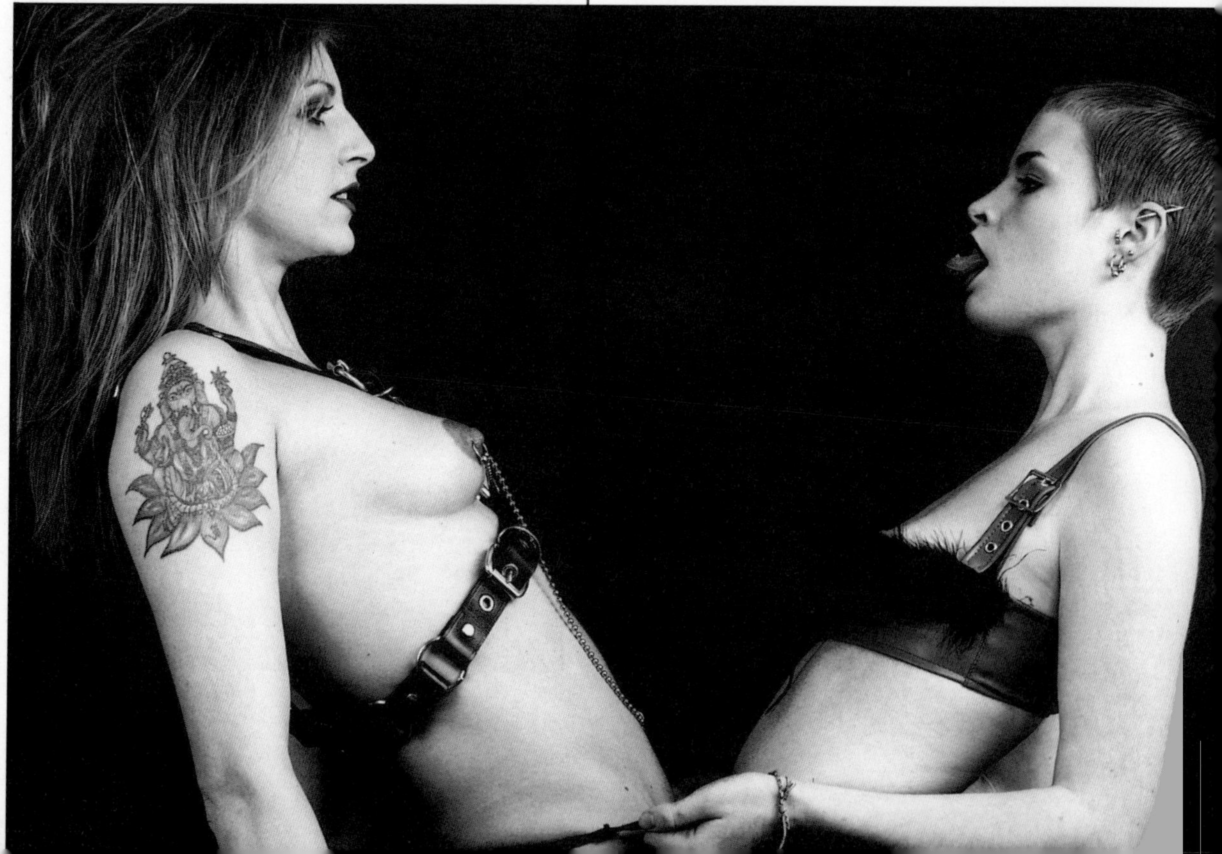

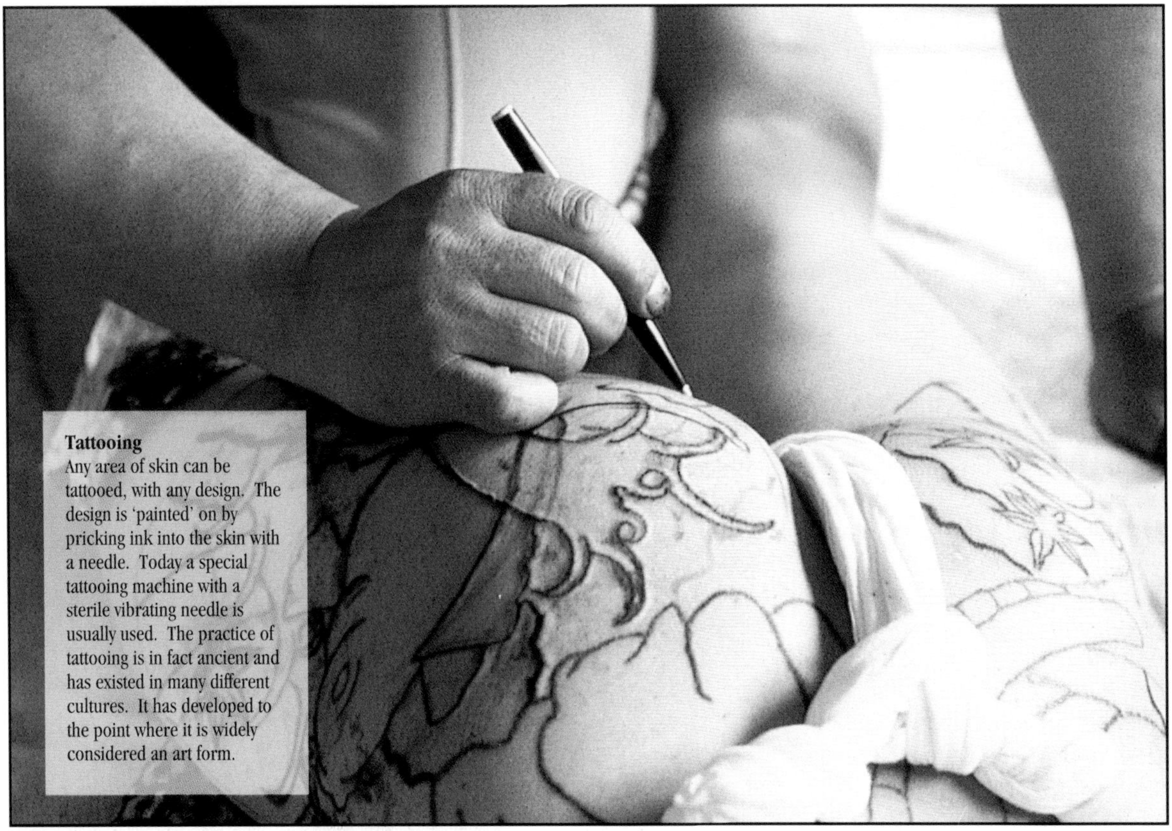

Tattooing
Any area of skin can be tattooed, with any design. The design is 'painted' on by pricking ink into the skin with a needle. Today a special tattooing machine with a sterile vibrating needle is usually used. The practice of tattooing is in fact ancient and has existed in many different cultures. It has developed to the point where it is widely considered an art form.

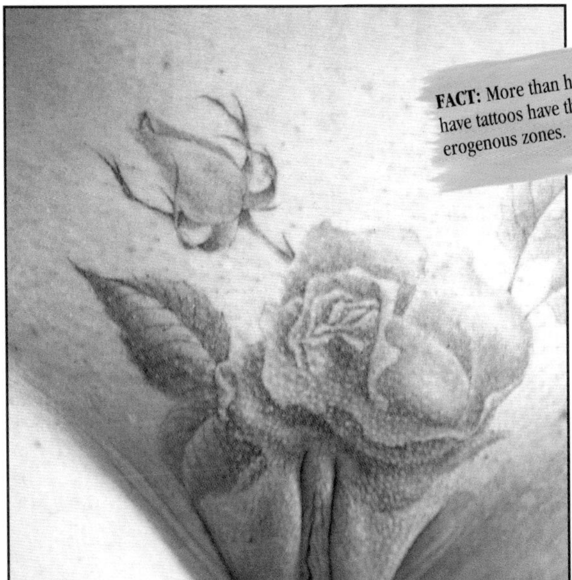

FACT: More than half of those who have tattoos have them on or near erogenous zones.

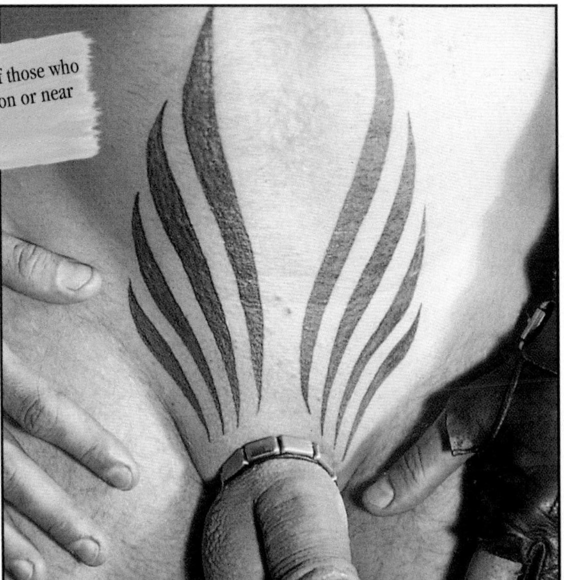

Body piercing

Like tattooing, body piercing is an ancient custom that has become more widely acceptable and even fashionable in some cultures, particularly over the past thirty years.

Ornamental body piercing has been carried out for centuries in cultures originating from Asia, North, South and Central America, Africa and Oceania. In the West only ear piercing is a well-established and widely accepted practice. However, noses, eyebrows, cheeks, lower lips, tongues, nipples, navels and sexual organs can all be pierced. Women can pierce the clitoris or the clitoral hood vertically or horizontally, and the inner and outer labia. Men can pierce various parts of the foreskin, the glans and the base of the penis, as well as the scrotum and the perineum.

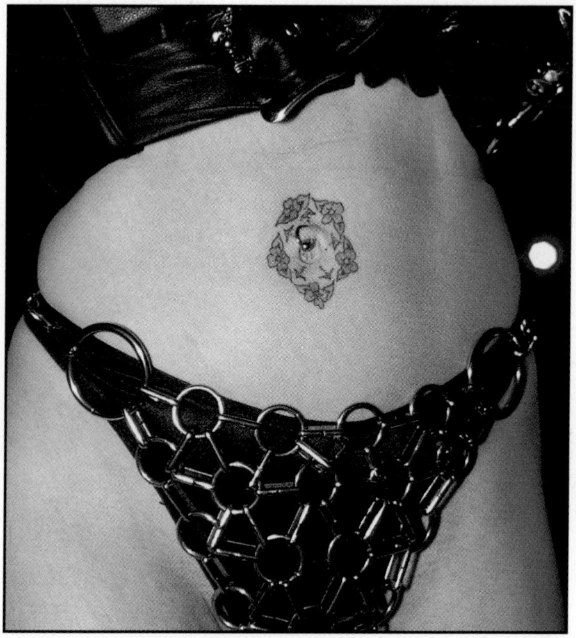

Male genital piercing

A number of specific terms are used for certain types of male genital piercing. The most common kind is the Prince Albert or dress ring, which refers to a ring which passes through the glans, into the urethra just below the frenulum and out through the tip of the penis, curving round underneath. It was originally used by Victorian men to hold the penis flat inside one or other leg of the tight trousers which were fashionable at that time. The ampallang is a rod which passes horizontally through the glans; the apadravya passes through vertically. A dydo pierces the rim at the edge of the glans: several of these are usually used together. The term hafada refers to the piercing of the scrotum, while the guiche is a ring in the perineum.

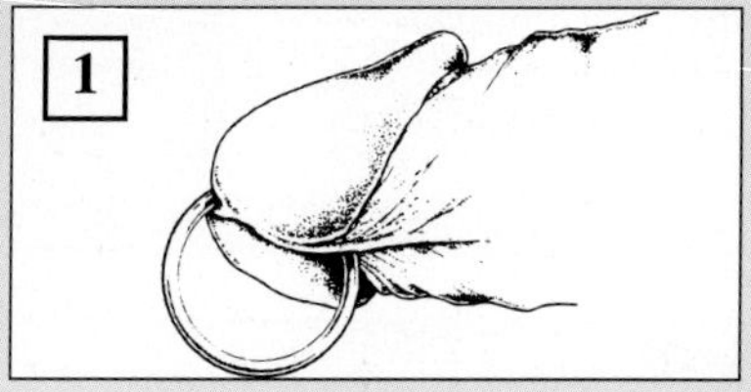

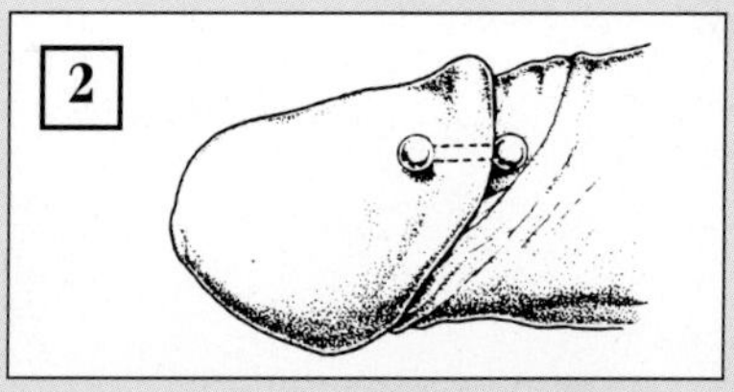

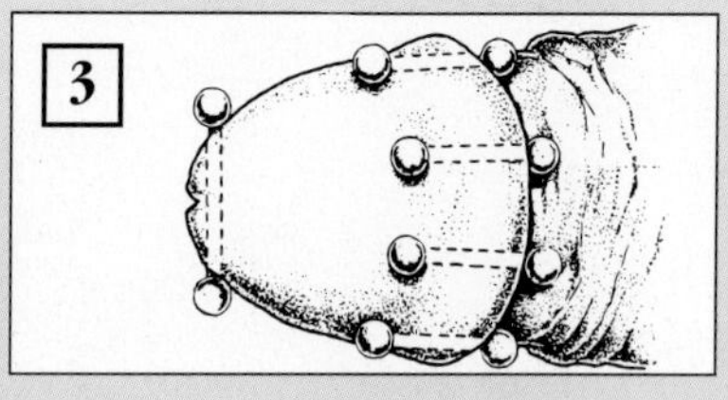

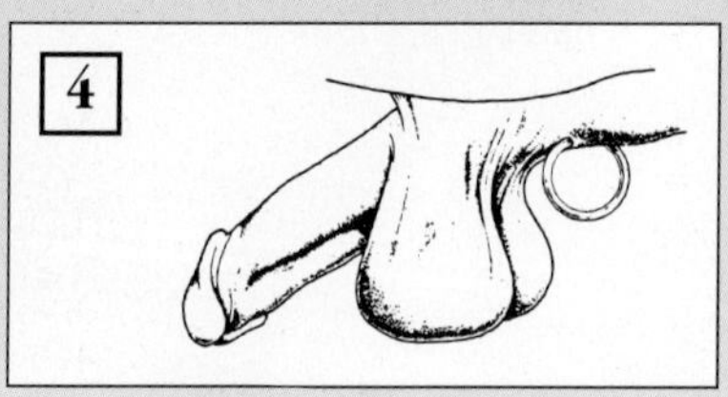

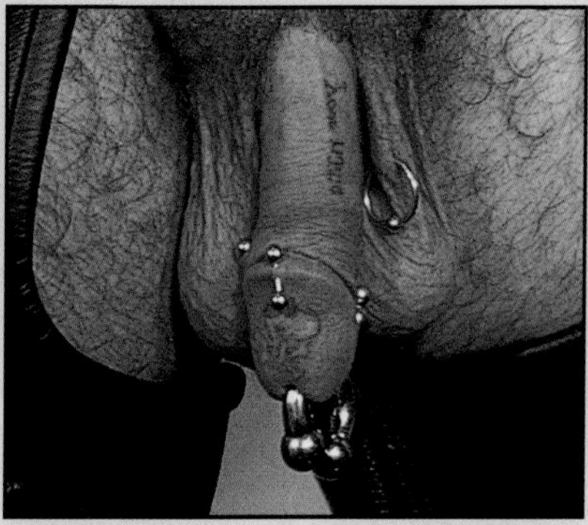

1. Prince Albert

2. Dydo

3. Dydoes with (left) an ampallang

4. Guiche

Genital jewellery – used by some people to embellish their genitals and enhance their sex play. Genital piercing is becoming increasingly common.

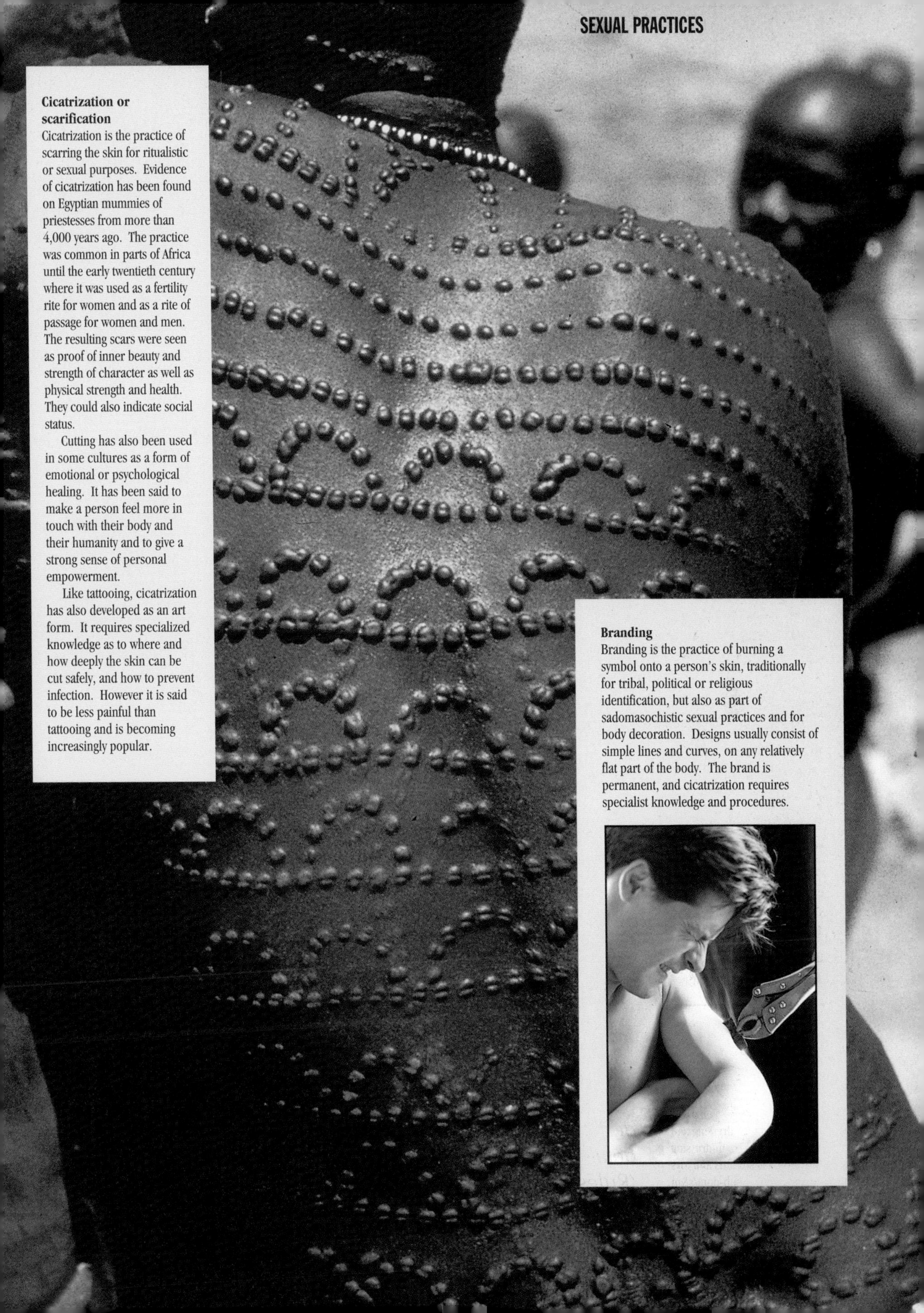

Cicatrization or scarification

Cicatrization is the practice of scarring the skin for ritualistic or sexual purposes. Evidence of cicatrization has been found on Egyptian mummies of priestesses from more than 4,000 years ago. The practice was common in parts of Africa until the early twentieth century where it was used as a fertility rite for women and as a rite of passage for women and men. The resulting scars were seen as proof of inner beauty and strength of character as well as physical strength and health. They could also indicate social status.

Cutting has also been used in some cultures as a form of emotional or psychological healing. It has been said to make a person feel more in touch with their body and their humanity and to give a strong sense of personal empowerment.

Like tattooing, cicatrization has also developed as an art form. It requires specialized knowledge as to where and how deeply the skin can be cut safely, and how to prevent infection. However it is said to be less painful than tattooing and is becoming increasingly popular.

Branding

Branding is the practice of burning a symbol onto a person's skin, traditionally for tribal, political or religious identification, but also as part of sadomasochistic sexual practices and for body decoration. Designs usually consist of simple lines and curves, on any relatively flat part of the body. The brand is permanent, and cicatrization requires specialist knowledge and procedures.

BONDAGE & FETISHISM

The forms of sexual expression are so many and varied as to be beyond count. Sex is the most personal of all human activities and the most intimate form of expression: it is therefore potentially an arena for forms of expression inappropriate in any other situation.

Bondage, dominance, submission and pain are rarely discussed publicly and when they are tend to receive bad press: the notion of 'deviancy' is frequently involved. However, they are forms of sexual expression which are enjoyed by many people.

All of these practices are deeply rooted in the human psyche. Aggression, domination and dependency, along with the sexual urge, are among the most basic human motivations in interpersonal relationships. These forms of motivation are linked with sex in that they, too, tend to be repressed. In many societies they are either seen as inappropriate except in specific situations, or considered appropriate only to one gender or the other.

The experiences of pain and resisting restraint result in a raised pulse rate, increased adrenaline and feelings of euphoria, all of which are also produced by sexual arousal.

This kind of activity can be practised at many different levels, according to the personal thresholds of those involved. Engaging in such activity does not mean forcing an unwilling person to comply with one's desires. However, when there is genuine consent and understanding, they can become a positive expression of desire and affection. For a guide to details and precautions see page 164 for 'Rules of the game'.

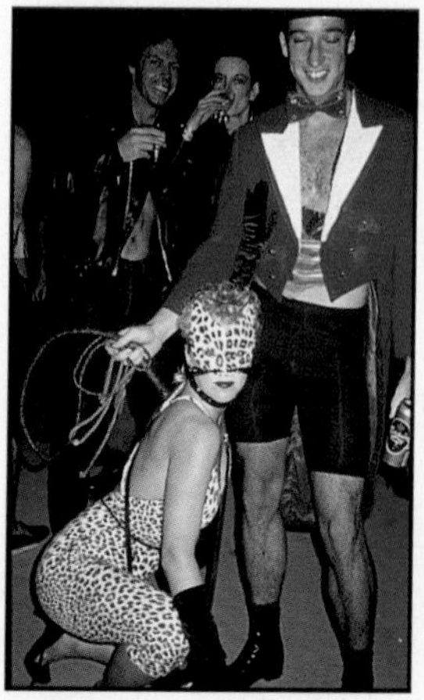

Bondage can include dressing up, costumes, role-playing games and any form of fetishism.

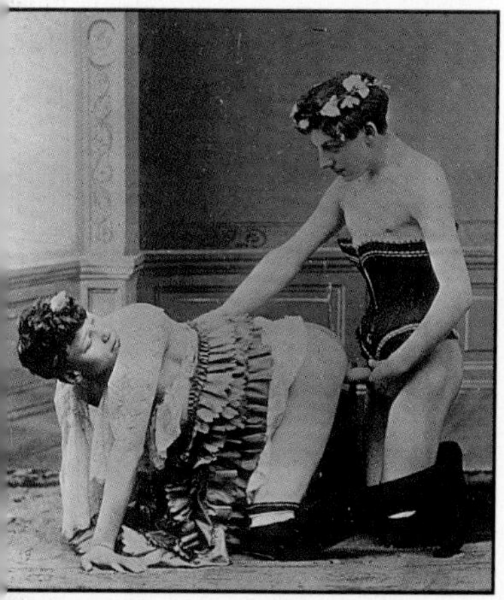

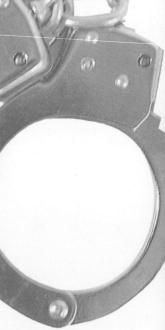

Far left: **Victorian photograph** depicting one form of fetishistic sex. Fetishism is probably the most varied facet of human sexuality – it is entirely personal and can range from the most commonplace to the most bizarre.

See also:
dressing and undressing
sex aids and toys
sub-dom/s&m

Bondage

Bondage means restricting a person's movement for sexual pleasure. Its most common use is to increase excitement for willing partners by defining active and passive roles.

Active and passive roles play a part in all sexual relationships. These can be expressed in the simplest ways, such as who is 'on top', or who is giving or receiving oral sex. The notion of giving and receiving can build a strong sense of security in any sexual relationship. That each partner is capable of giving a selfless demonstration of affection or desire, focusing particularly on his or her partner's pleasure, can reinforce the relationship.

Sex games and lovemaking involving bondage generally involve one partner being tied up by the other, who then devotes him- or herself to arousing, stimulating and teasing the tied partner and ultimately bringing them to orgasm. They can give or withold sexual pleasures as they choose. This can be highly arousing for both partners. The tied partner, unable to move, is relieved of any sense of responsibility, guilt or inhibition, and this may increase arousal.

Bondage can also be used as a part of submissive/dominant practices and games involving pain. Alternatively it can be used for physical support for certain positions and practices.

The most common bondage uses rope or handcuffs but many people simply use fabric or clothing such as scarves, hosiery and ties to tie a partner up or to tie them to a bed or chair. A certain amount of freedom of movement remains, but the restrained partner is sufficiently immobilized to enable the other partner to take a dominant role. Full-scale, purpose-made equipment is also available from specialist suppliers, some of which will make to order. This equipment can range from leather collars and cuffs to full body harnesses, chastity belts and chains. It often includes objects and materials to which the people involved have some kind of fetishistic attachment, such as fur, leather, rubber, shoes, gloves and so on. In some countries fully equipped dungeons are available for hire by those who do not have the necessary equipment.

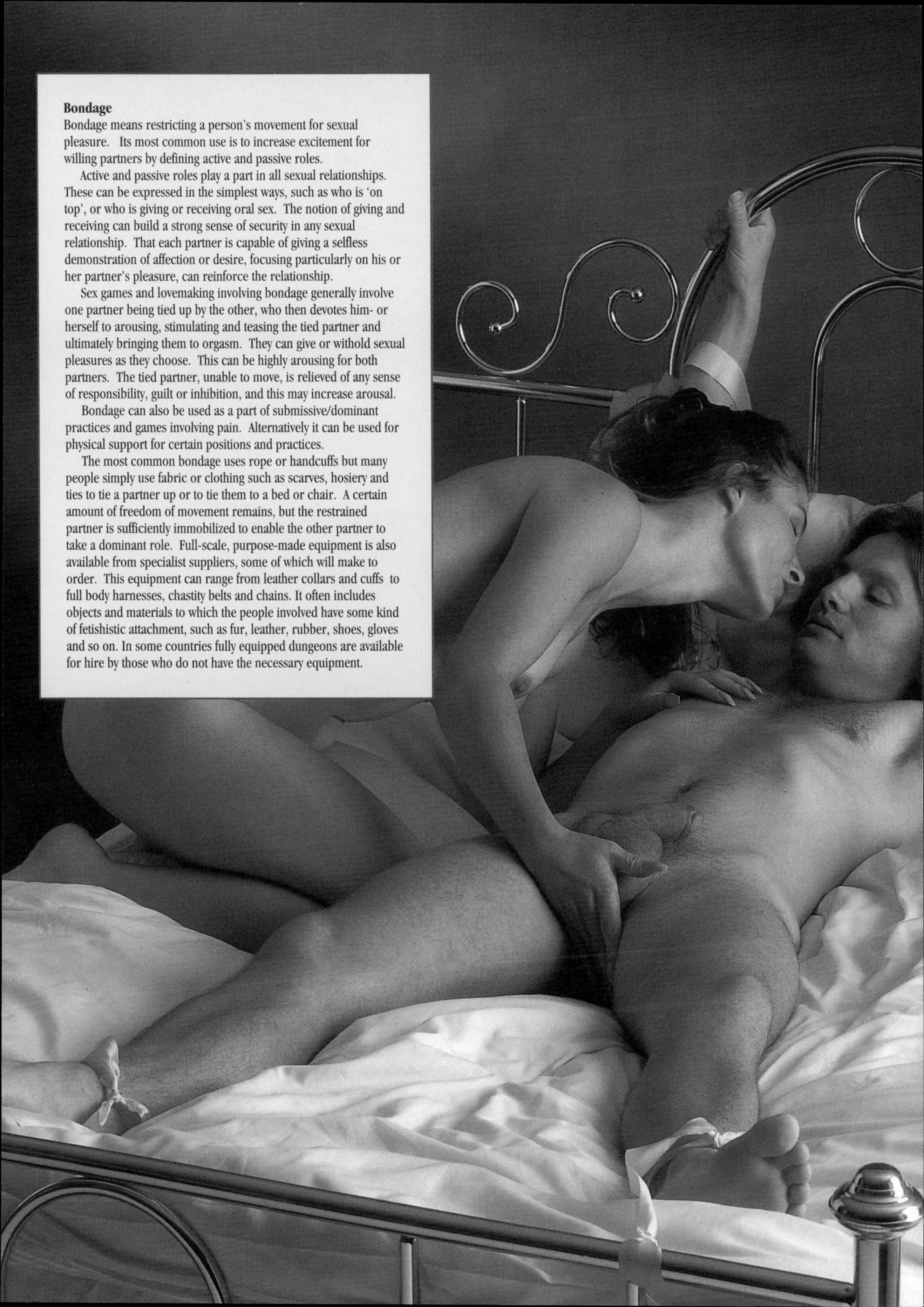

SUB-DOM/S&M

The need to dominate and to submit, to control and to be controlled, is present in most people: sometimes the non-fulfilment of either need in one area of a person's life can be compensated in another area, such as in their sex life. The popularity of submissive sexual practices recently exposed among high-ranking politicians and businessmen in some countries has been attributed to this concept, since they provide a complete removal of responsibility for decision-makings. Likewise those who are frustrated in their daily lives may find that dominant sexual practices boost their self-esteem.

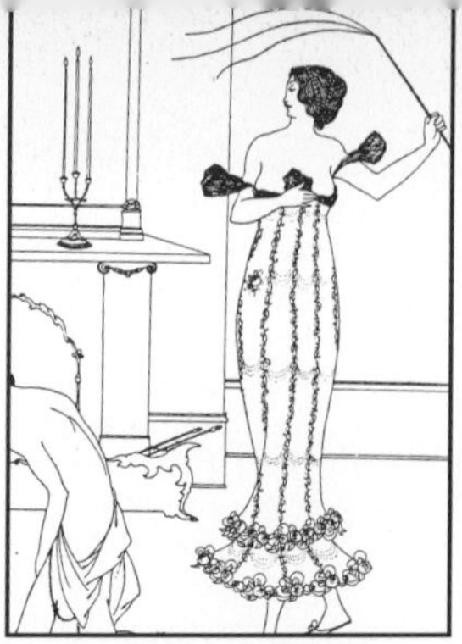

Illustration for the Earl of Lavender by Aubrey Beardsley (1896).

"I'm bringing back the birch, but only between consenting adults."
GORE VIDAL

Rules of the game

- The genuine consent of those involved must be established.
- Agreement should be reached in advance on any activities which either partner wishes to avoid.
- There should be an agreed release signal which will be honoured instantly.
- Only knots that are easy to undo should be used.
- Breathing should not be restricted.
- Nobody should be left tied up without supervision.

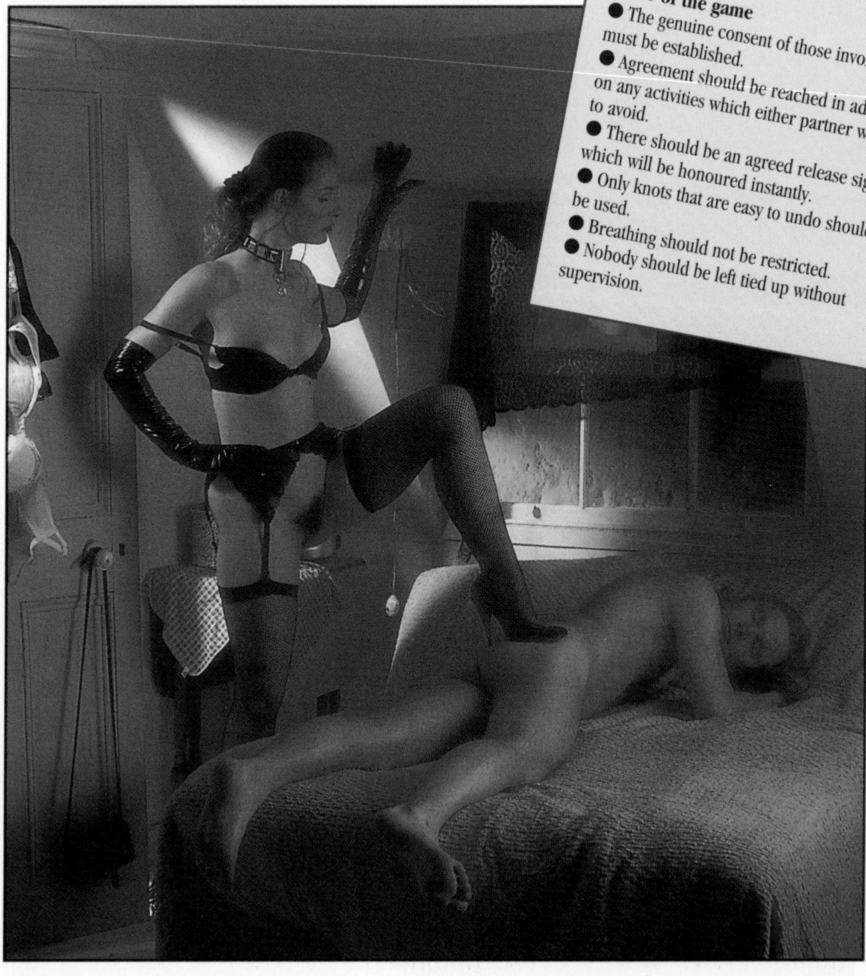

See also:
dressing up
body decoration
sex aids and toys
oral sex
masturbation
fantasy
pornography

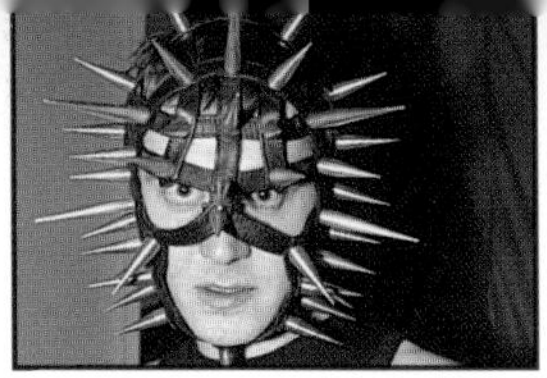

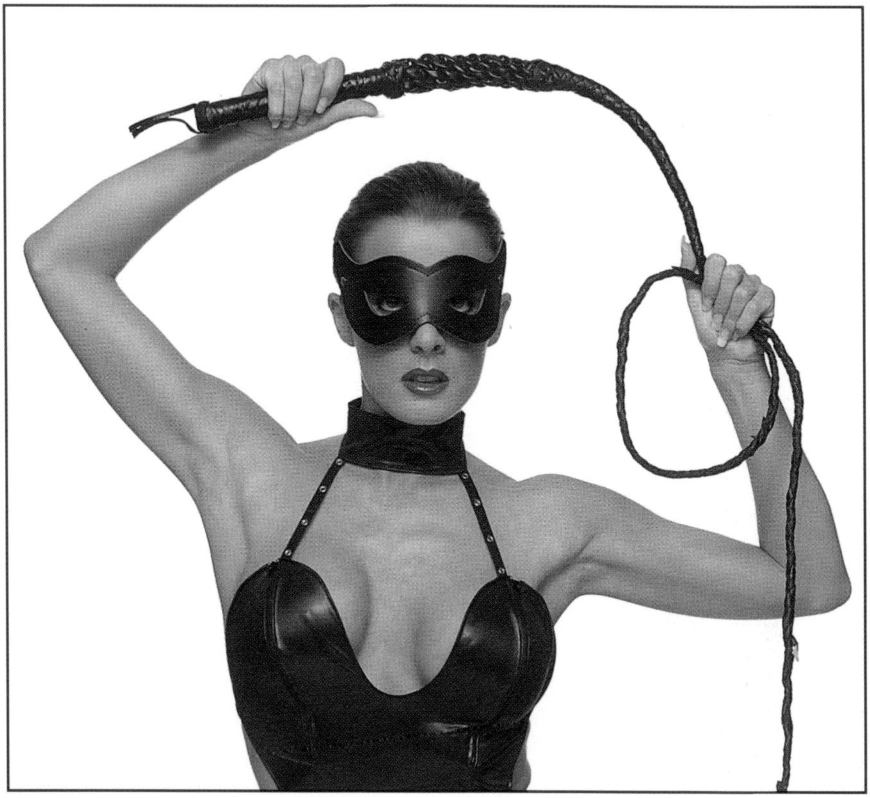

Domination and submission in sexual relationships can take many different forms. They are often part of role-playing games and fantasy: one of the most popular forms is taking the roles of master and slave. Exactly how control is manifested tends to be a very personal matter. Some of the more common or well-recognized forms are:

- Bondage
- Humiliation and degradation: insulting a partner, forcing them to do something menial or embarrassing, or using some form of defilement
- Infantilism: in this sense, being dressed and/or treated as an infant or child
- Coitus à cheval: in this sense, wearing a bridle-like harness and being ridden or 'trained' as a horse
- Defilement: the use of dirt, urine or faeces to humiliate
- Symbolic dress, including uniforms, lingerie and cross-dressing
- Flagellation
- Pain

Pain

The experience of pain can be close to the experience of sexual arousal. Slapping the skin causes it to become flushed and swollen, which is what happens to the sexual organs when they become engorged with blood. For many people the two are implicitly linked. Spanking, in particular, is popular using the hand or canes, whips, tawses and the like.

The terms most commonly used to describe this kind of behaviour are sadism, for those who enjoy inflicting pain on others, and masochism, for those who enjoy the experience of pain. Sexual practices involving pain are referred to as sadomasochistic or S/M. They can involve a partner or be part of solitary masturbation.

There is however a distinction to be drawn between S/M sex involving consenting partners, and sex play which involves physical pain and injury against a person's wishes. Consensual S/M is negotiated in advance and can be stopped at any time by either partner.

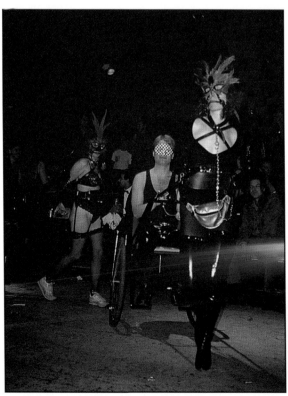

GROUP SEX

Sex with more than one partner has probably always been part of human sexuality, although the way it has been viewed by society has varied greatly from one cultural group to another and throughout time. Sexual freedom reached a highpoint in the late 1960s and early 1970s in Western society. Open relationships and sexual freedom were common until the discovery of HIV and the ensuing AIDS panic. Now, with safer sex practices and increasing social acceptance of different forms of sexual expression, group sex in general and partner swapping in particular are enjoying a minor revival.

FACT: Seventeen per cent of women in the West have engaged in some form of group sex.

"If God had meant us to have group sex, I guess he'd have given us all more organs."
MALCOLM BRADBURY

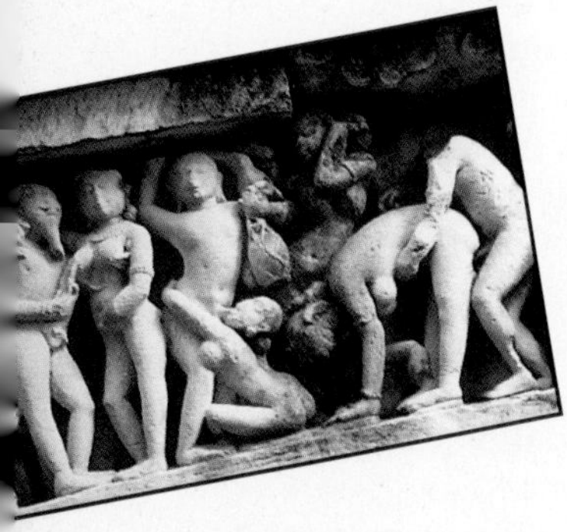

The attraction of group sex
Many people are aroused by the sight and sounds of other people having sex. But to be present while people have sex, to see, hear and smell them and even to be actively involved can be intensely erotic.

At the same time it can also be instructive to see how other people have sex: singles and couples alike can find the experience rewarding. It can provide a secure environment for experimentation with different kinds of sexuality and sexual expression. For established couples, group sex can add variety and boost each person's sense of his or her own attractiveness, without threatening the relationship. For others, at the heart of the attraction is the novelty and thrill of doing something which is in many cultures considered taboo.

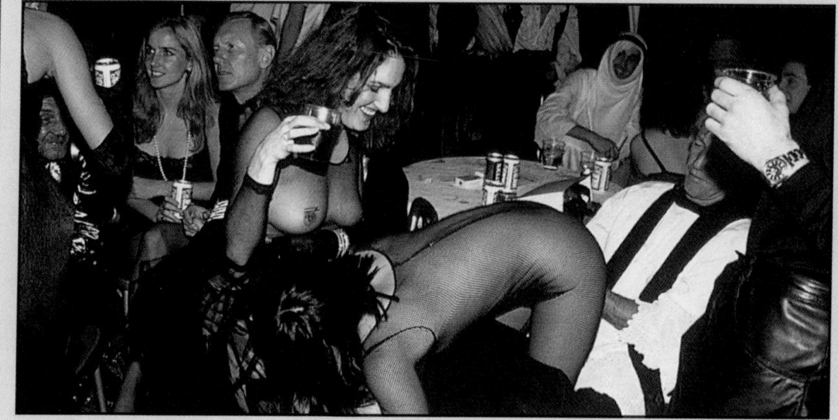

See also:
exhibitionism and voyeurism
fantasy
pornography
safer sex

Group practices

Group sex can take place through friends or acquaintances, through advertisements placed by couples or singles, or through group sex houses. Group sex houses usually have a strict code of behaviour pertaining to how individuals and couples are approached or refused for sex, what activities can take place and safer sex practices. The idea is to create a secure environment for free sexual expression.

Some people enjoy having more than one partner or making love with more than one person at a time. Others like performing for an audience. Any number of different people, positions and sexual practices may be involved. Certain terms are sometimes used for specific kinds of group sex: a rainbow and daisy chain are terms first used in the 1960s for – respectively – a group of people of different skin colours and a circle of people each performing oral sex on the person in front of them. The term 'gang bang' refers to a succession of people having intercourse with one person, usually a group of men with one woman, although this term may also be used to refer to group rape.

Swinging

Swinging is the term used for couples or singles having sex play in groups, in front of each other or with new partners, with mutual consent and usually together at the same venue. One of the older terms for this kind of activity was wife-swapping, which originated in Victorian times when husbands swapped keys to go 'home' in the evening. Today these practices can be arranged through swinging clubs or conferences, swinging parties or advertisements in specialist magazines; alternatively wife-swapping may occur between friends. Group sex and/or lesbian activity may be involved, although male gay sex is usually taboo.

The risks

The objections to swinging and group sex are moral, emotional and medical. The morality is very much a personal – and sometimes a religious – issue. The emotional side is more complex. Swinging as a couple requires a total commitment and absence of jealousy. If a relationship is unstable, swinging often does more harm than good, but experienced swingers find that it can strengthen relationships. Swinging is about sharing exploration and novelty, rather than having such experiences without a partner's knowledge. Safer sex guidelines should be followed to reduce medical risks. In some countries there are legal restrictions on group and/or homosexual sex.

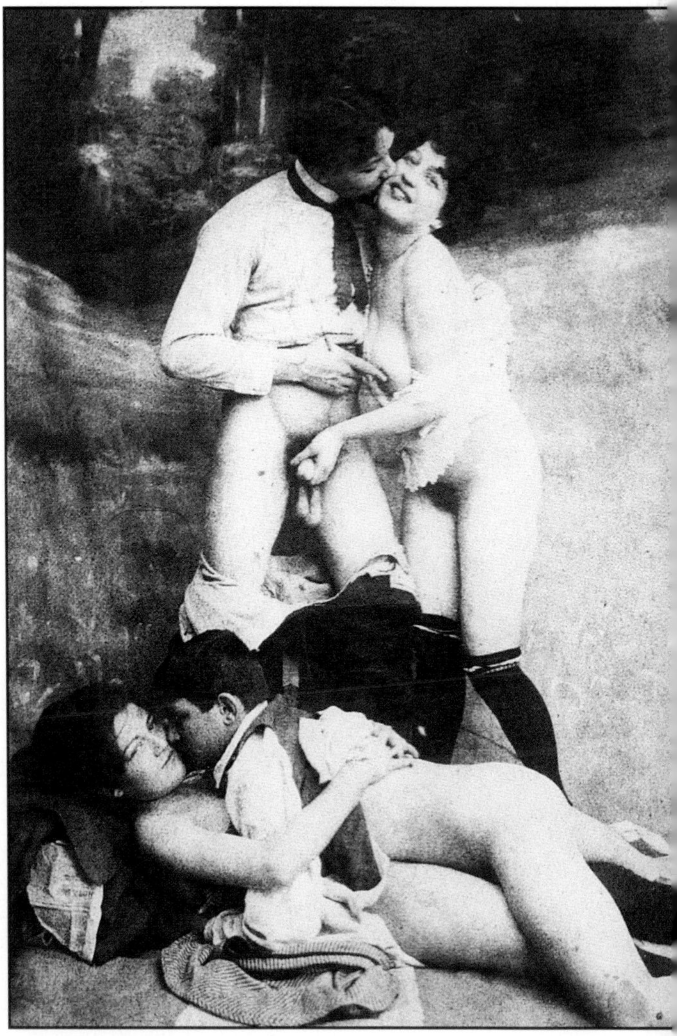

Group sex and swinging have been part of human sexuality in all cultures and throughout time. Right: **Swinging in the 1890's**; Far left: **Laksamana Temple**.

EXHIBITIONISM & VOYEURISM

Sexual display and visual stimulation play a part in most people's sex lives. They are a natural and instinctive form of sexual communication, both in the process of attracting a mate and within an established relationship. This aspect of sexuality is more prominent in some people than others and in some it can become compulsive. In certain cultures, if done in public, this may conflict with the norms of sexual and social behaviour.

Exhibitionism can be understood broadly as deriving sexual pleasure from displaying oneself. Voyeurism involves watching other people in order to become sexually aroused.

The desire to watch other people without their knowledge is also more common among men, although it has been reported among women. It may involve watching a person undress, spying on sunbathers or watching a couple engaged in any sexual activity. The fact that in many cultures this is a taboo and in some illegal may add to the attraction.

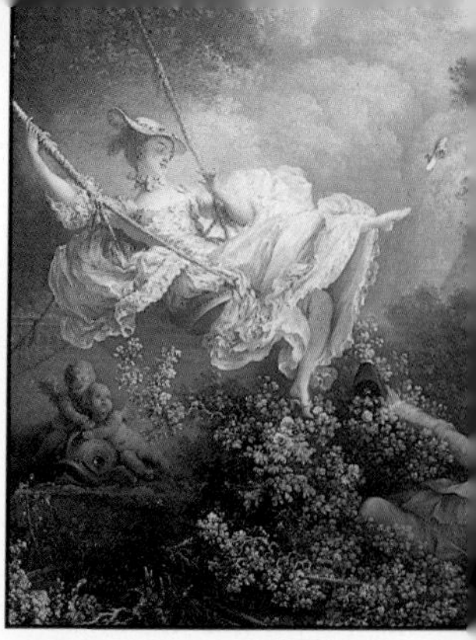

The Swing, by Jean Honore Fragnonard (eighteenth century). Showing and looking, in one form or another, are arousing for most people. In this case, both girl and boy seem to be equally aware – and equally enjoying themselves.

Forms of exhibitionism and voyeurism in the West ...

... IN DAILY LIFE

Most people engage in some mild form of exhibitionism and/or voyeurism as a part of daily life, in subtle forms of sexual display. These include, primarily, body language, clothing and other forms of body decoration, most of which have some sexual origin.

... IN A RELATIONSHIP

This occurs on a more open and conscious level in the context of a sexual relationship. While men tend to be more visually stimulated than women, many people of both sexes are aroused by the sight of their partner and the sight of themselves making love. Many people enjoy watching their partner masturbate, or making love in front of a mirror. Others are aroused by the thought of being watched. The two sides are closely linked: some couples make home videos of each other and their lovemaking, and enjoy performing for the camera and watching the result.

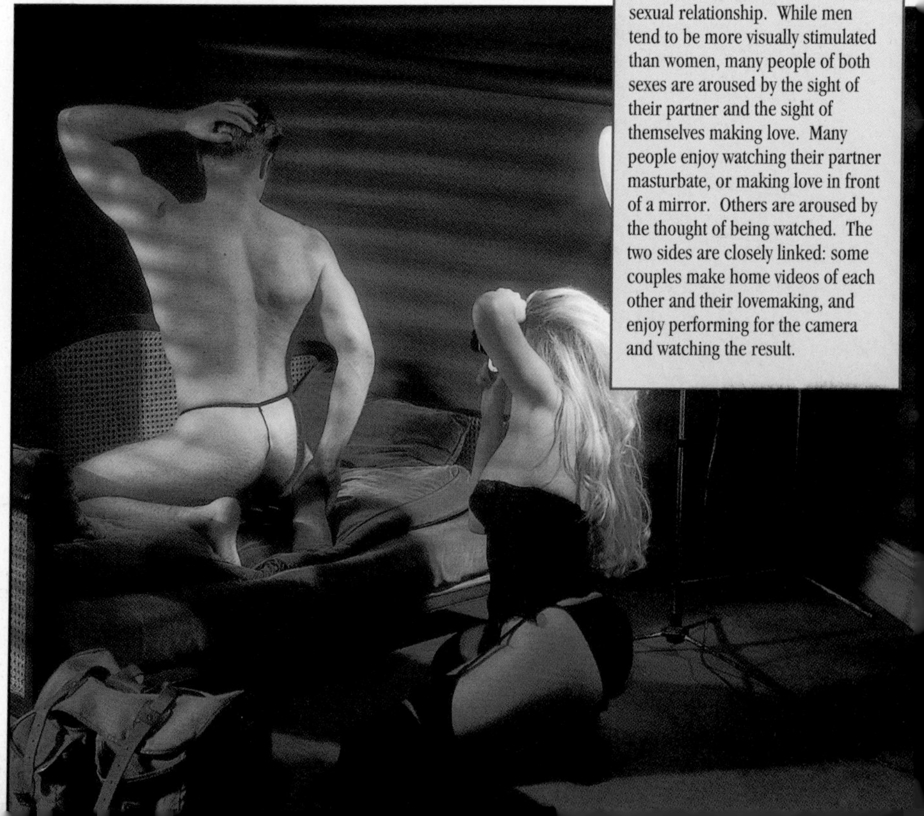

See also:
pornography
fantasy
body decoration
body language

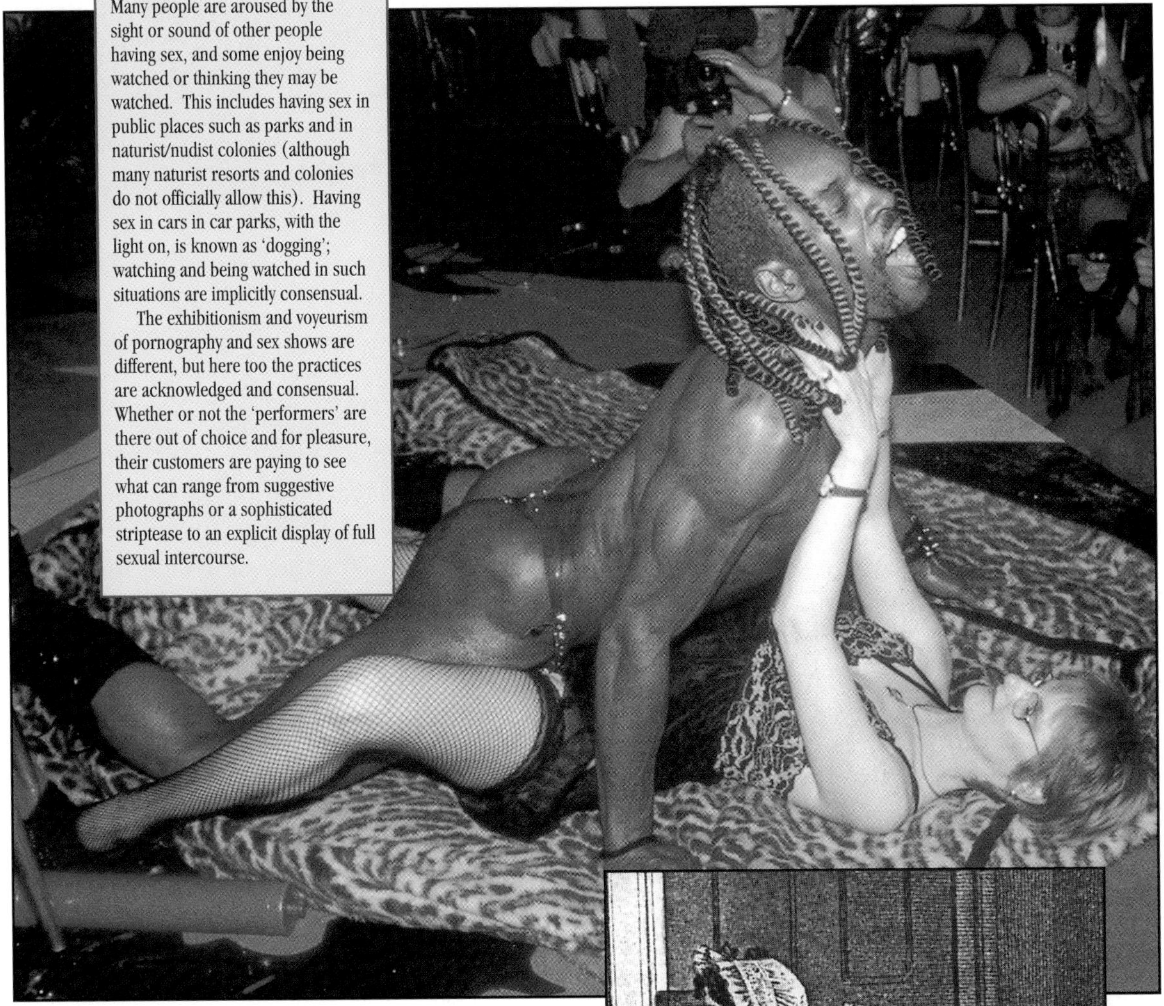

... IN PUBLIC

Many people are aroused by the sight or sound of other people having sex, and some enjoy being watched or thinking they may be watched. This includes having sex in public places such as parks and in naturist/nudist colonies (although many naturist resorts and colonies do not officially allow this). Having sex in cars in car parks, with the light on, is known as 'dogging'; watching and being watched in such situations are implicitly consensual.

The exhibitionism and voyeurism of pornography and sex shows are different, but here too the practices are acknowledged and consensual. Whether or not the 'performers' are there out of choice and for pleasure, their customers are paying to see what can range from suggestive photographs or a sophisticated striptease to an explicit display of full sexual intercourse.

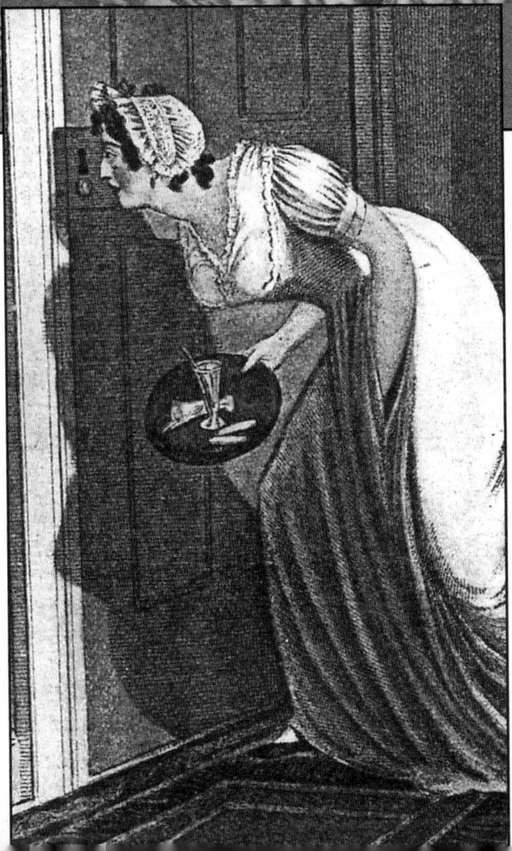

... IN SECRET

Lastly there are those who watch other people or expose themselves to strangers without anyone's consent; it is for these people that the words exhibitionist and voyeur are most commonly used, as well as other more disparaging terms like 'flasher' and 'peeping Tom'.

Those who expose themselves to others are, on the whole, male, and they tend to have little self-confidence, especially with regard to sex. Their intention is not to hurt but to shock: the pleasure derived from the experience is based on the shocked or horrified reaction of their victim. Being approached by a flasher may be alarming, but they are rarely involved in more serious sexual crimes.

PROSTITUTION

Prostitution is often known as 'the oldest profession in the world'. It seems to have existed in almost all cultures in one form or another. However, this is one sexual practice which is scorned in some cultures, and highly esteemed in others.

The reality is that few animals are naturally entirely monogamous, as the instincts for producing healthy offspring and ensuring their survival tend to overrule other considerations. Humans, and male humans in particular, are by nature promiscuous, and most are interested in sexual variation of some kind. This is seldom acknowledged, particularly in the West.

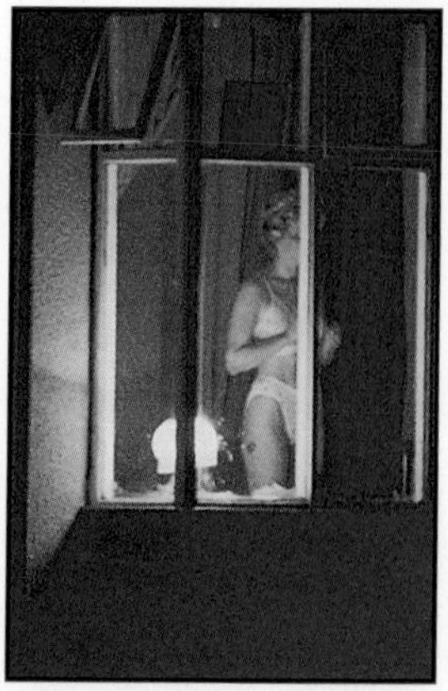

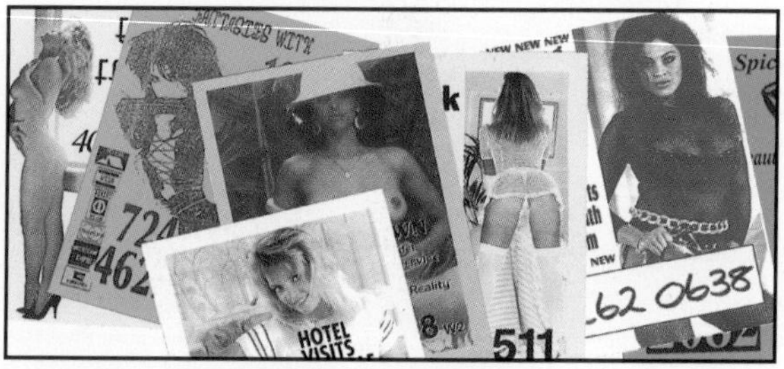

The professional relationship

Prostitutes can be female or male (usually female), adult or child, professional or amateur. A prostitute is described as professional if she (or he) makes their living from prostitution. The majority do not work as prostitutes from choice: money is the main objective.

In many ways the relationship between prostitute and client is a business relationship like any other. The activities involved are usually negotiated and paid for in advance, with any further activities requested paid for before they are performed. More importantly, the relationship is founded on mutual consideration and respect: once this is established the prostitute can take pride in providing the client's satisfaction. Consideration and reassurance are particularly important in those societies where prostitution is illegal or taboo.

See also:
pornography
fantasy
sex drive
safer sex

What is prostitution?
Prostitution is selling sexual services, usually for money although its forms may be as varied as any other sexual practice. It can provide sexual healing and sexual freedom, as well as straightforward sexual satisfaction. It caters to people who are single and people whose relationships do not satisfy their sexual needs; it can provide satisfaction for those who feel unable or unwilling to form a relationship. Where necessary, it can also provide sexual experiences for people with special psychological or physical needs or disabilities. The term 'sex worker' is now frequently substituted for the term 'prostitute'.

Prostitutes generally cater to a wide range of sexual preferences, although in each cultural group the sexual acts most commonly requested are those which are considered taboo. The same pattern may be seen in the demand for particular types of pornography or eroticism. Many people find release for their more far-fetched fantasies through prostitution.

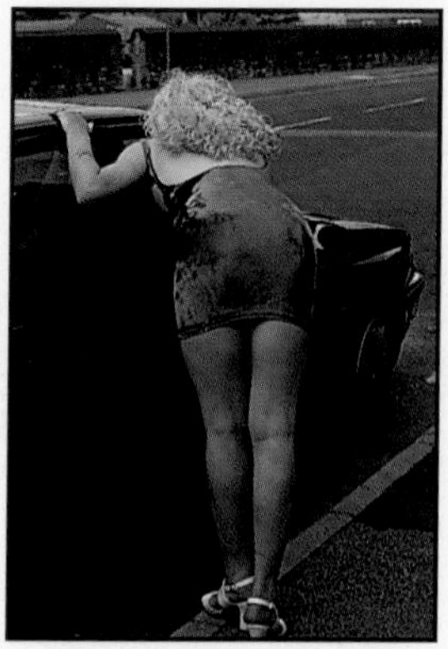

Prostitution and society

In many countries laws against prostitution have driven the profession underground. They have also made it potentially more risky for both prostitute and client and harder to monitor in terms of health and hygiene.

Prostitution may occur through street soliciting or legal or illegal brothels in any number of guises. Massage parlours, saunas, escort agencies or sex shows are all common 'fronts' for brothels (although many such businesses do not involve prostitution). Procurers or 'pimps' may find work for prostitutes, taking a cut of their earnings and sometimes offering a degree of security or protection. However, it is still potentially dangerous work which is not aided by social stigma, although support and self-help groups are becoming more common.

Recent changes

In the twentieth century, the number of male prostitutes has increased. The largest proportion of male prostitutes service male customers. Some may be transvestites, impersonating women very adeptly. The recent increase in child prostitution is concerning. Many children drawn into prostitution are runaways who have no other source of income. Child prostitution exists all over the world but trends show that the consumers tend to be from first world countries, and the suppliers are from developing countries. This partly explains the fact that tourism has generated a vast market for prostitution in certain countries, especially in the capital cities of Bangkok and Calcutta.

Attitudes toward prostitution in general have taken a more modern outlook. There are some who hold that eliminating prostitution would breed more forms of perversion and immorality, and that prostitution actually serves to reduce the instances of illegitimacy, abortion, rape and attacks on children. Contrary to previous belief, prostitution is not commonly linked to organized crime and in the West public health officials indicate that prostitutes are responsible for only a small percentage of sexually transmitted diseases. Strong arguments have been made in favour of legalizing prostitution, on the grounds that decriminalization would free the police and courts from dealing with victimless crime, allowing them more time for cases of a violent or more serious nature. The recognition of HIV and AIDS and the number of reports on the prevalence of HIV among prostitutes and their customers has generated new concerns and fears about prostitution.

A red light district – one of the most common ways in which prostitutes and their clients meet, but also potentially dangerous.

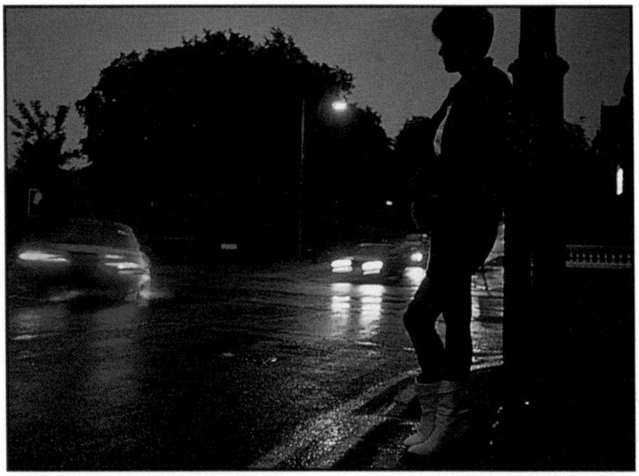

Prostitution and the law

In Britain, prostitution is not illegal, however soliciting for the purpose of prostitution is, as is living on 'immoral earnings'. It is also illegal to procure, or to take part in the management of, or to commit premises to be used as a brothel. Recent new legislation has meant that the police have been much tougher on 'street walkers', which in effect has pushed prostitution underground and given rise to many new guises for prostitutes, including such titles as call-girl, masseuse and escort. Brothels are now more commonly known as 'massage parlours'. America is one of the few countries in which prostitution is, to all intents and purposes, illegal (the State of Nevada is an exception). In most other countries the laws concerning prostitution try to control its socially damaging consequences and are aimed at restricting those who try to exploit prostitutes and at controlling public soliciting.

CYBERSEX

Cybersex is the term used to describe any kind of erotic experience involving a computer. Seen – and feared – by many as the future of sex, it has promised everything from the ultimate dating service to orgasms at the touch of a button.

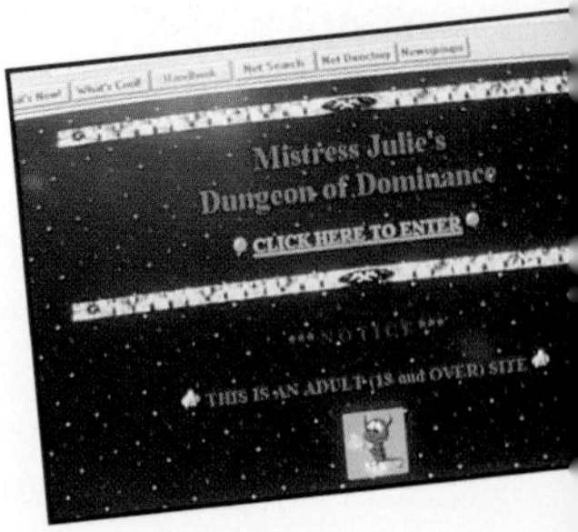

Sex on the 'net'

Electronic Mail and the Internet offer a number of sexual possibilities. As technology develops and the number of users grows, these possibilities can only expand.

Currently the best-known sexual use of the Internet is for pornography. Among the most popular Net sites are those which are used for pornographic text or images. In theory this has a valuable role to play, enabling people to explore their sexuality in new ways and in private. It makes sexually explicit material available to those who want it. There are even on-line sex shop catalogues. However, there are no controls over the kind of material distributed in this way or over access to it, and there is concern about the distribution of material deemed offensive or dangerous. This is particularly so when pornography involves – or is accessible to – children. The governments of Japan, the USA and other countries are already considering taking measures to monitor the Internet. Civil rights groups are preparing to oppose this.

The Internet is also widely used for making contact with other people, and this offers further possibilities for computer sex. Many people communicate through user networks or bulletin boards set up specifically for sexual communication: these are widely used for exchanging ideas, experiences or fantasies, or for looking for sexual partners. Many introduction services are already in existence, catering for singles, couples and all forms of sexuality and sexual preference.

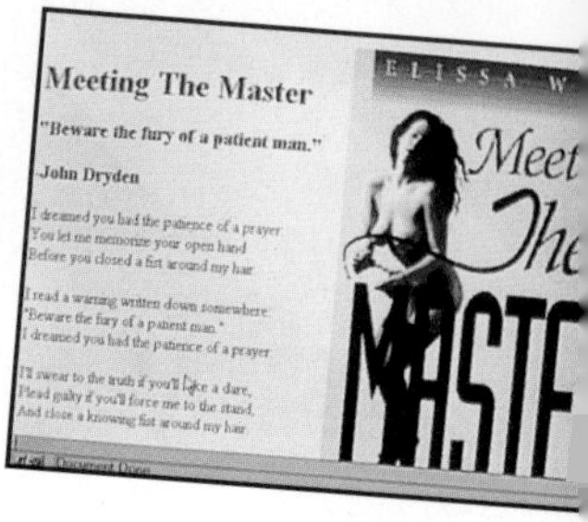

Sexual web sites proliferate on the Internet – from commercial erotica through to user discussion groups.

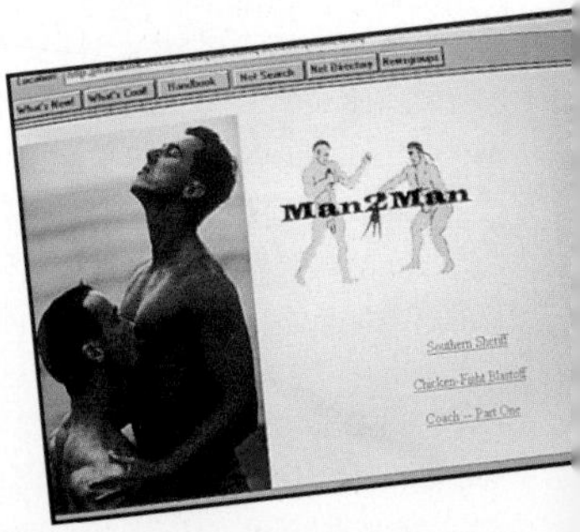

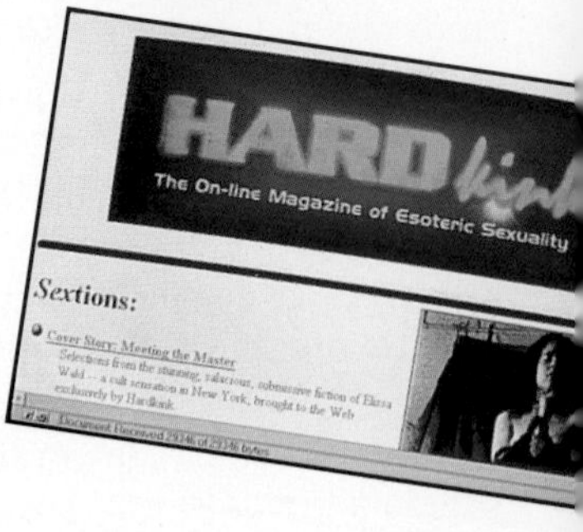

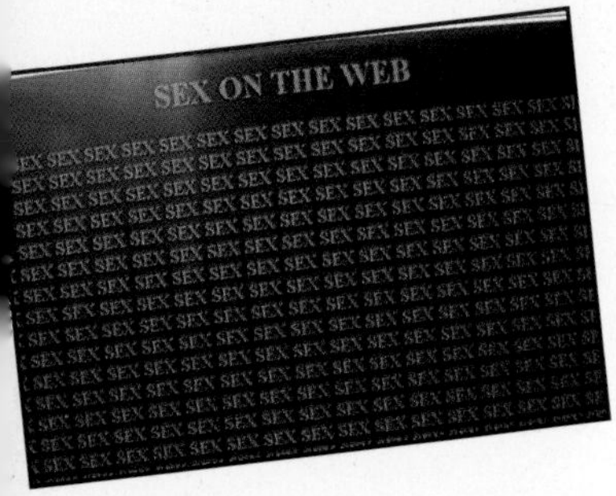

See also:
sex aids
pornography
exhibitionism and voyeurism

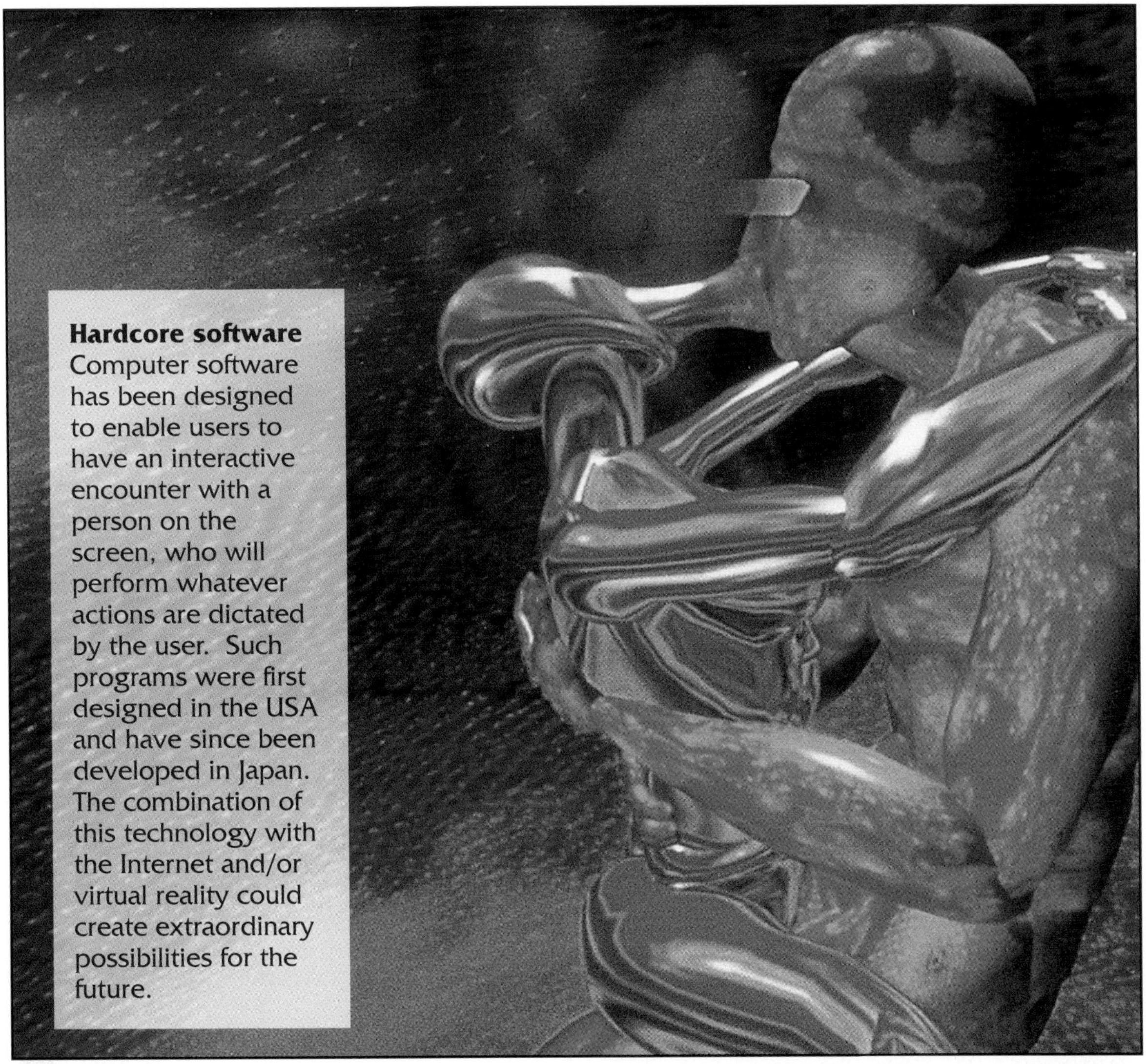

Hardcore software
Computer software has been designed to enable users to have an interactive encounter with a person on the screen, who will perform whatever actions are dictated by the user. Such programs were first designed in the USA and have since been developed in Japan. The combination of this technology with the Internet and/or virtual reality could create extraordinary possibilities for the future.

Virtual reality sex
The term virtual reality refers to the most realistic computer simulations. There are two sides to virtual reality sex. Firstly there is the idea of interactive computer software, in three-dimensional format, on screen. This has been referred to as 'teledildonics'. And there is the much-publicized idea – particularly in science fiction films and books – of the virtual reality suit. This would be a complete body suit to make possible lifelike simulation of sex, in three dimensions and involving all the senses. It seems inevitable that computer programming and technology will eventually turn even this idea into reality.

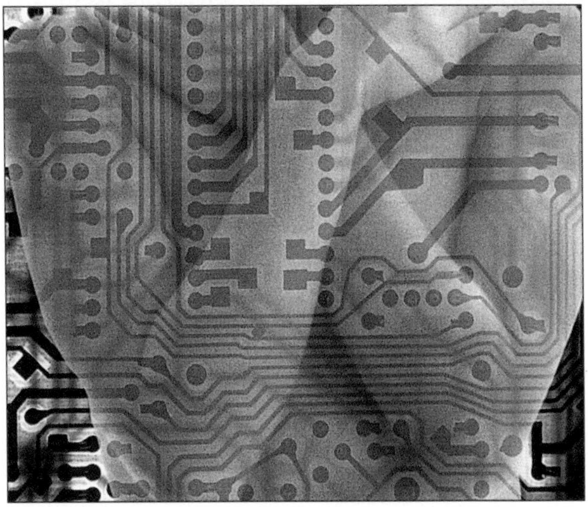

FANTASY

The most powerful human sex organ is the brain. Sex has been described as ten per cent friction and ninety per cent fantasy. The use of the imagination sets human beings apart from other mammals and is particularly important in the context of sexuality.

Most people fantasize, either frequently or occasionally, although the forms and subjects of those fantasies are so many and varied that the term may mean different things to different people. Fantasy reflects every aspect of a person's sexual psyche but potentially without any of the personal or social constraints which might be experienced in reality. Fantasy can be the truest form of sexual expression and has an important part to play in many people's sex lives.

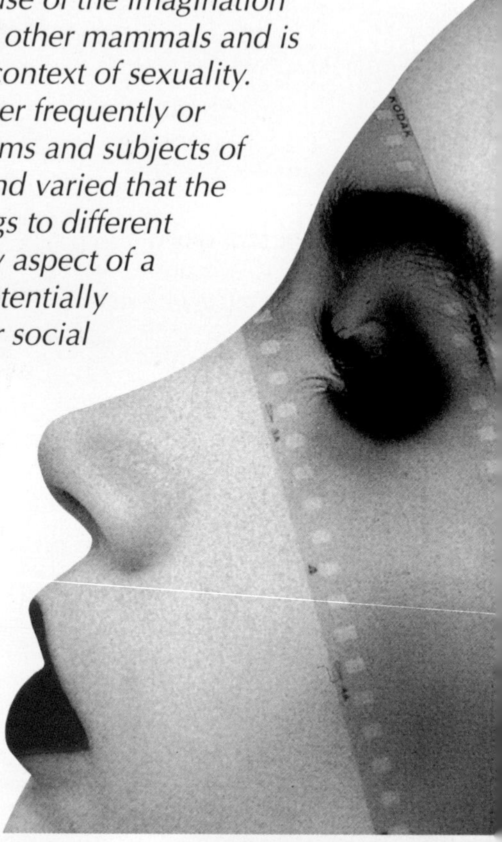

FACT: More than seventy per cent of men and women are reported to use fantasies while having sex.

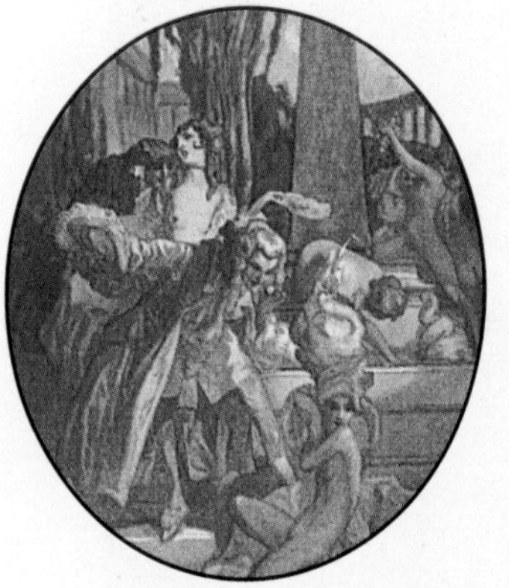

Eighteenth century fantasy, by Franz von Bayros.

See also:
pornography
masturbation
exhibitionism and voyeurism
sexual feelings

What is fantasy?

Sexual fantasy is the sexual use of the imagination. It means imagining situations, experiences, people or sensations for the purposes of sexual arousal. It can take the form of a long sequence of events or a story, or it may simply consist of isolated sensations or images. It can be conscious day-dreaming where the mind directs events, or the dreaming during sleep which is beyond any conscious control. It can last for several hours or a few brief moments.

Fantasy may or may not involve more tangible forms of stimulation. People may fantasize while masturbating, while making love with a partner, or while doing something completely unconnected such as working or travelling. The thought may be dismissed or, in a psycho-physiological merging, it may be carried through to orgasm. Fantasies are usually personal and private, remaining in the

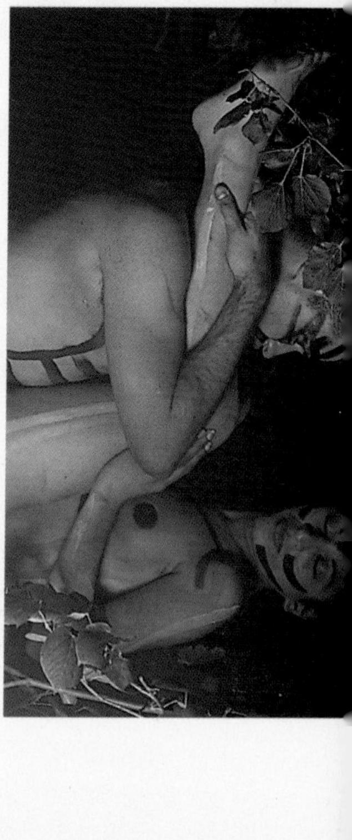

imagination of the individual, and many people prefer to keep their fantasies to themselves. However, they can also be shared, or acted out. Sharing a fantasy with a partner can add excitement to lovemaking, although some people may feel alarmed or even insulted by the nature of their partner's fantasies. Sharing a fantasy must be handled sensitively and, where appropriate, with a clear distinction between what is desired in fantasy and what is desired in reality. The decision to act out a fantasy is difficult, as the actual experience may be disappointing when compared with the imagined one. On the other hand, it can be the springboard to a thrilling way of exploring sexuality and experimenting with sexual practices.

Why do people fantasize?

A number of negative assumptions are often made about sexual fantasy. Having them has been said to imply that the person's real sex life is disappointing, or that they are not in love with or committed to their partner. However, this is not necessarily true. Surveys suggest that people who consider themselves and their partners to be good lovers are more likely to have fantasies. If anything, the extent to which fantasy is used reflects the strength of a person's libido. Equally, there is no correlation between use of fantasy and infidelity. Fantasy can take many different forms and serve many legitimate purposes. It is the safest form of sex.

During lovemaking

Fantasy can boost arousal at any stage of lovemaking. It can prepare the way for sex, arousing people before lovemaking even begins, or it can add excitement during sex. It can even help to bring on climax; this can be a key factor in enabling both partners to reach orgasm. It can also help to solve arousal or orgasm problems.

Emotional release

Fantasy is often used as a form of sexual release, as a substitute for sexual activity in reality. Many people, particularly women, are able to reach a high level of sexual arousal through fantasy, some even reaching orgasm. Like pornography, using sexual fantasy can be associated with masturbation.

A sense of guilt is one of the most common forms of sexual inhibition, generally produced by negative attitudes to sex in the family or cultural group. Fantasy can ease this in two ways. Firstly, people can fantasize about activities with which they would not feel comfortable in reality (see below). Secondly, fantasies such as those in which the person is compelled to be involved in sexual acts, can remove the fantasizer's sense of responsibility: in the fantasy he or she has no choice, leaving them free from guilt and thus able to enjoy themselves freely. This is the source of many masochistic, submissive or so-called 'rape' fantasies, which are quite distinct from desiring the use of force in reality. Equally, sadistic or dominant fantasies can be used as a safe outlet for pent-up anger or aggression.

Experimentation

The world of fantasy provides the ultimate safe environment for sexual experimentation. All guilt, anxiety, embarrassment and fear of consequences are banished; this is the one instance where full, free sexual expression is possible. This may be the most common use of fantasy.

There are two distinct kinds of fantasy experimentation. The first is largely based in reality, and takes the form of a kind of sexual rehearsal. The person can 'try out' a particular sexual practice without actually doing it; they can then decide whether or not they want to try it in reality.

The second kind is based more on the unobtainable, and can include anything from sex with a favourite film star to sex with one's partner on a desert island: this is fantasy as wish-fulfilment. However this category can also include activities that the person would not desire in reality, which could range from extramarital sex to some of the more extreme practices such as sadomasochism or bestiality. Such fantasies are not uncommon, and are harmless as long as they do not lead to illegal or dangerous activities.

WOMEN AND FANTASY

What do women fantasize about?
The most popular female fantasies include:

- Sex with usual partner
- Sex with a stranger
- Sex with a former lover
- Sex with another woman
- Sex with someone of a different race
- Sex in exotic or unusual locations
- Sex in imaginative or romantic circumstances
- Having sex in public and being watched
- Sex with two men or a man and a woman
- Group sex
- Watching a partner having sex with someone else
- Watching other couples having sex
- Working as a prostitute or stripper
- Being 'forced' to have sex
- Being tied up for sex
- Sexual activity with an animal
- Using a male sex slave

How do women use fantasies?
Women's fantasies tend to have more to do with atmosphere and circumstances than men's; they are more likely to involve a story or a series of events leading up to sex. Women are more likely to fantasize about their regular partner, albeit in different guises or situations. While men's fantasies tend to be more voyeuristic, women's are more exhibitionistic.

The process of sexual liberation is reflected in changes in women'ís fantasies, which have increasingly included dominant and assertive sexual practices. In many cases they have also become more overtly sexual and less 'romantic'. Women's sexual fantasies have always tended to be more varied and imaginative then men's and this continues to be the case: seventy-five per cent of women say that fantasy is an important and fulfiling part of their sex lives.

"In my sex fantasy, nobody ever loves me for my mind."
NORA EPHRON

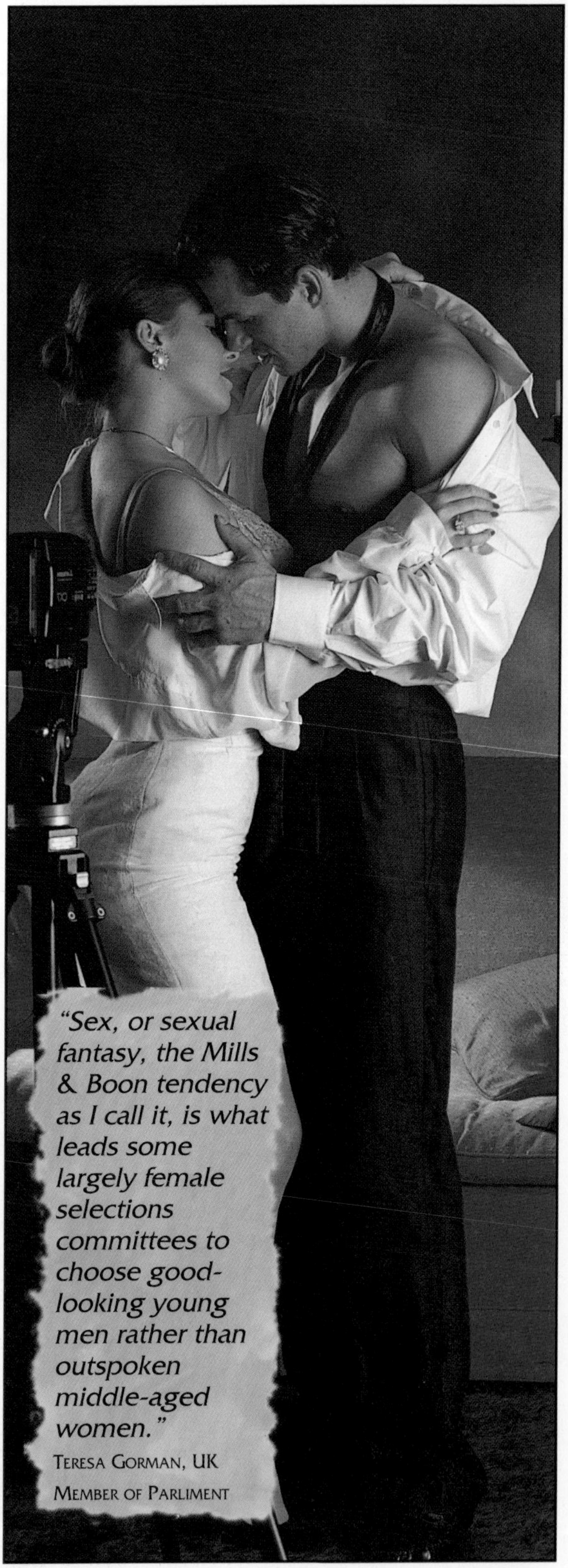

"Sex, or sexual fantasy, the Mills & Boon tendency as I call it, is what leads some largely female selections committees to choose good-looking young men rather than outspoken middle-aged women."
TERESA GORMAN, UK MEMBER OF PARLIMENT

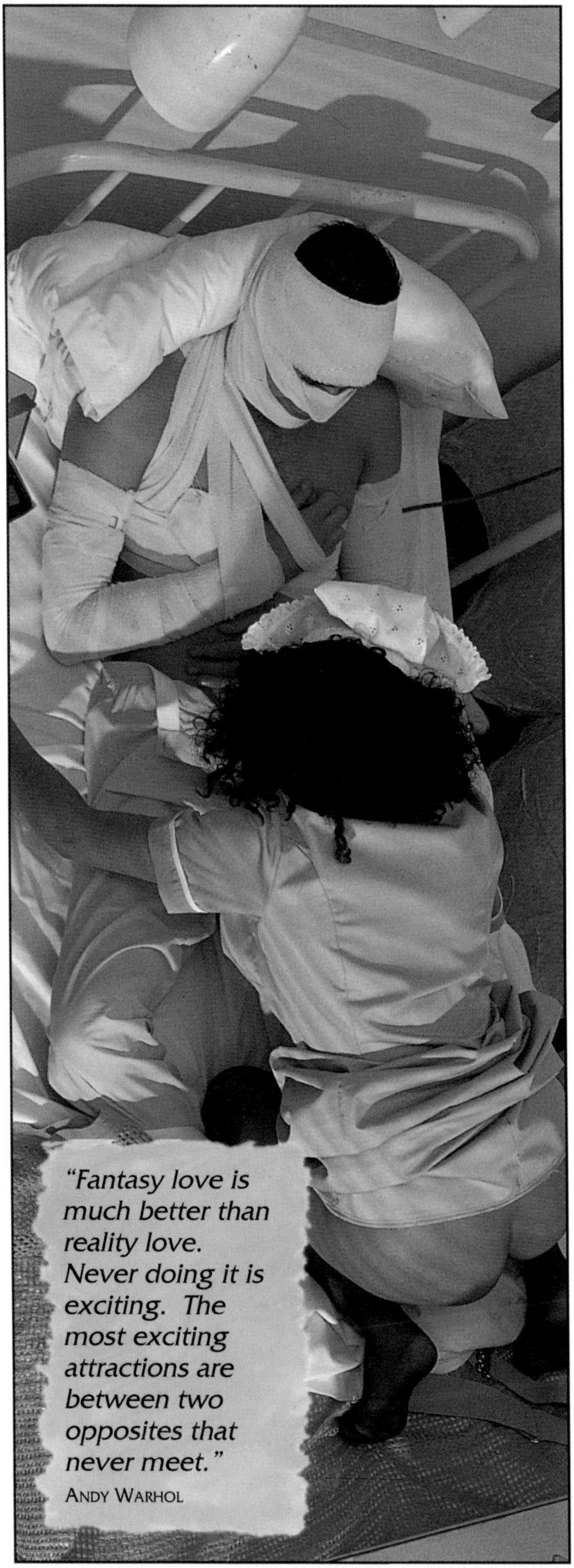
"Fantasy love is much better than reality love. Never doing it is exciting. The most exciting attractions are between two opposites that never meet."
ANDY WARHOL

MEN AND FANTASY

What do men fantasize about?
The most popular male fantasies include:

- Sex with a woman other than their usual partner, such as neighbour, colleague, friend, partner's best friend, past lover, stranger, celebrity
- Sex with someone of a different race
- Watching a woman masturbate
- Watching two women have sex, often a usual partner with another woman
- Watching other couples having sex
- Sex with another man
- Sex with two women or a man and a woman
- Group sex
- Watching other people having group sex
- 'Forcing' a woman to have sex
- 'Forcing' a woman to have oral sex
- Being made to have sex
- Sex in a public place
- Sex with a virgin
- Anal sex with a woman
- Having a woman use a dildo to perform anal sex on him

How do men use fantasies?
Men's fantasies tend to be more visual than women's, focusing on particular key images. They tend to be focused more on the person or people involved, and the sexual acts being performed, than on the situation or atmosphere. Men's fantasy partners may include acquaintances or a regular partner, but are often influenced by images from soft-porn magazines. Voyeuristic fantasies are more common among men than women.

All kinds of sexual activity can feature in men's fantasies, from the simplest and most straightforward practices to the more extreme and bizarre end of the scale. Dominant and sadistic practices may feature as an outlet for aggression, while fantasies about submissive practices can be used to relieve a sense of obligation to fulfil a stereotypical 'masculine' (active, dominant, aggressive) role.

3

SEX & YOU

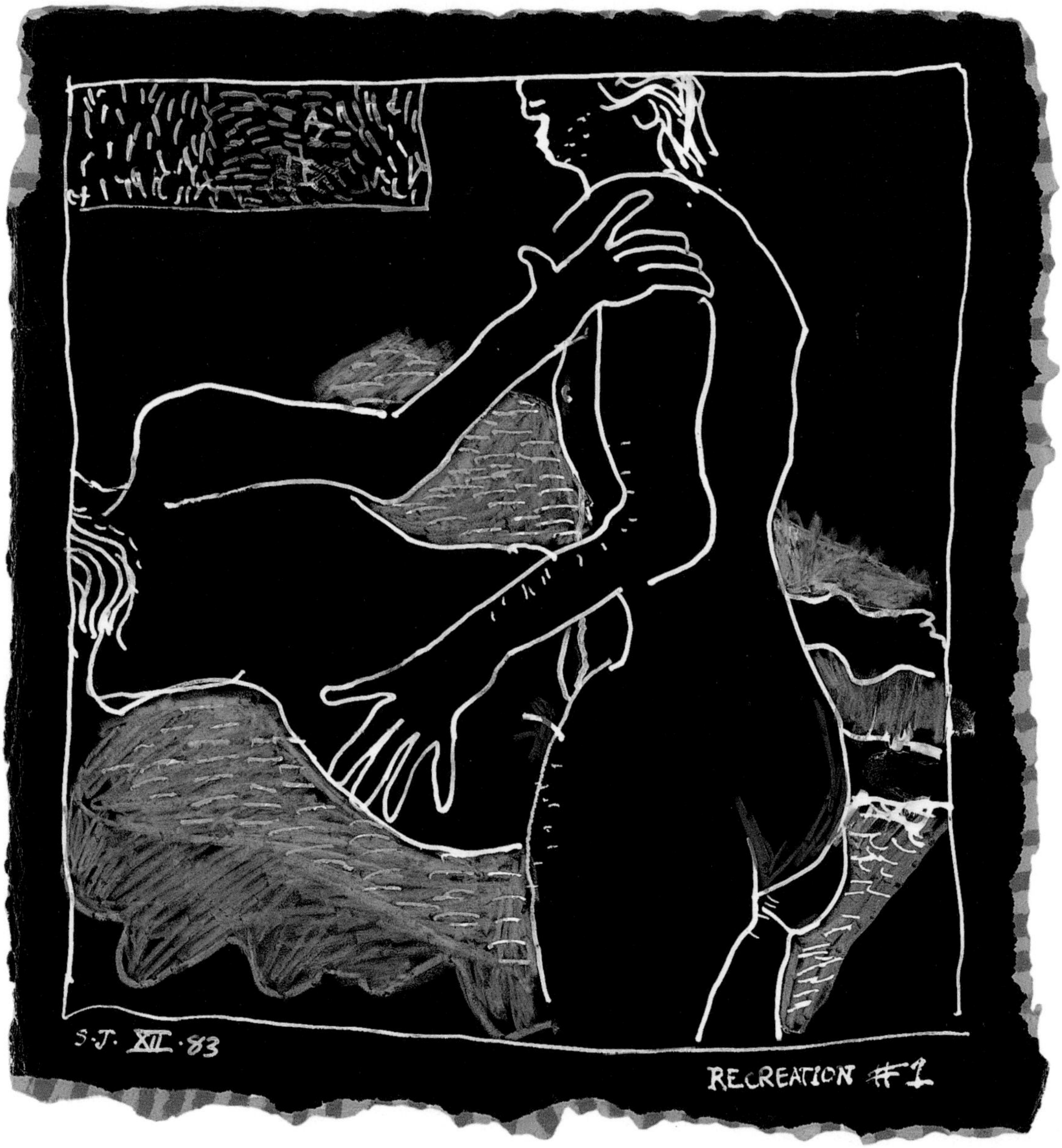

Relationships are important to most of us. It is likely that some relationships will be sexual ones and will vary according to sexual orientation, gender, upbringing and education about sex. Many people are anxious about sex and relationships and would like to improve their interpersonal skills. This section of the encyclopedia invites you, the reader, to use the information in the previous sections to develop your own sexual profile. It is designed to both advise and inform.

YOUR SEXUAL OUTLOOK

OVERCOMING INHIBITIONS

Inhibitions are feelings that can prevent you from enjoying sex to the full or, in extreme cases, even from becoming sexually aroused. Nearly always they are caused by feelings of guilt or anxiety about sex instilled by upbringing or by some traumatic sexual episode. We know, or we quickly learn, what makes us uncomfortable and we learn to avoid those situations or activities. But sometimes people are set in attitudes and patterns of behaviour that can make them avoid sex or suppress sexual feelings altogether.

Letting yourself be sexual

If it is hard for you to think of yourself as sexual, or to develop sexual feelings, start by using fantasy. In your imagination, you can safely experiment with feelings and sexual activities that you would find threatening in reality. Let yourself go. Become totally involved and concentrate on all the sensations you feel. If you practise this when you are alone and masturbating, this may help you feel less self-conscious about expressing pleasure with a partner.

Reassess old attitudes

Take a fresh look at your attitudes towards sex, and perhaps towards pleasure too. People who are sexually inhibited often feel that any sensual pleasure for its own sake is wrong. Making yourself more receptive to pleasure – good food, music, pictures, even a sauna or massage should make it easier for you to enjoy sex as another legitimate source of pleasure.

Learn to like your body

Some people are embarrassed about their bodies, not because they have any obvious blemishes or deficiencies, but simply because they have an image of how they would like to look and their body does not measure up. Until you learn to appreciate your body as it is, you may find it hard to believe that anyone else can really like it.

See also:
physical attraction
psychological attraction
masturbation
sexual learning

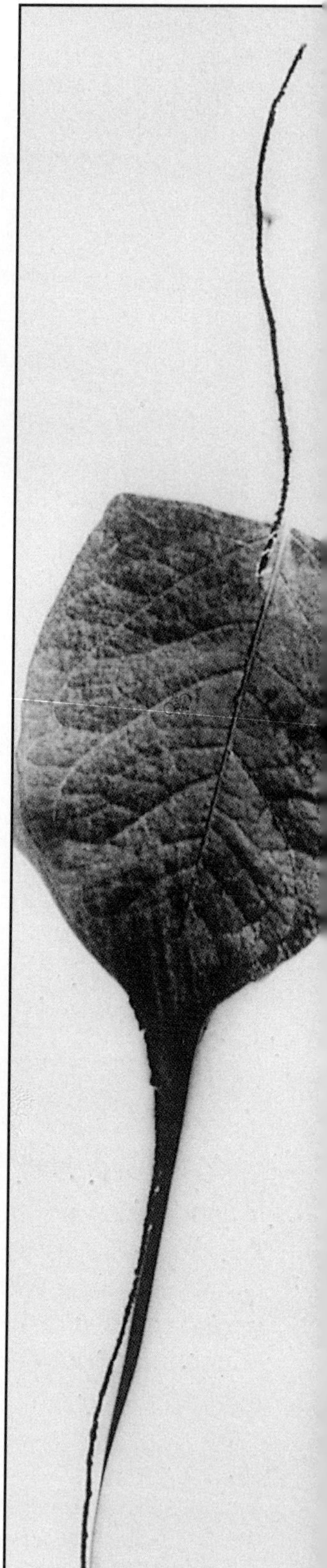

SEXUAL ANXIETIES

Anxiety about sex is as destructive to enjoyment as inhibitions. People may be anxious because they lack correct information. Ignorance about your own body and lack of opportunity to compare it with anyone else's can make you believe that your genitals are odd, or ugly, or even abnormal. Ignorance about sex itself means that 'first night nerves' are common, and anxieties about sexual performance, or about whether you will please your partner, are almost universal. Often you can dispel sexual anxiety by telling a partner how you feel. Discussing your fears helps put them into perspective, allows your partner to reassure you, and you to reassure them.

Fear of intimacy

When you are in a close sexual relationship, you should be able to tell your partner honestly what you want and how you feel without having to worry that you will be mocked or rejected. But to achieve this kind of intimacy demands trust and commitment. If you have been hurt in past relationships it may take time before you risk getting close to anyone again. And if you were raised in a family where feelings and emotions were seldom shown and never talked about you may find it hard to develop an intimate relationship in adulthood. To do so will involve changing fundamental aspects of your behaviour.

Building intimacy

Set aside time each day to talk about what has happened to you, or to discuss worries or problems. Try to talk about what matters to you, and don't avoid sexual or emotional issues even if they make you feel uncomfortable. Spend time together on leisure activities as well as in sexual encounters. And when intimacy builds up, don't back off or let pressure of work or other commitments keep you apart.

Choosing the right partner

If you find it hard to form intimate relationships, avoid choosing someone like yourself. Instead, go for someone who is unlikely to let you get away with shutting yourself off emotionally. When you sense that you are growing closer (perhaps closer than feels comfortable) don't back off emotionally. Don't try to put a distance between you by provoking a quarrel, or remembering past grievances, or by focusing on your partner's least attractive features. These are excuses to yourself to avoid involvement. Also, if you have a partner who is critical of you, it will be hard to think better of yourself. A loving and supportive partner is important for most people – and particularly for anyone for whom lack of self-confidence is a problem.

Learning to show your feelings

Affection needs to be shown. Touching your partner in an affectionate or loving way is one of the easiest ways of demonstrating it. You don't even need to say the words – 'I love you' – that people who fear emotional intimacy find so difficult to say (though it helps if you can do this too). Make a point of touching when there is no question of this being interpreted as an immediate sexual invitation. The lesson you are trying to learn is that physical affection can be built into a whole relationship, and should not be confined only to its sexual moments. When you are making love, spend time on loving foreplay, for example, kissing, touching and massage.

Giving up your emotional independence

The more self-contained you are, the more you shut your partner out of the important areas in your life. Give them the chance to do something for you occasionally. Ask for help, or advice, or a shoulder to cry on. Don't be afraid to show your vulnerability. It is important for you to learn to show your partner that you have needs, and to allow them to try to meet them. Of course you are running an emotional risk by doing this, by putting yourself into someone else's hands. But the rewards in your sexual and emotional life will be correspondingly great.

IMPROVING YOUR SELF ESTEEM

A poor self-image affects the way you behave towards other people – a fear of being rejected can make you shy or over-eager to please in social situations, and insecurity can induce jealousy, which may damage your relationships. It also affects the way other people behave towards you. By and large, other people will accept you at your own valuation. Your self-esteem has a direct bearing on your confidence in your own ability to attract and keep friends and sexual partners. When you have self-esteem, you feel you are worth something.

Causes of low self esteem

Most of the causes of low self-esteem stem from the way we were treated in childhood. Children accept their parents' view of them. Made to think they are good, loveable and successful, they will grow up believing this, and later unsuccessful experiences will be much less likely to induce feelings of inadequacy. However, even the normally self-confident person can suffer a temporary fall in self-esteem, and a consequent lack of sexual confidence, with the break-up of an important relationship, for example, or a set-back at work. When you have been dealt some major blow to your self-esteem, it is important to try to see it in perspective, as only part of your life, not the whole of it.

Avoid affairs on the rebound

After any loss of self-esteem, whether at work or in a relationship, it can be tempting to throw yourself headlong into an affair. This is certainly a quick way to soothe a bruised ego, and it may work for a while, but the risk is that rebound affairs seldom last long. It is usually wiser to rely on the support of friends, and wait till your emotional balance is restored before seeking another lover. If in two or three months you still feel a lack of sexual self-confidence, the problem may be a deeper one.

LEARNING TO ASSERT YOURSELF

Shyness is a label many people attach to themselves. Unfortunately, other people often call it being unfriendly, stand-offish, or, because you sometimes find it hard to say what you think, or indeed to say anything at all, boring or uninteresting. Have faith in your own likeability too. You may have to learn to be more assertive, to believe that you are a person worth knowing, with views and opinions that are worth listening to. Then others will believe it too.

Overcoming shyness

Shyness is an attitude of mind. The way to stop being shy is to change your attitude. You can start by thinking of yourself not as a shy person, but as someone who is only shy in situations in which most people feel at least a little shy – in large social groups, for example, or when meeting attractive strangers. When talking to people, direct all your attention outwards towards other people, not inwards towards yourself. It may help to become involved in some quite new situation with people who don't know you but with whom you have interests in common (a club or political party for instance). Here you can make a fresh start as an 'unshy' person.

Practise assertiveness

If you are shy and low in self-esteem you will tend to go to any lengths to make sure people like you. But you can't please everyone. If you are unable to risk offending others you probably make little effort to ensure that your own wants and needs are met. It is a good idea to practise being more assertive in your daily life. You should then gradually find it easier to tell others – including sexual partners – what you want. Practise saying no in situations where you would normally unwillingly say yes, for example. Learn to ask people to do small favours for you. You need not be aggressive about this. You are simply stating your views and preferences.

BUILDING SELF-WORTH

When you have a poor self-image, you will believe that this is the image you project to others, and may also believe that it can't be changed. Both of these notions are wrong. There is a lot you can, do not only to build up your own self-esteem, but to change the way other people see you.

Assessing your strengths and weaknesses
First, make two lists: your good points – character and personality as well as physical; and your bad ones – the things about yourself that you wish were different or could be improved. Try to be specific. Don't be tempted to minimize your strengths. Don't just do this from a sexual point of view – if you play soccer well, or are a good cook, or paint, include this too. If there are talents you admire in others and feel would add to your self-confidence if you had them (learning to drive or play an instrument for instance), put these down. If your list of weaknesses is by far the longest, you are probably being too self-critical, as people with a poor self-image tend to be, dismissing some of your good points as too trivial to include.

Analysing your strengths
Look at your list of strengths. Are you making the best use of the ones you've got? Do you try to put yourself in situations in which you know you can shine? If you have good eyes or a nice smile do you know how to use them? If you are tall, do you make sure your posture is good or do you slouch, round-shouldered? Finally, look at the 'weakness list'. How many items on the list are things you can do nothing about (no-one can make themselves six inches taller, for example)? Delete these from your list and resolve never to think about them again. As for the rest, make them the start of your self-improvement programme.

Improving your image
Start with your physical appearance. Don't be defeatist. Saying, 'I never bother with the way I look' often covers the fear that even if you did bother it wouldn't make any difference. But appearance can be changed. A new and more flattering haircut or colour, contact lenses instead of spectacles, or vice versa – there are endless ways to improve the way you look. When you are buying clothes, think about styles or colours you have never tried before but which could suit the way you'd like to look.

Make gradual changes
When you make changes, don't try to do too much too quickly. Introduce them gradually, one at a time, over a few months. This will make you less self-conscious about your new image and give you and everyone else time to adjust to it. It may also take time to get used to other people's changed reactions to you. When you have done what you feel is the best you can with yourself, learn to like yourself the way you are, even if you still fall short of your 'ideal' image.

Making yourself more flexible
The more qualities you require for someone to be attractive to you, the less flexible your 'blueprint' for a partner, and the less chance there is that anyone will ever satisfy it. Instead, it is better to try to change your expectations and develop a less rigid blueprint. The next time you meet someone you are interested in, don't worry too much about whether they match up to your ideal. Instead, concentrate on the things about them that appeal most to you. You may find they have qualities which you wouldn't have listed in your blueprint, but which seem special in this person. Focus on these positive qualities as much as you can. There are some qualities you will never be able to change in another person. But do the qualities outweigh the faults?

THE SINGLE PERSON

FORMING RELATIONSHIPS

Many people are perfectly happy being single, but for those who are not, finding the right relationship can be a central part of life. However, it is important to recognize that, while many people believe there is just one perfect partner for them, there are in fact many people with whom you can fall in love and have rewarding and lasting relationships. And if you are wondering whether someone better might come along, it will prevent you from making the most of the relationships you do have. Even if you think of yourself as an ordinary person, you can be sure that there will be some people who will find you attractive. As an initial friendship develops, you may want to transform it into a sexual relationship.

The first date

The aim on your first date is to get to know each other and make the other person feel you like them, without making it too 'heavy' and frightening them off. A casual date without too many sexual overtones may feel most comfortable – lunch or a drink after work perhaps. But don't be too familiar on a first date, or try to be too intimate – and don't talk about previous partners.

The importance of timing

Choosing the right moment to advance a relationship and knowing when to hold back, is crucial to sexual success. Moving too fast puts the other person under pressure. Move too slowly and they may lose interest. If you get it wrong, it is often because you have ignored or misread the other person's signals. Body language plays a part. If you find you are looking into each other's eyes for longer and longer periods, this is a definite 'come-on' signal, indicating that it is time to move on to a more overtly sexual stage. Start by taking the person's hand. If they don't draw away, move on to more intimate gestures such as kissing and hugging.

See also:
body language
physical attraction
touching
kissing

Taking too much for granted
If you are often rebuffed after your first sexual overtures it may be because you take it for granted that sex is on the agenda in any relationship. It isn't. Get to know each other. If the other person feels they are free to choose, not under pressure, they will be less likely to reject you. Never, ever, make someone feel they are under any obligation to have sex with you. Nobody ever is.

Sexual good manners
When you are both ready to make it sexual, be sensitive – you will be nervous, no doubt, but so will they. If you are both clearly tense, suggest a bath, shower or massage together first. Tell them how desirable you find them, and never criticize their looks. This first time you might both prefer just to lie and explore each other's bodies and cuddle. If you do have sex, always discuss safer sex beforehand.

MINIMAL DATING PROGRAMME

For many people, even taking the first steps towards a sexual relationship is hard, because they doubt their ability to make any kind of close friendship or sexual relationship. If you are in this position, this minimal dating programme will help you establish a normal social, and then sexual, life in gradual steps.

Step one: Making a neutral date
The first step is to make a neutral date that will cause you as little anxiety as possible. So it should be with someone you like, but don't find especially attractive, and don't care at all about making a sexual impression on. Make it casual, with no romantic overtones – lunch, or a visit to a concert or film or exhibition. Asking them at fairly short notice makes it appear even less of a formal date – and will give you less time to be anxious about it too. Repeat this kind of date a few times until you feel little anxiety.

Step two: Dating someone who matters
The next step is to date someone you do find attractive and if possible, someone who you think might find you attractive too. To begin with, keep to the same platonic, neutral dating you practised in the first step. When you feel relaxed with your date, start to make it clear that you find them attractive. Don't rush things, but don't let them stand still either. Make each occasion more romantic, involving a little more affectionate physical contact. Taking their arm, holding their hand, a goodnight kiss – these are all recognized steps on the way to a sexual relationship.

Step three: The final move
Once you feel you have got close to the person, and you think there is a real sexual spark between you, you can make the final move. Here you have to take a risk, but don't hold back for fear of rejection. The only way you can succeed is by risking failure. You also have to decide whether to be open and tell them of your sexual anxiety, or whether you simply go ahead and trust to luck. In fact you may find that because you've already established a close relationship, there is no failure. Even if things don't go well, it should be easier for you talk about your situation, and enlist their help in trying again.

Step four: First times
'First night nerves' are probably universal. Whether it is love, lust or simple curiosity that has got you into this situation, it is an unusual person who doesn't feel at least a little tense or nervous. It's best to be open with your partner – they'll probably be relieved that you are as nervous as they are. If you're a virgin, or have less experience than your partner, then they can reassure you. Don't expect the first time to be a great experience – it seldom is, and sex improves with practice.

RELATIONSHIPS

LEARNING TO COMMUNICATE

Talking about sex in general is easy, but talking about your personal sexual feelings and preferences is difficult for almost everyone. It isn't only that it makes you feel vulnerable to reveal your intimate thoughts and feelings; because your sex life is a concern shared with your partner, you need to consider their feelings too. Learning to communicate the way you feel, to make suggestions or request changes, without making your partner feel hurt, rejected or criticized, is a real art. But if you want a relationship that is able to grow and develop so that it can meet both your needs, it is a necessary skill.

Talking about sex

However close you are, your partner cannot read your mind. There is no substitute for straight talking if you want to discover each other's sexual needs and preferences. It is often easier to talk about sex with a new partner, when sex is very probably on both your minds. So take advantage of any new relationship to set up a pattern of good communication. At this stage you know little about each other, so it seems natural to ask them what they like, and to tell them if there is any sexual activity you particularly like or dislike. Be as specific as you can. Then when you get to know each other better it will be easy to continue the same pattern.

The right time to talk

Most people find it is easiest to talk about sex when they are actually making love. It's easy to say 'I love what you're doing', or 'Am I pressing hard enough?'. However, for couples in well-established relationships who have never been in the habit of talking about sex, it is hard suddenly to alter the pattern and start – it may seem too much like an accusation that sex hasn't been great up until now. It may be easier to broach the subject of sex on more neutral ground – perhaps over a relaxing drink or meal.

See also:
sexual feelings
making love
sex positions
sexual practices

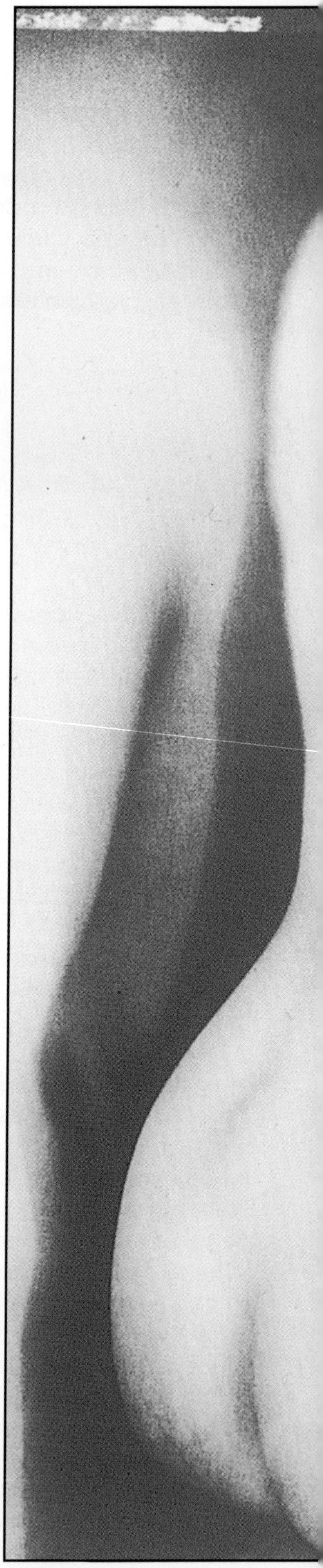

Reassuring your partner
Stress what you like rather than emphasizing what you dislike. Remember, everyone is sensitive about their sexual performance, and anything that can be taken as a criticism probably will be. So try saying, 'I love it when you stroke me just there,' rather than 'Why can you never ever find the right place?' If there is a really delicate matter to be raised – personal hygiene for example – try suggesting it's a problem you share. 'I haven't had time for a bath for a couple of days – I'm sure I must stink. Let's take a shower together.' Don't expect too much self-disclosure too soon, or ask a question you wouldn't want to answer yourself, or one that you know would embarrass your partner.

Saying no
At times, one of you will want sex and the other will not. It's important to find a way of saying no without hurting the other person. The secret is to make it clear that it is not the person who is being rejected, only the invitation, and that only temporarily.

DEALING WITH ANGER

Anger and good sex are incompatible. Two people who set out to live together have to learn to talk their problems out without letting anger get out of control and destroy their relationship.

- Say what has upset you at the time, don't bring it up days or weeks later.
- It causes less resentment to say how your partner's behaviour makes you feel than to criticize them as a person.
- In an argument, stick to the point at issue. Don't say '...and another thing' and bring up past grievances.
- Don't let yourself go out of control, or start an argument when you are blazingly angry. It is too easy to say wounding or destructive things that can't easily be forgiven or forgotten. Cool down a little first.
- Make up before you have sex.

SUSTAINING RELATIONSHIPS

No-one can predict with any degree of certainty whether a relationship will last. The most unpromising-looking partnerships often survive, while others, which seem to have everything going for them, fail. What we can say is that a relationship works best when both partners satisfy most of each other's needs for much of the time, and that the most important ingredient for success is your own determination to make it work. Certain other factors also seem to be particularly important in determining a couple's chances of making a successful long-term partnership.

Timing
Don't commit yourself too young. Commitments made before the age of nineteen are least likely to survive, simply because the two people involved will change as they mature and may grow apart. It's also sensible not to make a relationship permanent too soon. It probably takes at least several months to get to know the best and worst of each other. However, if commitment is postponed for longer than about two years, it is a sign that you may not want to commit to that person, or that you are not ready to lose your independence.

Similarity
It is probably easier for a couple who have similar interests and attitudes, and want much the same sort of things out of life, to live together without friction. It may help if you are both of similar intelligence, and if there is not more than ten years' age gap between you. It's important to have the same feelings and attitudes towards sex too. Sexual compatibility is not just a question of technique – that can be learned. What matters is that sex should not be much more (or less) important to one partner than the other, and that you are truly attracted and aroused by each other.

Flexibility
Look for a partner who is flexible, receptive to new ideas or willing to try out new activities. Neither relationships nor individuals remain the same. Everything changes and a partner who is very inflexible and uncompromising may find it hard to adapt to the inevitable changes in any long-term partnership. However, it is equally important not to assume that a partner will change, or that you can change them. The chances are that a partner who is jealous, moody, alcoholic or wildly extravagant will not change substantially under your influence. If you cannot put up with them as they are, you'd do well to steer clear of long-term involvement with them.

Emotional maturity
A stormy courtship is a bad sign. It will be difficult to have a fulfiling and happy relationship with a partner who is angry, domineering, aggressive or critical. On the whole, people change very little, and a pattern of courtship quarrels is likely to continue. Be wary, too, of making a lasting commitment to someone who is very insecure or over-dependent, unless you are prepared for an unbalanced relationship in which you always have to be the supportive and reassuring partner. Finally, for most people it is important to have a partner who is capable of giving and accepting physical affection.

JEALOUSY

Everyone who has ever been in a close relationship has experienced jealousy and recognizes the pain that it can cause. It is one of the most powerful and destructive of emotions. Jealousy is often assumed to be a sign of love. If you are insecure in your relationship, you may even try to make your partner jealous, as if this would somehow 'prove' he or she loved you. In fact, what jealousy really demonstrates is not love, but a fear of loss.

When is jealousy reasonable?
Sometimes jealousy is a reasonable response to a relationship under threat. How much you show is a matter of judgement, and control. It's reasonable to be jealous if a partner sets out to flirt with someone else in your presence, for example, or if you have solid grounds for thinking that they are involved with someone else. Under these circumstances a flash of jealousy may serve a positive purpose. It can either act as a timely warning to a partner that their behaviour is going beyond the bounds of what you are prepared to tolerate, or force hurt and angry feelings into the open that need to be acknowledged if the relationship is not to be permanently damaged.

Unreasonable jealousy
Jealousy is not always justified. It is unreasonable to be jealous of lovers your partner had before you met, for example, or of old friends who have long been part of their lives. You cannot rewrite anyone's past and if you try to destroy it, or insist that all ties with the past are cut, your partner will inevitably feel resentful. Jealousy that arises from your own feelings of insecurity causes deep resentment too. Unless you have solid grounds for thinking a partner is cheating, it is a mistake to cross-examine them about what they do in your absence, or to look for clues to infidelity amongst their belongings.

Rebuilding trust
When you have once had good cause for jealousy, it is natural to worry that the same thing may happen again. It takes time, sensitivity and self-discipline to rebuild trust, and to repair the damage to self-esteem that is inevitable when you find a partner has, even temporarily, preferred someone else to you. It's important that the 'wronged' partner tries to let their grievances go, and does not show their lack of trust by monitoring their partner's every move. It is equally important for the partner who has strayed to give the relationship priority and offer extra reassurance and affection.

INFIDELITY

Most affairs are with colleagues and close friends. Affairs that are based only on sexual attraction are usually self-limiting, lasting on average only a few months, and probably do least damage to a long-term relationship. More damaging is the affair that satisfies an emotional need to be more deeply loved or valued in the unfaithful partner.

Why do affairs begin?

Most people convince themselves that their affair was a spontaneous and irresistible 'falling in love'. In fact, it nearly always involves a conscious decision. It may begin out of curiosity or a need for sexual excitement, or because their regular partner has a problem that makes sex difficult or unsatisfactory. An affair may be a morale booster, or entered into as revenge on an unfaithful partner, or a way of finding the 'ideal' partner with whom (it is believed) a perfect love would be possible. It may have the relatively positive aim of precipitating a crisis in a relationship that needs a thorough overhaul. Whatever the reason, there is always the risk that continuing the affair may seem to be an easier option than solving the problems in the relationship.

Running a successful affair

An affair probably causes least grief and gives most pleasure when it fulfils a simple sexual need for both partners, neither of whom makes additional demands on the other. But few relationships are as simple as this. If you want to have a successful affair without jeopardizing your primary relationship, you need to make a commitment to both, which means compartmentalizing your life and your emotions. Don't neglect your partner or try to justify what you are doing by dwelling on their failings, even to yourself. Make the most of your time with your lover – most affairs have to be conducted with one eye on the clock, and grievances can build up quickly when there is no time to resolve them.

Whether to confess

Confession is bound to affect, and may destroy, a relationship. If you do confess, or are found out, your partner's reaction will depend partly on how long the affair has been going on. It is easier to understand and forgive a casual brief fling than to accept that they have to view a large part of your life together quite differently. It can take a long time to rebuild trust. The unfaithful partner, too, runs the risk that the affair may be too successful, becoming more important to them than was ever intended so that they have to examine their commitment to their partner.

Discovering a partner's infidelity

If you suspect your partner is having an affair, should you confront them? Before you do, be sure that you really want to know and have considered the implications. Remember that most affairs last only a few months at the most. If you do confront, decide on your aim. If you are trying to save the relationship, however bitter you are, try to get your emotions under control first so that you do not say too many things that will be unforgivable or unforgettable. You want to know why it happened, so give your partner the chance to tell you. Ask questions only if you want to know the answers. It will probably hurt more than help you to know, for example, the sexual details of the affair.

Working out a solution

Once an affair is out in the open it is essential that you both make time to talk about it. It will be tempting to want to give vent to your own feelings, and of course you must have the opportunity to do this. But it is actually more vital to the survival of the relationship that you understand why your partner went into the affair and how they feel now. If they were looking for something in the affair that was missing in your own relationship you both need to recognize and acknowledge this, and work out what can be done to meet the need they evidently felt. Many couples survive the discovery of an affair and emerge with a stronger mutual understanding.

ENRICHING YOUR SEX LIFE

What makes a good lover? Sexual happiness depends on more than technical ability. The good lover is confident in their own sexuality but, just as important, they have the ability to make their partner feel good about themselves – sexy and responsive. The best sexual relationships are equal, so that neither partner has to feign enjoyment or enthusiasm and both have a real affection for each other that makes them able to satisfy each other's emotional as well as sexual needs. Finally, there is no substitute for sexual chemistry, which no-one can explain or understand.

Attraction and affection

Love-making should be sensual as well as sexual. Foreplay is important because it is the way both partners express their sensuality and delight in each other's bodies. Use touch to show affection as well as to ask for sex. After sex a man tends to feel all his needs have been satisfied, but a woman's need for affection is often intensified by sex. For her, afterplay – a hug, a cuddle, a few intimate words – may be as important as foreplay. Don't be afraid to show that you like sex. Sex should never be something that is 'done' by one partner to the other, either performed or received as a duty. It is for your mutual pleasure.

Imagination and innovation

One way to keep a sexual relationship exciting is to explore a range of sexual activities. Use your imagination to introduce variety into your sex life. A different time, or place, or position, or having music to make love to – if sex is beginning to feel boring there are innumerable ways to spice it up. Make time for sex so that there is no need to rush. Pause every now and then and let your arousal wane, perhaps talk for a while, and then have the added pleasure of arousing each other all over again.

SEXUAL BOREDOM

Sex doesn't have to become boring if the couple involved are flexible enough to change and adapt as the years go by. The reality is that things change. The excitement and intensity that mark the early stages of an affair give way to a calmer, less frenzied phase. Passion diminishes, but long-term lovers know each other's bodies and needs and preferences, and accept and trust each other, and this can more than compensate for anything that may have been lost.

Enjoying a life together

Sex is only part of a relationship, and if the relationship as a whole bores you, the chances are that sex will do so too. Try giving each other more attention, spending more time together, having more fun together, flirting with each other. Shared activities or new interests can give you points of contact and something to talk about, perhaps even make you more stimulating and interesting for each other. Try occasionally doing something nice for your partner, for no special reason except just to please them. It doesn't have to be anything spectacular – just something to make them feel that they enhance your life.

Breaking your sexual routine

Introducing change into a long established sexual routine is often difficult, but it is a good way of combating sexual boredom. If you suggest making changes, be careful not to make it seem as though you are criticizing your partner. If your partner views the idea with suspicion, make the changes small and subtle at first. You might suggest simply that you leave the lights on instead of making love in the dark, or go to bed on a Sunday afternoon if yours has always been a bedtime-only sexual routine. Later you might want to make more dramatic changes, adding a new position or even a new activity to your sexual repertoire.

Valuing your relationship
One way of dealing with boredom is to look for new levels of excitement or new experiences you can share together. Another is to try to feel more positively about your present sex life and your present partner. Start by looking at all the things you've enjoyed about sex with your partner. When you are making love, concentrate on the physical sensations. Remember, these don't change – there is really nothing new out there. All that really changes is your attitude to sex with your partner. Even if you don't feel like sex, keep up the habit of affectionate contact, spontaneous hugs and kisses: don't withdraw physically from your partner. Above all, discuss your sex life with your partner and decide what is good and what might need changing.

Being open to change
At the time of the Kinsey report in 1953, fewer than half the women interviewed had ever had sex in anything but the missionary position. Couples now are generally much more innovative, but many people are still resistant to change, sometimes because they feel anything that isn't 'normal' (i.e. what they are used to) is wrong, or because they feel embarrassed about looking or feeling ridiculous if they try anything new. Don't approach a new sexual activity as a challenge, it's meant to be a pleasure and if you don't both enjoy it, drop it. And remember that most human sexual activity is reassuringly ordinary. Anything too unusual or acrobatic is usually also too uncomfortable for most people to enjoy.

ACCEPTING SEXUAL REALITY

The early stages of a sexual relationship are magic – but they have little to do with real life. No-one can live at that level of passion, excitement and intensity for long, and it is these very qualities that tend to fade the fastest. If this sexual high is what you crave, then you are bound to be disillusioned. Unless you are realistic enough to accept that intense passion is bound to fade, and learn to value the calmer waters of the next, less frenzied stage of the affair, you may write off a perfectly good relationship as boring.

Don't reach for the unattainable
Sometimes disillusion sets in because you have a fantasy view of sex that could never live up to your expectations. The danger of these unrealistic expectations is that you may go from one affair to another, each time convinced that this will prove to be the ultimate sexual experience, and each, time as familiarization sets in, you will be disappointed. Instead, try to feel more positive about the way things actually are.

Living in the present
Learn to value your relationship as it is now. Don't compare things as they are with past experiences. Sex may not be as exciting now, but it is probably much more reliable. Neither of you are as likely to suffer sexual or performance anxiety, and each of you knows what the other likes, and how best you can arouse and satisfy each other. And because your excitement and arousal are not quite at the peak they used to be, you can probably prolong your love-making.

Increase the pleasure
All satisfying sexual activity is a two-way process. Your partner's evident pleasure in your love-making will be satisfying to you. And the more pleasure you give, and the more they enjoy sex with you, the more they will want to give pleasure to you. Make use of the fact that you can intensify any physical sensation by focusing on it. Everyone has experienced this with pain, but it works just as well with pleasure too. Learn (and teach your partner) not to equate physical affection with sex. It is a pleasure and a comfort in its own right, and helps keep your relationship alive. When you feel affection for someone, you will enjoy making love to them more.

SEXUAL PROBLEMS

MALE AND FEMALE PROBLEMS

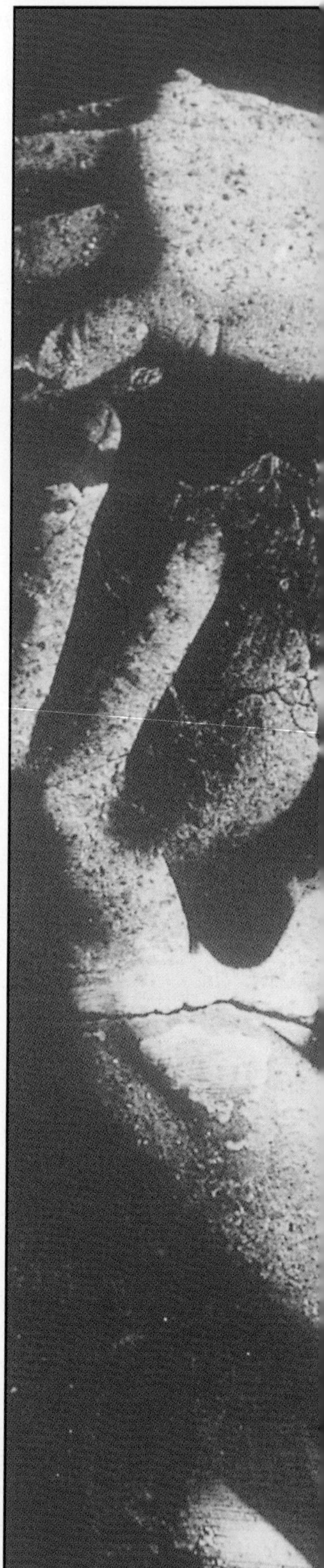

UNRESPONSIVENESS

It is quite possible for a man to have sex with a woman who is unresponsive and unaroused, but it almost certain not to be a fully satisfying experience for either of them. Your partner sees your sexual excitement as a direct response to them and proof that they are desirable and you desire them. 'Frigidity' may sometimes be used as a term of abuse for someone who has failed to respond, implying some permanent sexual deficit. This is rarely the real reason for unresponsiveness.

Occasional unresponsiveness
Your sexual response is very much affected by circumstances. If you are on bad terms with your partner, for example, you won't readily respond sexually – and may feel used and very resentful if they want to have sex to patch up a quarrel without having resolved the issue properly first. Sheer exhaustion can make you unresponsive; too many demands in other areas of your life can leave you with no energy or enthusiasm for sex. A busy couple may have to make sex a priority in their lives and plan for it if their sex life is not to disappear altogether. Lack of privacy or a fear of interruption can make you unresponsive too.

Long-term unresponsiveness
A few people have such a strong and permanent mental resistance to sex that they cannot respond sexually to anyone. In this case, professional therapy will probably be needed to overcome the problem.

More often, however, unresponsiveness develops because of some long-standing problem or disappointment with sex in a relationship, which has made the person 'switch off' sexually. A programme of exercises designed to reawaken your sexual feelings may be helpful, provided you have

See also:
health and hygiene
oral sex
anal sex
sex drive
orgasm
anatomy of sex

the co-operation of a sympathetic partner. If they are to be successful it is important that there should be no unresolved issues between you which may have contributed to the problem in the first place.

Learning to enjoy pleasure

Sexual responsiveness is impossible if you are unconsciously blocking out all sexual feeling. You have to learn to accept and enjoy these feelings, and to begin with it is easier for you to do this if you are under no pressure to have sex. Avoid the genitals and intercourse at first to give you a chance to explore the sensual responses of your whole body. You and your partner simply take turns in caressing and exploring each other's body, focusing on what you feel and enjoying the sensations. Ideally both of you should be naked, and you may want to have a warm bath or shower together first to relax you. Try to practise this exercise for at least two weeks before moving onto the next stage. Sexual responsiveness may develop faster than this: if this happens, let things take off instinctively. However, beware of feeling pressurized into genital contact too early, and retreat from it if either of you feels that you have moved too far too fast.

Genital pleasuring

When you and your partner feel comfortable doing the previous exercise, move on to the next stage of the programme, which involves exploration and caressing of each other's genitals – but still no intercourse. It is important for you to tell your partner when they touch you in a way which feels good. If you feel tense or anxious doing the exercise, erotic fantasies may help to distract you. Although orgasm isn't the aim of the exercise, if either of you do become highly aroused, you can continue stimulation to orgasm. Finally, if you wish, you can move on to having intercourse with your partner. Once again, experiment to discover the movements and positions that produce the most intense sensations before attempting to reach orgasm. It is important to share your feelings and emotions during these experiments.

CONFLICTING SEXUAL TASTES

Very often some new activity or approach to sex can give a real boost to a sexual relationship, and if you both enjoy it, it will strengthen the sexual bond between you. If your partner suggests a new sexual activity that you feel unenthusiastic about, try not to reject it out of hand. Don't think of it as something designed to test you, but as a possible new source of pleasure. Be guided by your own instincts. It's fine occasionally to do something you don't particularly like just to please your partner. But if you really dislike the idea of something, don't do it. And if you try something new and discover that you don't enjoy it, let your partner know how you feel.

SEXUAL GUIDELINES

The rules for any sexual activity should be:

- Don't do it unless you both enjoy it.
- Don't put pressure on each other to do anything that one of you finds distasteful
- Don't do it if it is harmful.
- Practise safer sex to avoid infection.

Oral and anal sex

These are among the most common areas where men's and women's tastes conflict. Men, on the whole, tend to enjoy them more than women. The idea of anal intercourse, especially, arouses strong negative feelings in many women. It can be painful, unless it is performed gently, with plenty of lubricant. There is also a risk of infection being carried by the penis to the vagina unless it is washed well afterwards. Reluctance to try oral sex is also often because it is thought 'dirty'. A person may feel happier about giving it if their partner agrees to withdraw from the mouth before ejaculation, and if only the tip of his penis is taken into the mouth to avoid any fear of choking.

SEX-DRIVE DISCREPANCY

Individual sexual needs vary widely – there is no such thing as a 'normal' sex drive. Sex is not a competitive sport so it doesn't matter how often a couple make love. What may matter is when their needs do not match. If this happens it does not mean that one of you is 'over-sexed' or that the other is 'under-sexed'. A man's sexual drive is at its height in his late teens and twenties. Women usually find their sexual needs increase as they grow sexually more experienced and confident, probably reaching a peak at around forty. In everyone, sexual drive decreases somewhat with age.

BRIDGING A SEX DRIVE GAP

If there is a substantial difference in a couple's sexual appetites, they will need to evolve various strategies to cope with this to minimize tensions in the relationship.

- Masturbation is the most obvious and easiest solution to a sex drive gap.
- When your partner suggests sex and you don't feel like it, don't reject the idea out of hand. Let your partner try to arouse you – stimulation can often sharpen sexual appetite.
- If you are the low-drive partner, make the first move whenever you do feel like sex. Don't feel that this will only encourage your partner to make even more demands on you. Your initiative is more likely to make them feel they can back off a bit.
- Use psychological stimulation – erotic books, videos or magazines – to increase arousal.
- Never use sex as a weapon – either refusing it as punishment, or demanding it when you know your partner is not interested.

MALE SEXUAL PROBLEMS

ERECTION PROBLEMS

Almost every man, at some time or another, has failed to get an erection when he wanted to, or lost it at a critical moment. This can happen because he is tired, or has drunk too much, is not in the mood, or has lost interest in sex or in his partner. Very often, because erection is a reflex process over which a man has very little control, it fails because anxiety interferes with the natural process. Nervousness in a new relationship or guilt in an illicit one can often induce 'performance anxiety'. Occasional failures are quite unimportant – unless they cause anxiety that perpetuates the problem.

Coping with occasional erection failure
Things will improve if you resolve only to have sex when you feel in the right mood and really want to have it. Avoid casual encounters, at least until your sexual confidence improves. You may be less anxious with a partner you know and trust. If you lose your erection, don't overreact, but simply reassure your partner that it is nothing to do with them. Meanwhile, stay close and intimate – there's plenty you can do to give you and your partner sexual pleasure without an erection.

Physical causes of erection problems
Until fairly recently it was thought that erection problems were all in the mind. Now it is recognized that, especially amongst older men, they sometimes have a physical cause. Diseases that affect the blood supply or nerves in the penis can cause erection problems. So too can some drugs and operations. And whatever the cause, anxiety that it might happen again can intensify the problem. If your erection fails frequently, even when you are masturbating, or if you have never at any time had an erection, see your doctor, as there may be a physical cause.

TREATING A LONG TERM ERECTION PROBLEM

Exercises alone

When 'performance anxiety' has built up over a long period, you may lose all confidence in your ability to keep an erection. This exercise is designed to reassure you that even if you lose an erection, gentle stimulation will bring it back.

1. Stimulate your penis by hand until you achieve an erection.
2. Stop the stimulation and let the erection subside completely.
3. Masturbate again until you have a full erection. Then deliberately lose it again.
4. Repeat this a third time, and then ejaculate if you feel like it. Use a lubricant to enhance sensation if it is difficult to regain your erection.
5. Repeat this exercise every day until you feel confident that, at least when you don't have to worry about satisfying a partner, you can achieve an erection, lose it, and then regain it.

Exercises with a partner

Stage one: for this stage of treatment you need your partner to be willing to forego intercourse until you have gained more confidence.

1. Spend time in bed together simply caressing, without worrying about whether or not you get an erection.
2. Let your partner stimulate you manually (or orally) to erection, but not to orgasm.
3. Let the erection die away, then have them stimulate you again. Repeat this until you are confident that you can lose and regain an erection in your partner's presence. Then they can bring you to orgasm.

Practise stage one three or four times a week for three or four weeks, then move on to stage two.

Stage two: the next stage of the exercise is to learn to feel comfortable having intercourse.

1. Your partner caresses your penis till you have a full erection.
2. Your partner then guides your penis inside them. Begin moving gently, but if you feel you are nearing orgasm, withdraw.
3. When you feel you can enjoy just being i nside your partner, start to thrust more v igorously. If you lose your erection, or feel anxious, withdraw so that your partner can again stimulate you manually.
4. As your confidence grows, experiment with other positions. Slow down and just enjoy being contained any time you feel anxious. Ejaculating inside your partner is the final step.

DELAYING EJACULATION

Men often worry because they feel they come too soon. Maybe their partner doesn't always reach orgasm, maybe they feel they would enjoy sex more if only they could hold off a little longer.

Learning to last longer

Make sure your partner is fully aroused before you enter, and during intercourse, try to make less stimulating movements than thrusting. Even simpler is to ejaculate then try again. This time the edge will be off your excitement and you should be able to last longer.

The stop-start technique

Premature ejaculation usually occurs because the man has not learnt to recognize the sensations that lead up to orgasm. In fact, he may even have taught himself to deliberately ignore them, believing that he will have more control if he switches off and thinks about something else during intercourse. Focus on the sensations you feel during masturbation, so that you learn to recognize the point at which orgasm is inevitable. When you feel close to orgasm, stop masturbating, let your arousal die down, then start masturbating again. The aim is to try to stave off ejaculation for about fifteen minutes.

FEMALE SEXUAL PROBLEMS

OVERCOMING FEAR OF PENETRATION

Many women have the expectation that losing their virginity is a painful experience. It need not be. If it is, it is almost certainly because the expectation of fear has made you tighten up and this reaction makes intercourse more difficult. It may even, when a woman's fear is extreme, make it impossible. Nearly all of the fears a woman has about penetration are unfounded. Consult your doctor if intercourse really is painful, because there is nearly always some medical reason for it.

Fears about the hymen

Many women imagine that the hymen forms a complete barrier across their vaginal entrance. In fact it is a thin membrane with an opening through which the menstrual flow can pass. If a woman uses tampons the opening will stretch, and by the time she has vaginal sex, the hymen has usually virtually disappeared. Even if it is still intact, it is nearly always thin and elastic enough to rupture easily without causing much pain or bleeding. In older women the hymen may be less elastic, which may be a problem for the woman who first has sex late in life. Occasionally it may not rupture completely, but leave small strands that can cause pain during vaginal intercourse.

Worries about vaginal size

It's very common to worry that your vagina may be too small. In fact, the vagina is rather like a concertina, with folded, elastic walls lined with ridged and folded skin. Normally the vaginal walls are collapsed in on themselves, with no space between them, but they can stretch as much as necessary, so that the vagina distends and shapes itself to whatever it contains, whether during intercourse or childbirth.

Fear of pain

Intercourse should not be painful. The inner two-thirds of the vagina are sensitive to pressure, but is so insensitive to pain that a minor operation can be carried out in that area without an anaesthetic. If there is some discomfort when your partner enters you, it is probably either because your vaginal entrance has never been stretched by a finger or tampon and is still tight, or there is too little vaginal lubrication because you are not fully aroused. If you stretch your vaginal opening with first one, then two fingers before intercourse begins, and use an artificial lubricant when you make love, there should be no discomfort. In some cases, pain may be caused by a vaginal infection.

Vaginismus

Very rarely a woman has such an intense fear of penetration or even of being touched in the genital area, that the muscles around her vaginal entrance tighten up and make intercourse difficult or impossible. This reaction, which is quite beyond the woman's control, may be the result of a sexually repressive upbringing, or it may develop after some painful or traumatic sexual experience. It is natural for someone who has been hurt to tense up against expected pain, and it is easy for this reaction to become a reflex. The following exercise will show you that penetration need not be painful and your anxiety should disappear.

Overcoming vaginismus

First, examine your genitals with the aid of a hand mirror. Part the inner lips so you can see the vaginal entrance. Touch it gently. Now lubricate a finger and insert just the tip. Bear down as you do this, as though trying to push something out of your vagina. Now push the finger in as far as the first joint, again bearing down. Relax with it inside you. If you feel the urge to tighten up, do so deliberately, tightening around your finger then relaxing again. When you are used to this, go on to insert the whole finger, and, finally, two fingers. Use plenty of lubrication and progress gradually, pushing the fingers in a little further each time you do the exercise.

ACHIEVING ORGASM

Understanding orgasm
Orgasm is a reflex reaction, and like any reflex it can be inhibited, and its intensity will vary according to your psychological state. It is usually triggered by contractions of the clitoris and felt as a series of intense pulsations within the vagina. Nearly every woman can reach orgasm through stimulation of the clitoris alone, and very few can reach it with no clitoral stimulation.

Faking orgasm
A great many women find it much easier to fake orgasms than to admit that they do not have them. They may feel sexually inadequate if they had to admit it, or they may be protecting their partner's ego. If you want things to change, you need to develop your own responses through masturbation, or if you have orgasms alone only, ask your partner's help and tell them what you need.

Learning to let go
Orgasm depends on your ability to 'let go', to relax and let sensations take you over. Tiredness, anxiety and tension can all make it more difficult for you to concentrate on your own feelings and reach orgasm. Feelings of resentment or anger towards your partner that make you hold back emotionally and inhibit your sexual responsiveness, can make it almost impossible. There are other emotional obstacles to orgasm, for example negative feelings about sex and, for some women, a fear of losing control. If you are the kind of person who likes to stay in control of yourself and your emotions, the idea of being carried away by orgasm can seem very frightening.

The right mood for orgasm
If you are in the right frame of mind, orgasm is much easier to reach. Give yourself time and privacy so that you are not rushed or worried about being interrupted. Try not to discuss worries, or topics that usually cause friction, before having sex. If you are feeling tense, relaxation exercises may help.

Avoiding tension
Tension, often quite unconscious, is a common cause of a woman's failure to reach orgasm. Deep breathing exercises can help to overcome this. Practise taking slow, deep breaths, letting each one out slowly as a deep sigh, without forcing it. When you have practised this so often that it begins to feel natural, try doing it during masturbation. It will stop you holding your breath and tensing your muscles, and make you more likely to enjoy your sensations.

Fantasy and masturbation
If erotic fantasies have always helped you reach orgasm when you masturbate, they will probably do so during intercourse. Try making your partner the central figure in your masturbation fantasies, and then begin to carry these over into intercourse. This may make you more sexually responsive to your partner.

Experimenting with positions
It is worth experimenting to find a sexual position in which orgasm is easier – for many women being on top is effective because it enables them to have some control over the movement. For some women, stimulation of a small pressure-sensitive area about half way up the front wall of the vagina – known as the G-spot – produces very intense sensations which may trigger orgasm. You may need to experiment with your partner to find this G-spot and the kind of stimulation that works best for you.

The 'bridge' technique
If you are not having orgasms during heterosexual intercourse, but you can reach orgasm when you masturbate, direct stimulation of the clitoris by your partner during intercourse may be enough to tip you over into orgasm.

A variation of this is the 'bridge' technique. This method requires that either you or your partner stimulate your clitoris till you are close to orgasm while his penis is inside you. Then penile thrusting gives the final trigger.

4

SEX & CULTURE

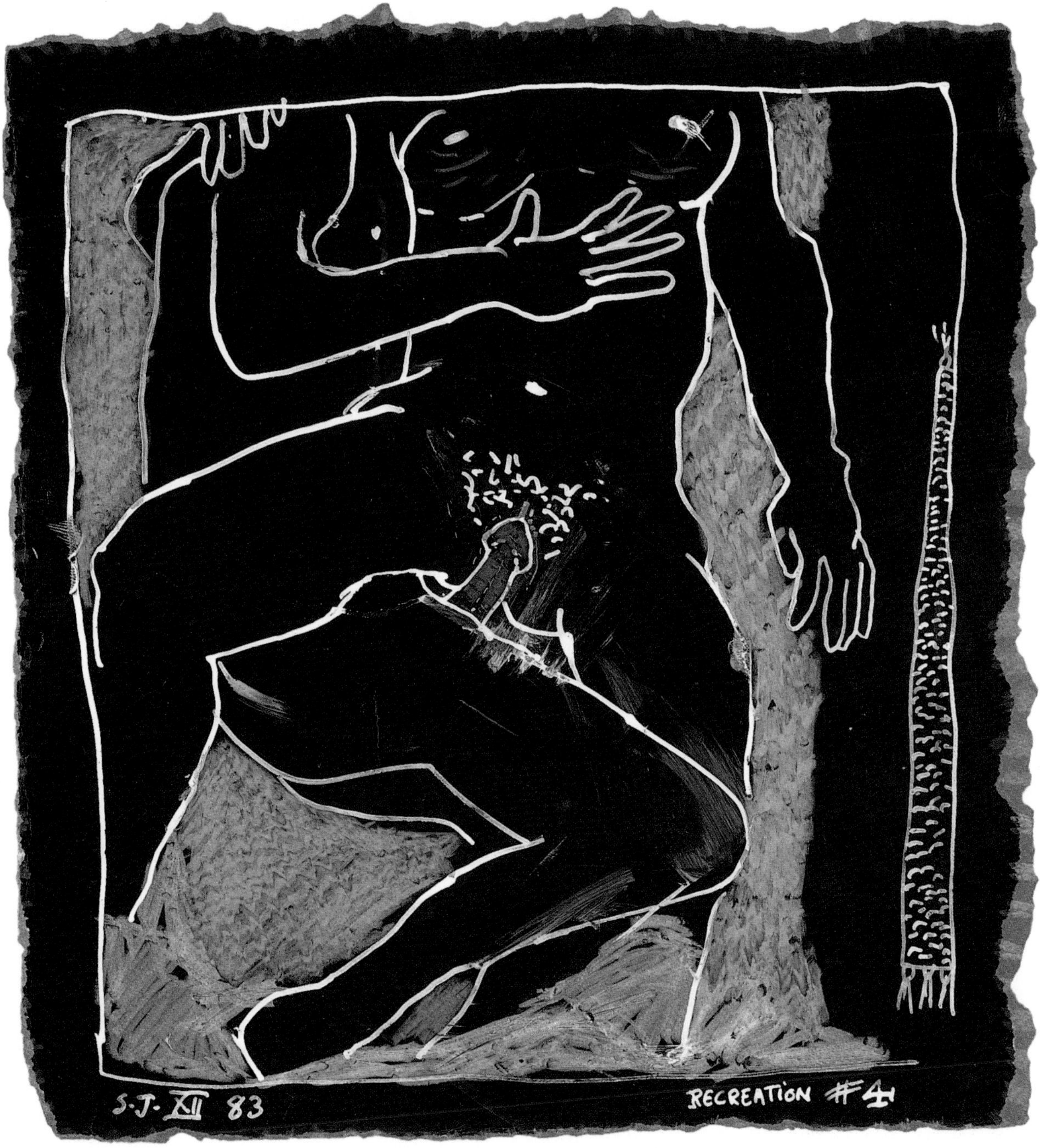
S-J-XII 83
RECREATION #4

SEX THROUGH THE AGES

Where sex is concerned, there is nothing new under the sun. Every sexual act, every sensation, every emotion has been experienced by millions of people since the world began.

Some 5000 years ago, disciplining sexual relationships was one of the most fundamental and reliable ways of disciplining people. This was important in the early days of civilization: a stable society could not exist without rules. Initially, the state's interference in sexual matters was limited to areas of public concern – legitimacy, inheritance, and population control – and this was as true in China and India as in the ancient Near East.

Religion brought about a change. In religions that had many gods, those gods were rarely in total agreement about what was right and what was wrong. It was only when the idea of 'one god' emerged that ideas of absolute right and absolute wrong became entrenched, so that religious morality and secular law became inseparable. This was what happened to the ancient Hebrew society. Like every other tribe of the Near East, the Hebrews needed to increase their numbers for their own security. Since the Lord also required them to 'Be fruitful and multiply' (*Genesis* 1:22), the laws they passed to help them achieve this end took on the sanctity of Holy Writ. When they banned all forms of unproductive sex, the ban had the force of religious, as well as social, law. The result was that when Judaism, and later Christianity, developed, the basically practical bans imposed for a specific purpose at a specific point in time, were carried forward through the centuries as part of a religious package. That is why, until only a few decades ago (until today, in the case of the Vatican), contraception was regarded as morally wrong; homosexuality as unnatural; masturbation as a sin.

It is salutary to remember that even today's most emancipated lovers are still, to some extent, conforming to – or breaking – rules laid down thousands of years ago for reasons that had very little to do with the most intimate and personal of human encounters.

Nothing new under the sexual sun...

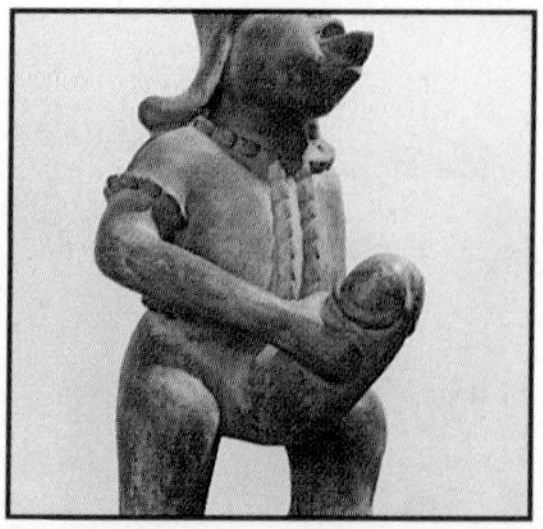

...masturbation

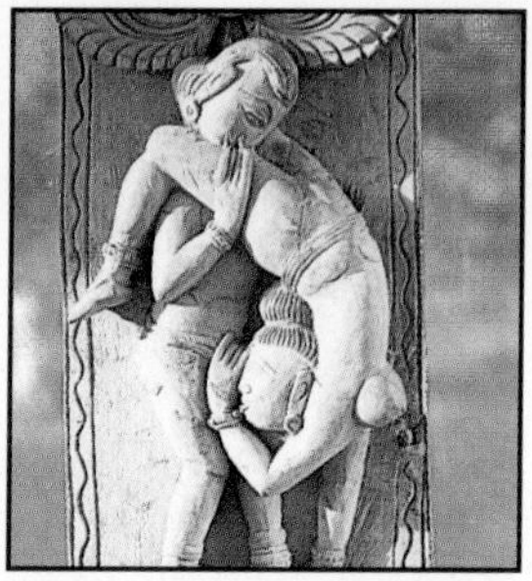

...69 / *soixante-neuf*

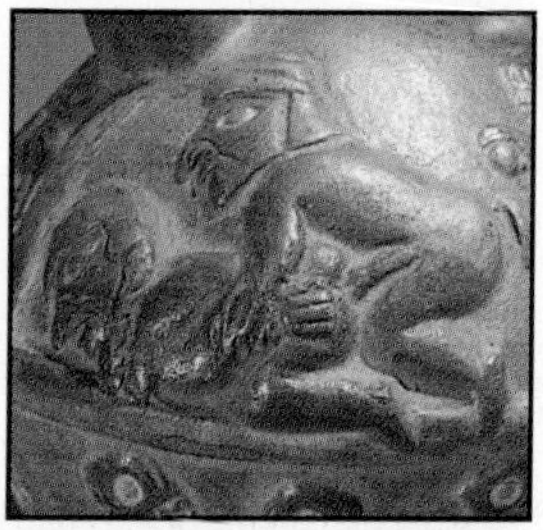

...anal sex

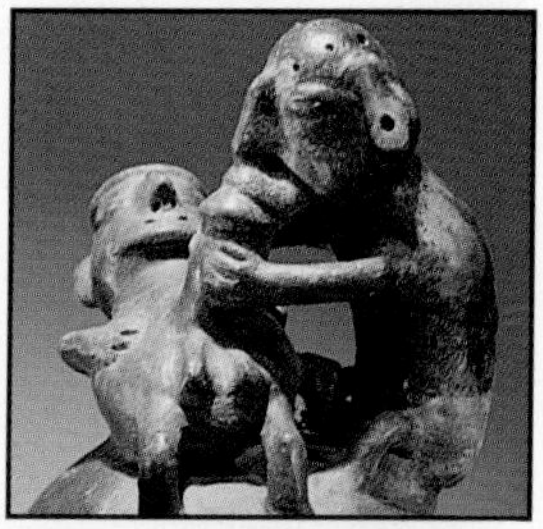

...homosexual fellatio

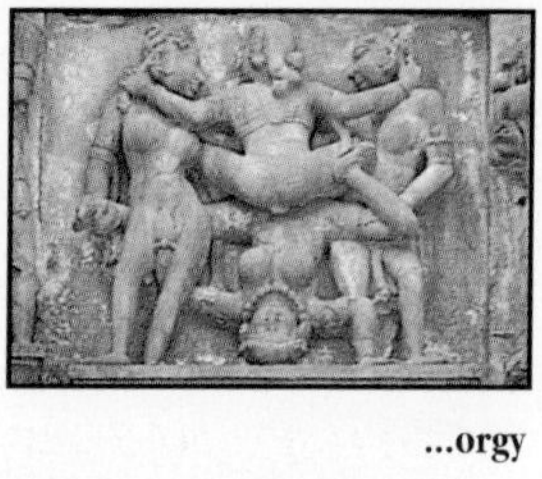

...orgy

BEFORE RECORDS EXIST

Before recorded history, men and women seem to have been more or less equal. In the thousands of years leading up to the Neolithic revolution – between about 10,000 BC and 3000 BC – man had been the hunter, and woman the gatherer of plants and small, living edibles such as snails, turtles and crabs. Location and climatic conditions dictated whose contribution to the food supply – and therefore whose tribal status – was superior at a given time.

It was the woman who gave birth to children, of course, but there is no evidence to suggest that prehistoric human beings knew anything about the biological role of the father. This was a role that could not easily be deduced from the communal pattern of everyday cave living, when the only calendar was the moon, and nine months in relation to life expectancy almost as long as two years today. It was a simple fact of life that the human female, like the wild mare or the reindeer cow, should be either pregnant or nursing for most of her adult years; it was natural for man and woman, stag and hind, ram and ewe, to enjoy the act of sex without seeing in it anything but the physical fulfilment of the moment.

Then came the neolithic revolution, when the sheep and the goat, the cow and then the pig, were tamed and brought into the farmyard; when man no longer had to hunt them but instead watched over them anxiously, waiting for them to drop the lambs or kids that would increase or replenish the flocks, the same individual animals day after day, all year round. Now, for the first time in human history, man had the opportunity to sit and observe closely, to think and to make connections.

What must have been traumatic was not only the discovery of the male contribution to procreation, but its potential scale. A single ram could impregnate over fifty ewes.

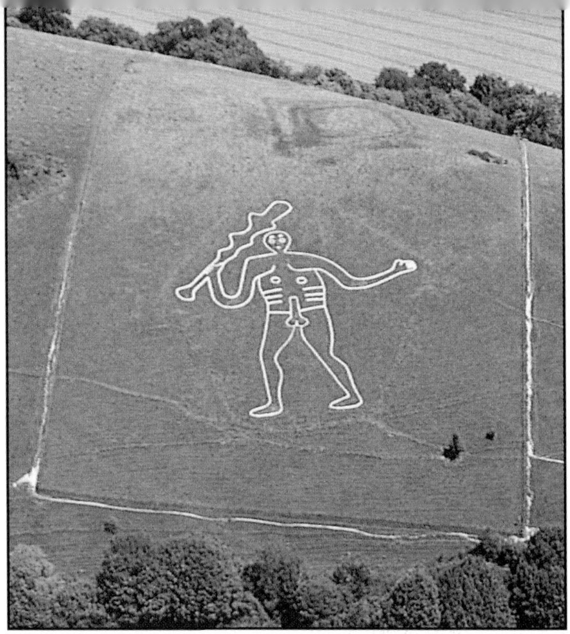

The Cerne Abbas Giant, Dorset UK.

With comparable power, what could man not achieve?

The men who emerged from the Neolithic era into the period of recorded history were very different from those who had gone before, those who had believed woman to be the creative force. There may have been other reasons for this change – archaeology offers no answers to what went on in the prehistoric mind – but these new men had the kind of assurance, arrogance and authority that spring not from useful toil nor knowledge of a good job well done, but from the kind of revelation – beyond argument, beyond questioning – that makes men feel like gods.

It was now possible for a man to look at a child and call him 'my son'; to look at a woman and call her 'my wife'. By Biblical times, when civilization had developed and it had become necessary to make laws, and to write them down and enforce them, those laws made it clear that even the 'free' woman, whether she was Egyptian, Babylonian or Hebrew, was little more than a slave, the property of her father during childhood and of her husband from adolescence on. It was a situation that was to persist throughout the world almost until the twentieth century.

SEX AND THE HEBREWS

Virtually all the Hebrew laws on marital fidelity, legitimacy, incest and prostitution were designed to satisfy the requirements of fertility. By the first century BC, it could be said that, 'The law recognizes no sexual connections except the natural union of husband and wife, and that only for the procreation of children.' (Josephus, quoted in S.W. Baron, A Social and Religious History of the Jews *(1967) vol. II, p. 219).*

Prostitution was practised in the Near East and there were even 'male cult prostitutes' in early Judah, but as time passed the Jews came to hate prostitutes with a feeling that was at best intemperate, at worst obscene. The problem, of course, was that, when a woman slept with many men, no man could lay claim to her sons.

There were numerous measures designed to reinforce the principle, and they were accompanied by thundering denunciation of all kinds of non-productive sex. In Babylon, homosexuality was perfectly acceptable, but the Lord had told the children of Israel, 'If a man lies with a male as with a woman, both of them have committed an abomination; they shall be put to death, their blood is upon them.' And, without any perceptible change of tone, 'If a man lies with a beast, he shall be put to death; and you shall kill the beast. If a woman approaches any beast and lies with it, you shall kill the woman and the beast' (*Leviticus* 20:13, 15–16).

Viewed from the perspective of fertility, abortion was also considered a crime and contraception a sin against holy writ. To strike a pregnant woman might bring anything from a simple fine to a 'life for life, eye for eye, tooth for tooth' (*Exodus* 21:22–24).

As in most societies, all Hebrew law had logical beginnings. But in most societies, the laws are amended to suit changing times. Hebrew law, however, could not change since it was divinely inspired and therefore not open to amendment. As a result, as the centuries passed and Christianity emerged from Judaism, the ancient taboos were transmitted to the Western world in the form of articles of faith.

A Jewish wedding in Portugal, from an eighteenth century engraving.

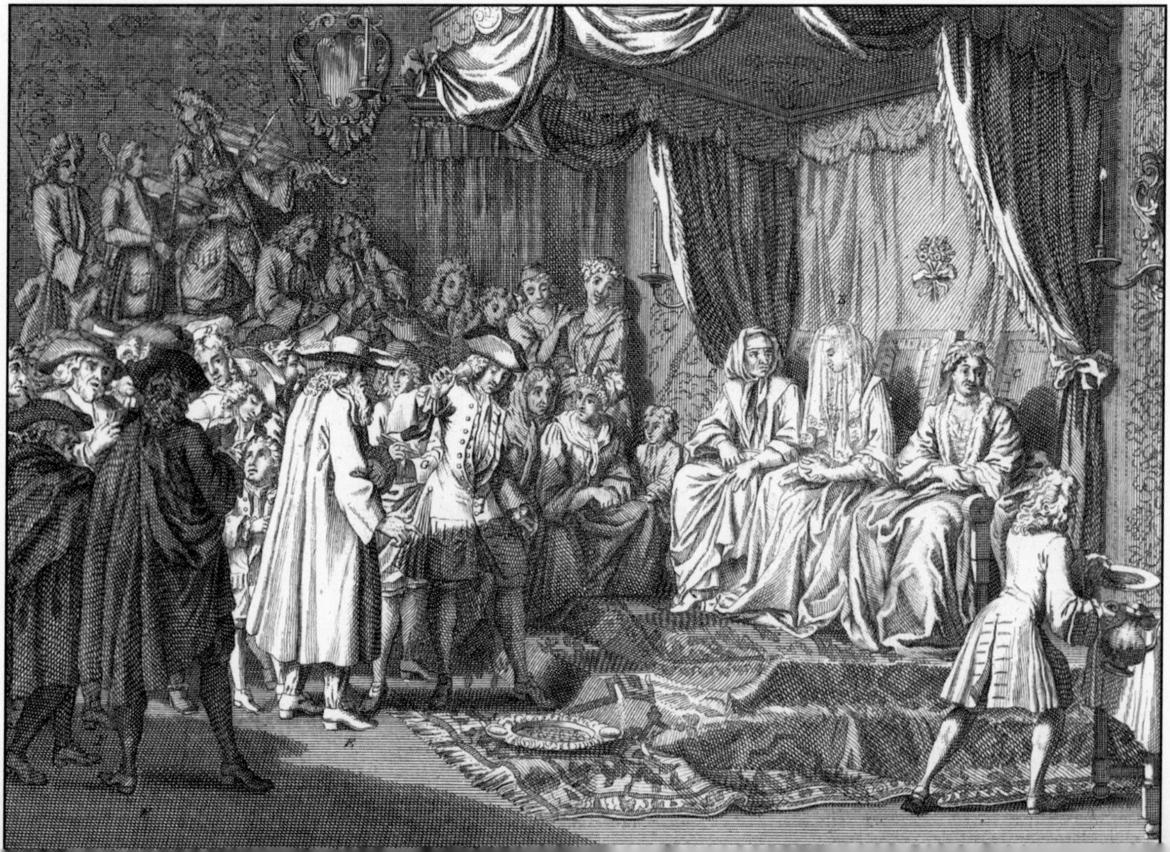

‘A good wife who can find?’ asked the Book of Proverbs 3000 years ago (*Proverbs* 31:10ff), and, given what the men of the Near East expected of ‘a good wife’, it was an understandable question.

What they did not require were beauty, charm or sexuality. Beauty was vain, charm deceitful and sexuality actively dangerous. What they wanted was fruitfulness. ‘Like arrows in the hand of a warrior are the sons of one’s youth. Happy is the man who has his quiver full of them!’ (*Psalms* 127:4–5). In addition to ensuring the succession, a wife’s duties included seeking wool and flax and food, rising before dawn to care for her family and instruct her servants, buying fields and planting vineyards, keeping accounts, helping the needy, spinning, weaving and clothing her household in scarlet and herself in linen and purple, making and selling linen garments, working late into the night when the need arose. In addition, said the Book of Proverbs, she had to look on the future with optimism and to be unfailingly wise, kind and conscientious.

As a reward, she was entitled to share her husband’s favour with his secondary wives and concubines. Most Hebrews had several of these, although none approached the record of King Solomon, who ruled from c.955 to 935 BC and was said to have had 700 wives and 300 concubines. In Babylon, by contrast, a man was not allowed to have more than one fully accredited wife at a time, though he might have any number of concubines; if his legal wife turned out to be barren, it was up to her to supply him with a substitute childbearer.

Like the ‘good wives’ of Egypt and Babylon, the Hebrew wife could also look forward to being divorced out of hand if she offended her husband. And she could be stoned to death if she was even suspected of taking a lover.

In every way that counted, all were unequivocally inferior to their husbands.

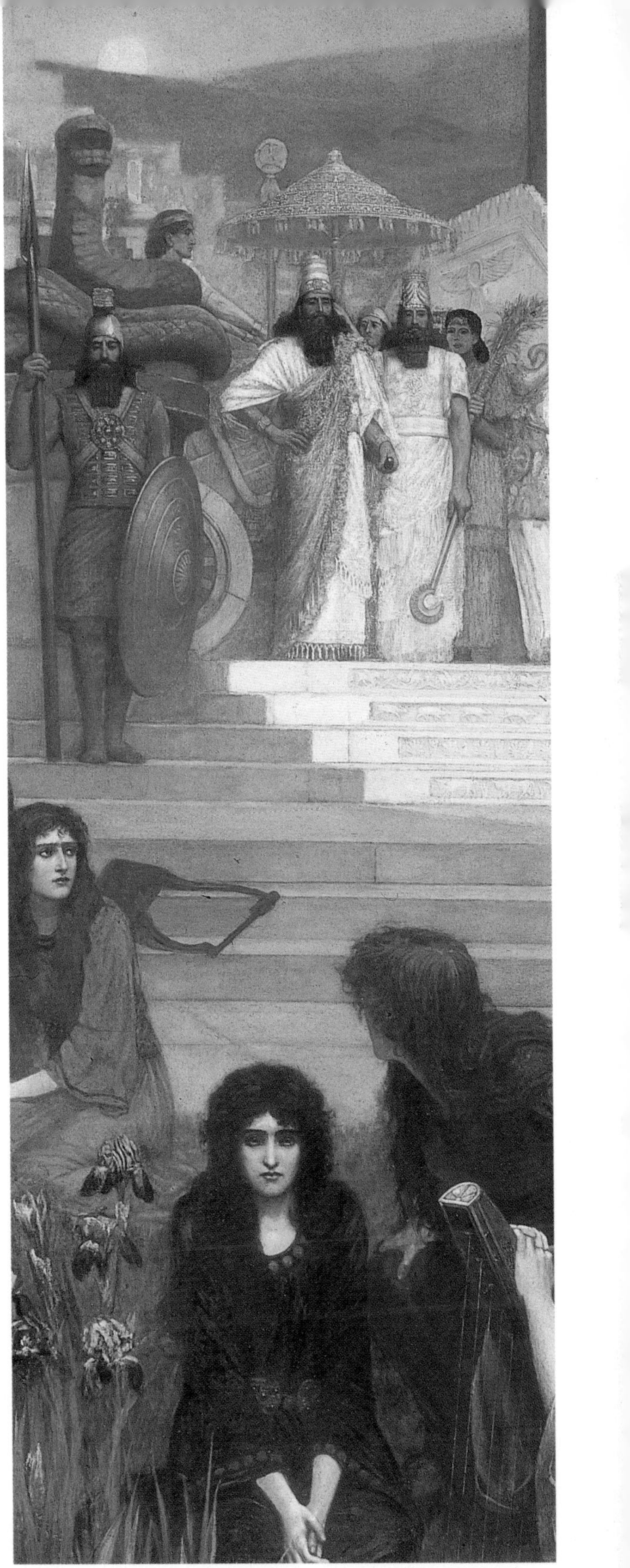

The Daughters of Judah in Babylon (detail), by Herbert Gustave Schmalz (nineteenth century).

SEX AND THE GREEKS

The Athenians, almost contemporaries of the Hebrews, had different problems. Athens was over-, rather than under-, populated, and more concerned with discouraging than encouraging fertility. It did this less by discriminatory legislation than by attitudes of mind.

One of the most noticeable traits of sexual life in Athens from the sixth to the fourth centuries BC was the Athenians' dislike of women, whom they regarded as irrational, oversexed and morally defective. Many Athenians would have preferred not to marry at all but, as the poet Hesiod put it, 'He who evades, by refusing marriage, the miseries that women bring upon us, will have no support [children] in the wretchedness of his old age....On the other hand, he whose fate it is to marry may perhaps find a good and sensible wife. But even then he will see evil outweigh good all his life.' (Hesiod, *Theogeny* 585–612)

In such a climate, it was hardly surprising that women had no more civil or political rights than slaves, having to submit throughout their lives to the absolute authority of their nearest male relative. A woman received little serious education and spent her days in the women's quarters; she rarely ate with her husband and never when he had guests. If it was necessary to beget an heir in a hurry, she was expected to have intercourse with him at least three times a month until she became pregnant. A husband could repudiate his wife with the greatest of ease, and was legally obliged to do so if, by some miracle of ingenuity, she contrived to commit adultery.

Toward the end of the fourth century BC, however, and with more conviction in the third, Athenian men began to rediscover an interest in women, though not in wives, and turned instead to *hetairai*, or courtesans. 'We have *hetairai* for our pleasure,' said one statesman, 'concubines for our daily needs, and wives to give us legitimate children and look after the housekeeping.' (Demosthenes (attr.) in *Nearam* 122)

One of the special charms of the *hetairai* was that they excelled in all the things the Athenians had spent centuries in preventing their wives from learning about: not only sex but also culture, literature, art and politics. The *hetairai* were successful women in a man's world and that was to be true of their successors, worldwide, for most of the next 2000 years. Courtesans have always had a better time than wives.

The well-educated Greek male found the company of adolescent boys much more to his taste. This was a socially acceptable preference during the two centuries when pederasty flourished, since the Greeks sturdily maintained that it was a branch of higher education, with an older man making himself responsible for his protégé's moral and intellectual development. Such relationships had three virtues in Greek eyes: they helped to channel and control the homosexual phase common in adolescent boys the world over; they gave grown men experience of the tenderness that they rarely found within the matrimonial home; and they delayed the time when younger partners began to think of marriage and making their own contributions to the overpopulated state. Scholars cannot agree whether this 'pure love' was, or was not, wholly spiritual but all the indications are that, as with the Courtly Love of later times, Greek pederasty was one of those sentimental ideals that are pure in theory but a good deal less so in practice.

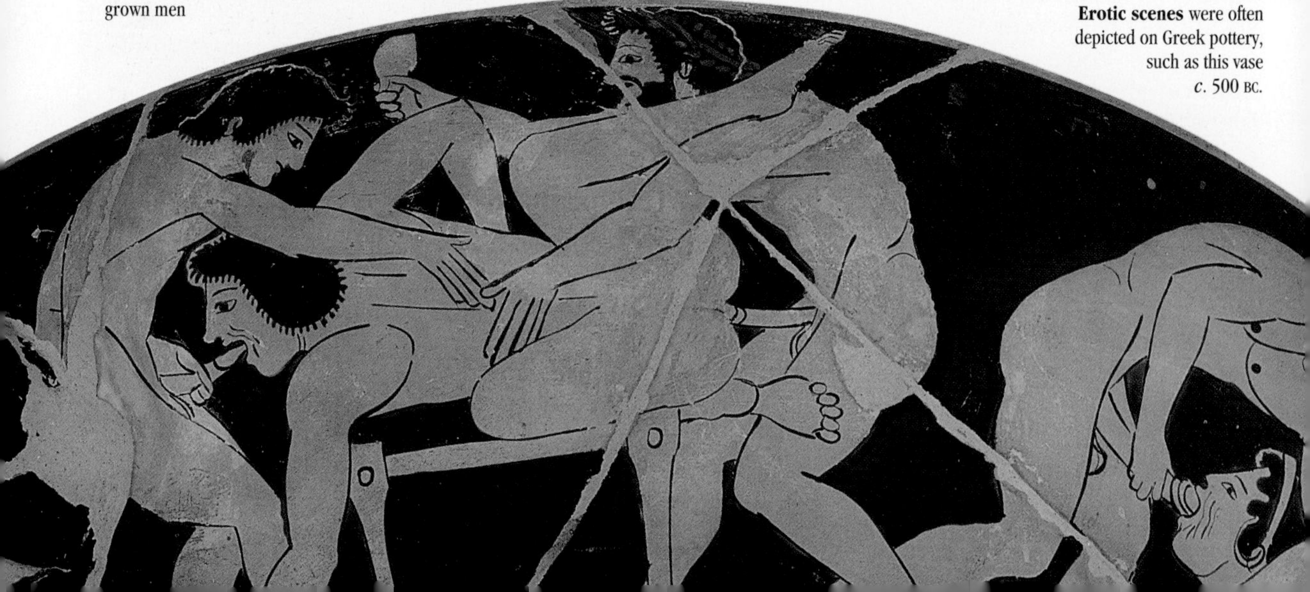

Erotic scenes were often depicted on Greek pottery, such as this vase *c.* 500 BC.

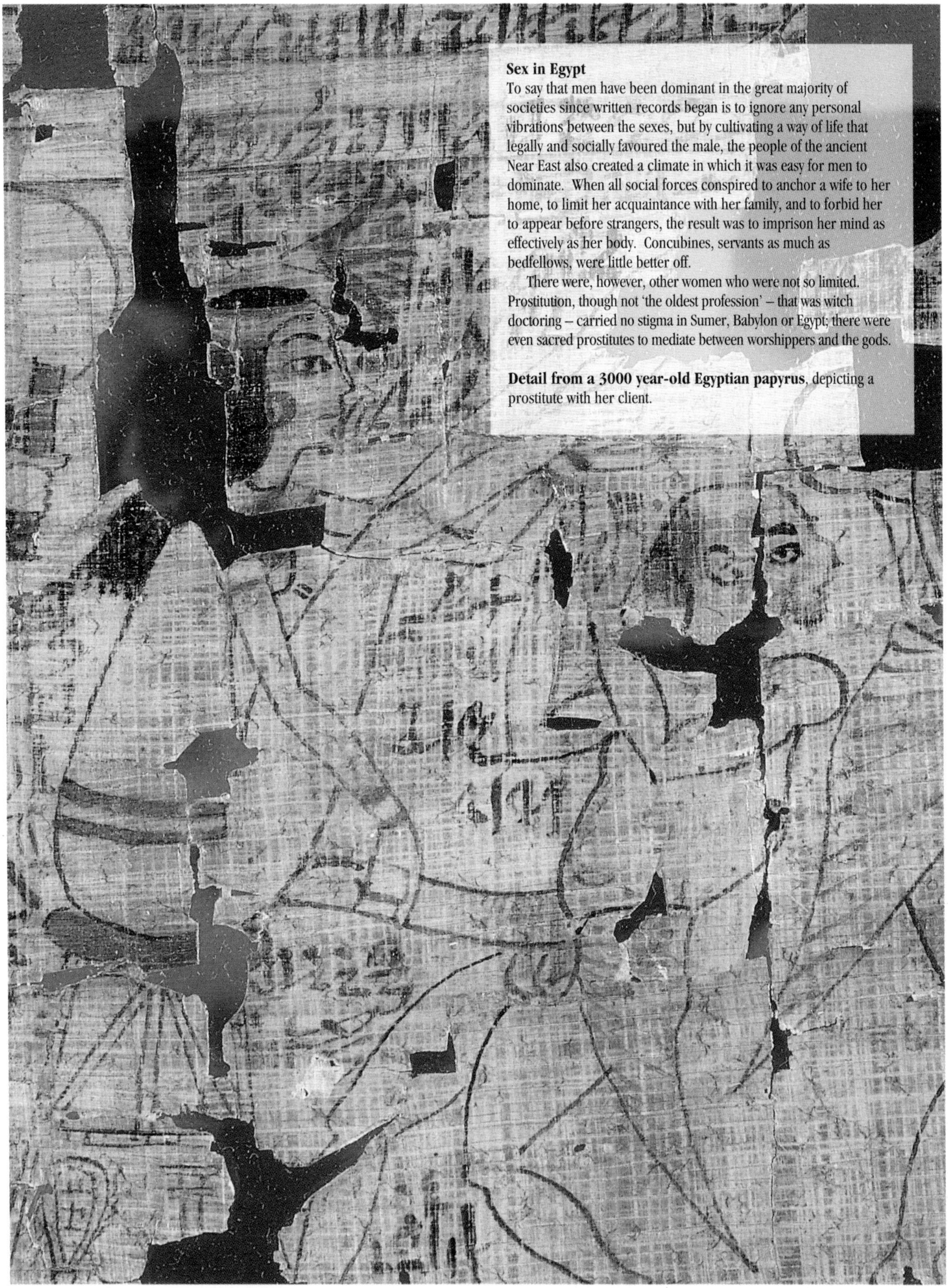

Sex in Egypt

To say that men have been dominant in the great majority of societies since written records began is to ignore any personal vibrations between the sexes, but by cultivating a way of life that legally and socially favoured the male, the people of the ancient Near East also created a climate in which it was easy for men to dominate. When all social forces conspired to anchor a wife to her home, to limit her acquaintance with her family, and to forbid her to appear before strangers, the result was to imprison her mind as effectively as her body. Concubines, servants as much as bedfellows, were little better off.

There were, however, other women who were not so limited. Prostitution, though not 'the oldest profession' – that was witch doctoring – carried no stigma in Sumer, Babylon or Egypt; there were even sacred prostitutes to mediate between worshippers and the gods.

Detail from a 3000 year-old Egyptian papyrus, depicting a prostitute with her client.

SEX AND THE ROMANS

Ironically, it was the success of the hetairai *in Greece that encouraged wives in Rome to take a hand in their own emancipation. Facing the same generalized dislike on the part of their menfolk as the* hetairai *had overcome in Athens, they had, however, neither the inclination nor the talents to use sex as a means to their own ends. They chose instead to declare war, turning themselves into perhaps the most obstreperous group of women in all history.*

Rootless and restless, the women of Rome's upper classes had a freedom rare in the ancient world, but which was also of little use to them. They were permitted to do a great deal as long as they did nothing constructive. Legal disabilities and social pressures combined to build round them a kind of intellectual rampart within which they could think and act almost as they wished. But they could not break it, in case they tried to influence others, to trespass on man's preserves, even – unthinkably – to shape the political and imperial policies of Rome itself. They contented themselves, therefore, with spending money, beautifying themselves (not for their husbands but for their lovers), taking to one of the fashionable new religions, or suing for divorce.

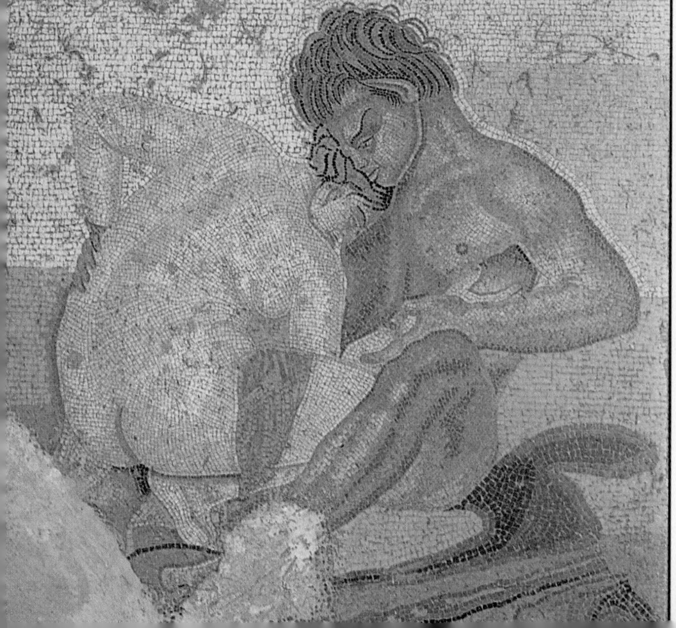

'Her score is mounting,' remarked the poet Juvenal sourly of the dashing divorcee of his day. 'She has had eight husbands in five winters. Write that on her tombstone!' (Juvenal, *Sixth Satire*, 227–8).

The Roman wife's right to part from her husband, unmatched in the ancient world, was not the product of considered legislation but had evolved from the fact that Rome recognized three types of marriage: the grand, ceremonial one; the simpler, civil ceremony; and marriage by *usus* or simple cohabitation. After a year of living together in continuous association the couple legally became husband and wife, the woman only then ceasing to be a member of her father's family and entering into that of her husband.

There was a loophole that proved large enough for independence to slip through. To the literal Roman mind, 'continuous association' meant precisely that; if a woman absented herself from her common-law husband's house for three successive days and nights the qualifying period had to begin all over again. With careful timing and a little ingenuity, a woman could postpone almost indefinitely the moment when she became legally subject to her husband instead of to her more sympathetic father. It suited the wife, and it suited her father, too, because for as long as his daughter remained 'in his hand', he also retained control over her assets and was able to reclaim a substantial portion of her dowry if the marriage failed. To the property-conscious Roman, the temptation was irresistible.

There is little doubt that many well-educated, intelligent, bored women did run wild, and the question is why, in a society that was essentially masculine, were they allowed to get away with so much for so long? Perhaps the main reason was that there were not enough women to go round. Rome, like most of the ancient world, was obsessed with sons. Girls were a burden, and the fate of all too many girl children was infanticide. It was a shortsighted policy, since it meant that the competition for wives was stiff. A man attracted to marriage by the prospect not only of a son and heir but a useful transfusion of money in the form of the dowry, was forced to recognize that, no matter how he subsequently felt about his wife, if he wanted to keep the dowry the only sure way of doing so was by keeping her too.

Where children were concerned, the economical Roman husband had no desire for more than two or perhaps three. There was plenty of contraceptive advice available for those who wanted it, but in view of the general tenor of relationships between husbands and wives, it is possible that the most widely used form was the simplest and most reliable of all – abstention. As the centuries passed, the birth rate among citizens fell and continued to fall to such a dangerous level that it became necessary for the Senate to pass laws designed to stabilize family life and fertility.

They had no effect. The Romans' failure to raise families had as much to do with involuntary as with voluntary factors. Mortality rates were high and childbearing years correspondingly few. Most Romans, like the people of the Palaeolithic era, could expect to die before they reached the age of thirty. Ten per cent of the population of Italy was crammed into Rome itself, helpless prey for any marauding virus. Even when a woman did conceive, she frequently suffered miscarriage, difficulties at parturition or postnatal infections.

There were also other, invisible hazards directly related to sterility and/or impotence THAT, ironically enough, affected not the poor but the free-living rich, who almost certainly suffered from chronic lead poisoning, which can cause sterility in men and bring about miscarriages and stillbirths among women. The Romans absorbed lead from the water that ran through their lead pipes, from cups and cooking pots, from cosmetics such as the white lead women used for face powder, and from their wine, which was often sweetened with a grape syrup boiled down in lead-lined pots.

They drank a lot of wine but almost certainly to no avail since alcohol may increase sexual desire but detracts from

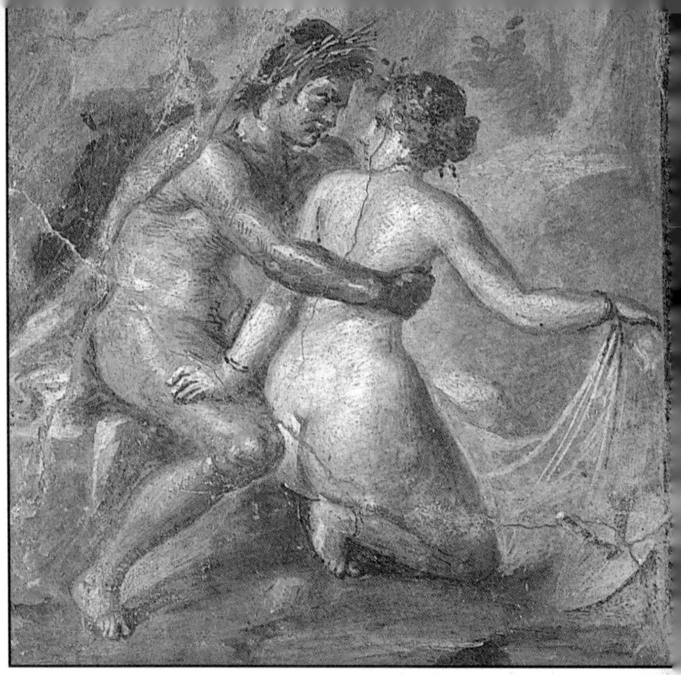

Above and left: **Erotic scenes from Pompeian wall paintings.**

sexual performance. Scientists today have shown that excessive alcohol also has a direct toxic effect on the testes, bringing about a substantial decline in secretion of the male sex hormone, testosterone.

That was not all. Every time a Roman went to the public baths (which he did daily) he further endangered his sex life and his fertility. The water at the baths was sometimes so hot, said Seneca, that one would scarcely condemn an erring slave to be washed alive in it. The normal temperature of the testicles is lower than that of the rest of the body, and modern research shows that a temperature raised only to normal body temperature (36.9°C or 98.6°F) is enough to inhibit sperm production. (Long cold baths rather than long hot ones can double an infertile patient's sperm production in a matter of two to three weeks.)

Too much wine, too many hot baths, unsatisfactory and unproductive sex...these are not usually considered factors that might bring down an empire. But it was shortage of manpower that, combined with a devalued currency, opened the gates of Rome to the barbarians and destroyed what had once been the most elegant and logical political edifice yet devised by humankind.

SEX AND THE CHINESE

In Asia, as in the West, society was male dominated. Here, too, man was concerned with fertility but, instead of discouraging any sexual practices that might interfere with it, he took the more constructive approach of actively encouraging those that might promote it. Sex was part of the pattern of life, and – in its perfected form – made a contribution to the expansion of the spirit.

In China, the philosophy of Taoism held that long life and happiness depended on living in perfect harmony with nature by balancing – in the individual as in the cosmos – the complementary forces of yin (yielding) and yang (thrusting). Taoism held that humanity had been led away from the natural path by its concentration on mind and will, and the disciplines that led back to it were necessarily disciplines of the body.

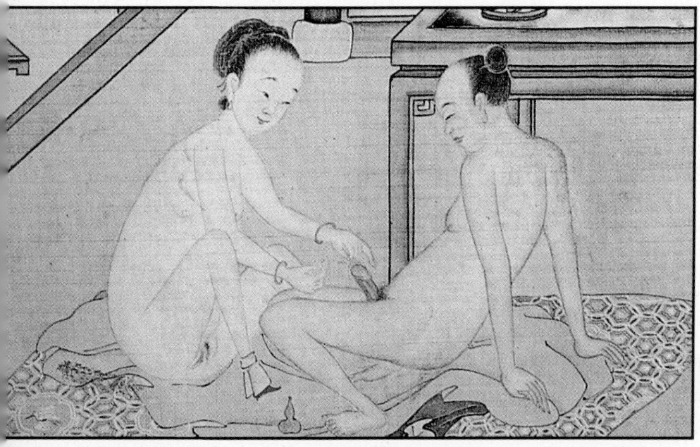

The Chinese actively encouraged sexual practices to promote fertility. Here, a young wife or concubine stimulates her lover's penis with a feather to develop or prolong his erection.

Sexual intercourse was the human equivalent of interaction between yin and yang, even though the parallels were drawn not in the direct fleshly sense of vagina and penis, but more subtly as yin essence (the moisture lubricating a woman's sexual organs) and yang essence (man's semen). These were interdependent; to absorb yin was to strengthen yang.

Since intercourse was one of the main highways to heaven, there was good and valid reason to offer guidance to travellers. The Chinese did so in the world's earliest (dating from about 200 BC onward), most comprehensive and most detailed sex manuals, which were intended as much for women as men and, indeed, often given to a bride before her wedding. They covered every aspect of the subject and proved that here, as in many other areas of human life and experience, the modern world has little to teach the ancients.

A woman's yin essence was believed to be inexhaustible, whereas man's yang essence was limited in quantity and precious: it had to be regularly strengthened by a woman's yin and was on no account to be squandered. The average man was recommended to allow himself a climax not more than once every three days in spring; twice a month in summer; never in winter.

There were special yin-yang rules to be followed when a man wished to father a child. His yang essence had to be at peak potency, built up over a number of sexual encounters without ejaculating until the final, all-important occasion. The handbooks emphasized that the preliminary yin nourishment should come from several different women. 'If in one night he can have intercourse with more than ten women it is best.' (Yu-fang-pi-chueh, *I-shin-po* 28 XIX) It was essential that he aroused each and every one of them to orgasm, when a woman's essence reached maximum potency. To the Chinese, uniquely, a woman's orgasm was as important to her male partner as to herself.

Unsurprisingly, perhaps, in view of all the sexual activity required of a man, aphrodisiacs were much in demand, notably the 'bald chicken drug' and the 'deer horn potion'. And the brothel trade flourished to service those polygamous husbands who were unable to afford more than half a dozen wives. The 'green bowers', however – havens of calm and relaxation, of good food and entertaining company – served another purpose. The conscientious Chinese husband very often went to them, not for sexual intercourse but to escape from it.

SEX IN THE ISLAMIC WORLD

The Chinese, until flexible Taoism gave way to straitlaced neo-Confucianism in the later Middle Ages, rejoiced in as many wives and concubines as they could afford. In India, too, polygamy was practised, though mainly by the rich. But it was the caliphs and, later, sultans of the Muslim world who were to supply the West with the most enduringly exotic of the Arabian Nights dreams – the harem.

In the seventh century AD, the Prophet Muhammad preached a visionary, composite of Arab, Jewish and Christian beliefs, that brought unprecedented unity to the nomadic peoples of the arid peninsula between the Red Sea and the Persian Gulf. Within thirty years, the armies of the Prophet had conquered not only much of the Mediterranean coast of Africa but all Persia, too. From desert Arabs to rulers of one of the most sophisticated empires the world had ever seen, this was an enormous step in little more than a generation. From both choice and necessity, the Arabs adopted many of the customs of their predecessors and also of the empire of Byzantium, their cultured (and hated) new neighbour.

The Byzantine habit of keeping women veiled and segregated, imported into polygamous Islam, overturned the Prophet's original desire to improve the lot of women, and made them virtual prisoners. Soon, polite society knew only two kinds of women: the courtesan, usually a singer, usually a foreigner, witty, beautiful, talented and inconstant; and the respectable lady, visible in public as no more than a pair of downcast eyes in a sea of black draperies.

Although such a situation sounded the death knell of romantic love, it had the opposite effect as far as the *idea* of romantic love was concerned. The Arabs had a strongly poetic streak and there soon developed an idea of 'pure love' that turned segregation into a positive benefit. The real woman within the robes, within the prison of her harem, scarcely mattered. To the poet she was a creature of the imagination, untouchable, unreachable, a dream. Her (enforced) chastity became so important in the idea of 'pure love' that it would have been a betrayal for the lover to satisfy his passion, even if he could.

In truth, if there had been the remotest likelihood of the opportunity arising, the whole concept of 'pure love' would have collapsed. It was, in effect, a masculine game, designed to satisfy intellectualized masculine emotions, but it came to be seen as something ennobling, a love that was a creative, spiritual source of inspiration. By one of the more entertaining quirks of history, it was a dream that was to be imported, somewhat amended, into the West during the later centuries of the Middle Ages, with very odd results.

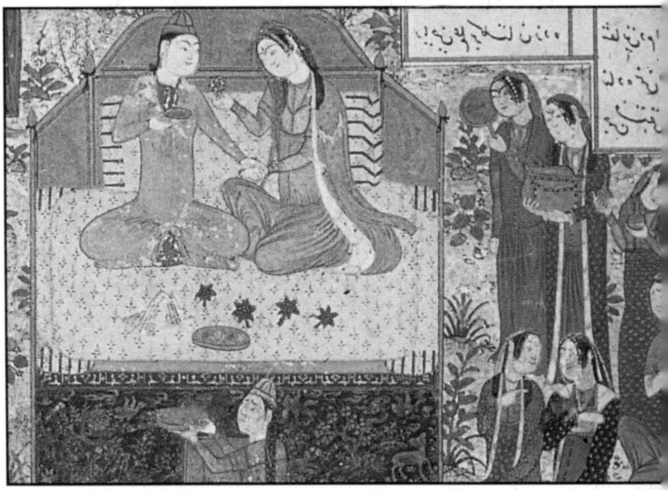

Humay and Humayan (detail), from the *Shahname* (1396), a Persian literary text.

A vision of the harem was also imported into the West by returning pilgrims and Crusaders. This was another kind of dream, a dream of perfumed air, tinkling fountains, soft music, seductive and submissive beauties, idyllic sex – and it resembled the real thing not at all. This time, it was a dream that was to remain a dream, wistfully cherished by northern knights bound by the chill fetters of their own loveless and monogamous marriages.

SEX IN INDIA

India, like China but unlike the West, recognized that pleasure was important to the human spirit. Indeed, the Hindu ethos identified it as one of the 'four aims' in life, integrally related to the concept of correct behaviour. Success in the first three – morality, material wellbeing and pleasure – was believed to advance the individual toward the fourth and ultimate goal, release from the cycle of rebirth.

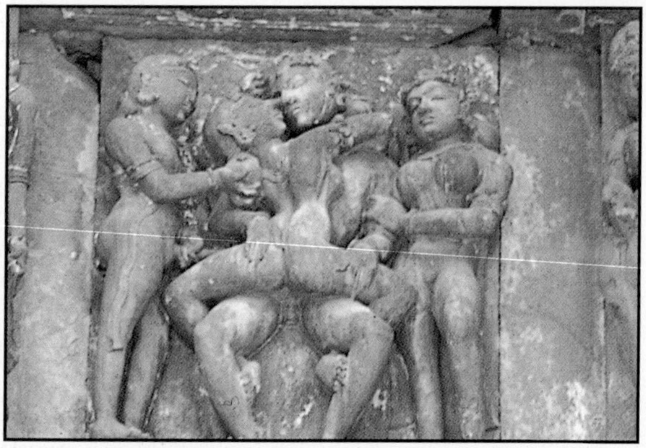

Erotic carvings cover the surviving Khajuraho temples built in the tenth century.

For Hindus, therefore, as for the Chinese, sex was akin to a religious duty, not one that would put him straight in tune with the infinite, but one of the least taxing and most enjoyable ways of improving his spiritual rating. And again like the Chinese, Hindus had sex manuals, the best known of which is the *Kama Sutra* (*c.* third century AD), but there was one distinct difference. Although early Hinduism was a sophisticated and fatalistic religion that often appeared callous to outsiders, the *Kama Sutra* acknowledged something that had been largely ignored by the Chinese – the possibility of there being more to sex than simply the mechanics of foreplay and intercourse.

Love was a recurring theme. The *Kama Sutra* identified four different varieties of love and the author frequently interrupted himself in the middle of one of his lectures on the nine different ways of moving the lingam (penis) inside the yoni (vagina), or the steps a man with a small lingam could take to satisfy a woman with a large yoni, to remind his readers that true lovers needed no rules to govern them, no teacher but instinct.

Even so, there was little poetic or romantic about the *Kama Sutra*. The ruthlessly self-centred nature of the Hindu concept of karma (fate) saw to that. Hindus were no more enthusiastic than anyone else about one man seducing another man's wife, but according to the *Kama Sutra* it could be justified by love. It was acceptable for a woman to influence her husband on her lover's behalf. It was acceptable, too, that if the woman could be relied on to help her lover kill her husband, they would both inherit his riches. But lacking motives of self interest that could be defined in terms of the second of the four aims, mere sexual appetite was no excuse.

The very existence of the eternal triangle in India at this time was almost certainly a product of the marriage system. The law books decreed that a bride should, ideally, be one-third of the age of her husband, because Indians, in common with many other peoples, regarded girls as naturally libidinous and preferred to marry them off at the earliest possible moment. Eight for a girl and twenty-four for her husband were the ages suggested, although the bride did not go to live with her husband until she reached puberty and was then introduced to the sexual side of marriage with care.

Even so, a wife was still only in her thirties when her sons were grown up and her husband an old man in terms of the time. When he died, she would be doomed to the hell of Indian widowhood, forbidden to remarry, forced to sleep on the ground, allowed only one savourless meal a day, and expected to devote all her waking hours to prayer and religious rites. The *Kama Sutra* was probably right to assume that, in the brief intervening spell of relative freedom before this fate overtook her, a woman would be tempted to succumb to the lure of a lover.

A Prince taking part in group sex, described by Vatsyayana in his *Kama Sutra*, Bundi Style, *c.* 1800.

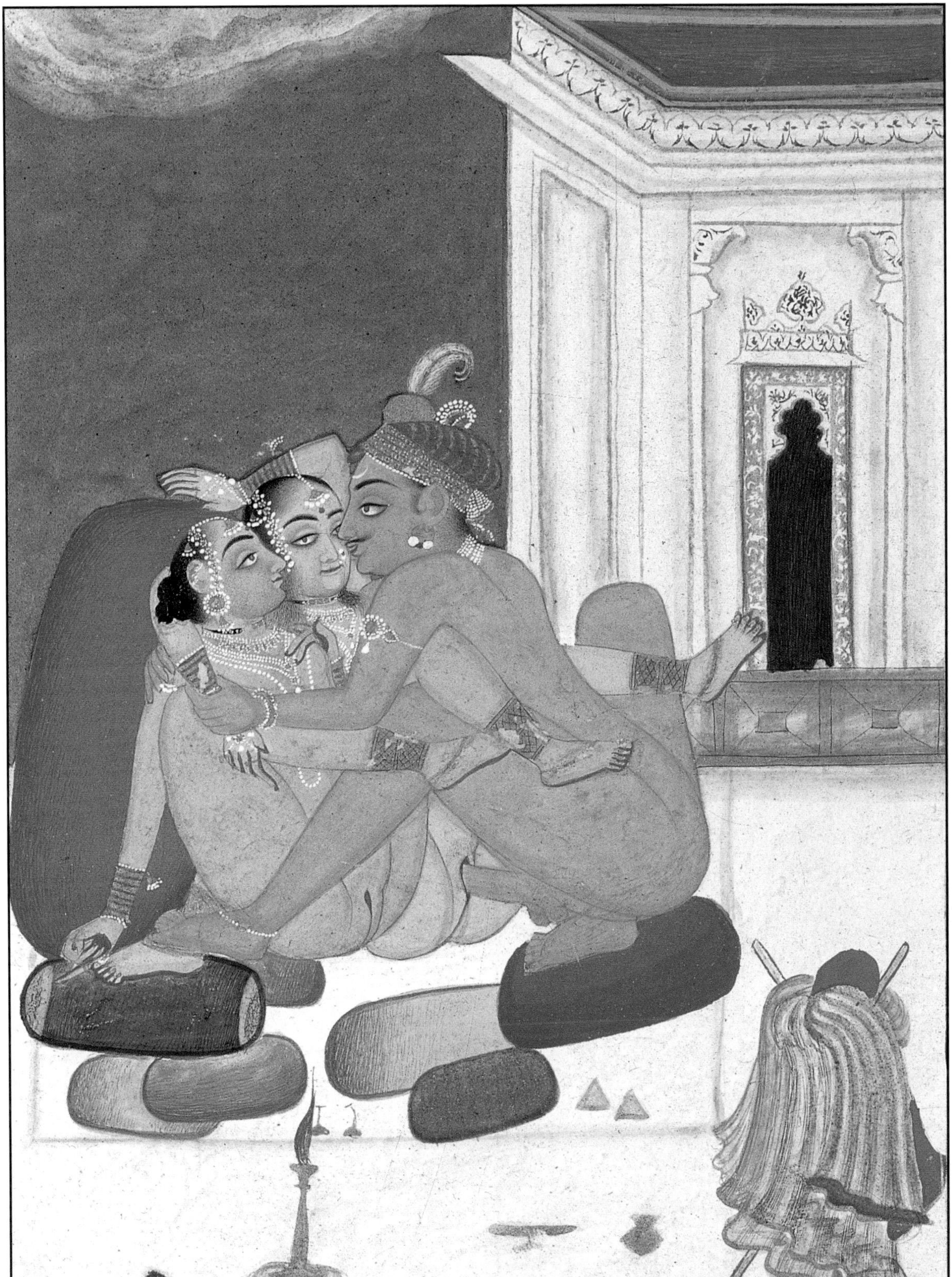

THE EARLY CHRISTIANS

Although Christianity, in most senses, was gentler and more tolerant than the Judaism from which it developed, the attitude of the Christian church towards sexuality developed into one of the most repressive in history.

Other societies had condemned, with varying degrees of severity, adultery (usually), contraception (rarely), abortion (sometimes), homosexuality (sometimes), female infanticide (rarely), zoophilia (sometimes), masturbation (never). The Christian church proscribed them all. Other societies had suggested suitable frequencies for marital intercourse. 'Three times a month', said the Greeks; 'Every day for the unemployed', said the Jews, 'Twice a week for labourers, once a week for ass drivers'. The Christian church said never, unless children were desired. Other societies had regarded sex as pleasurable, in any position. To the Christian church, pleasure was sinful and only the missionary position acceptable.

Because after the fall of Rome, reading and writing became the preserve of the monasteries, much in the way of doctrine that would otherwise have been discussed and argued over passed straight into the realms of orthodoxy. As a result, the words of the Church Fathers – dedicated but arrogant men who knew that what they said was right, because it was they who said it – took on an aura of revealed truth. Much of what the modern Western world still understands as 'sin' stems not from the teachings of Jesus of Nazareth, nor even from the tablets handed down from Sinai, but from the early sexual vicissitudes of a handful of such men as St Jerome and St Augustine who lived in the twilight days of imperial Rome.

Sex, however hedged by prohibitions, had never been sinful until St Paul advanced the theory that celibacy was superior to marriage because, then, no worldly obligations intervened between the worshipper and his

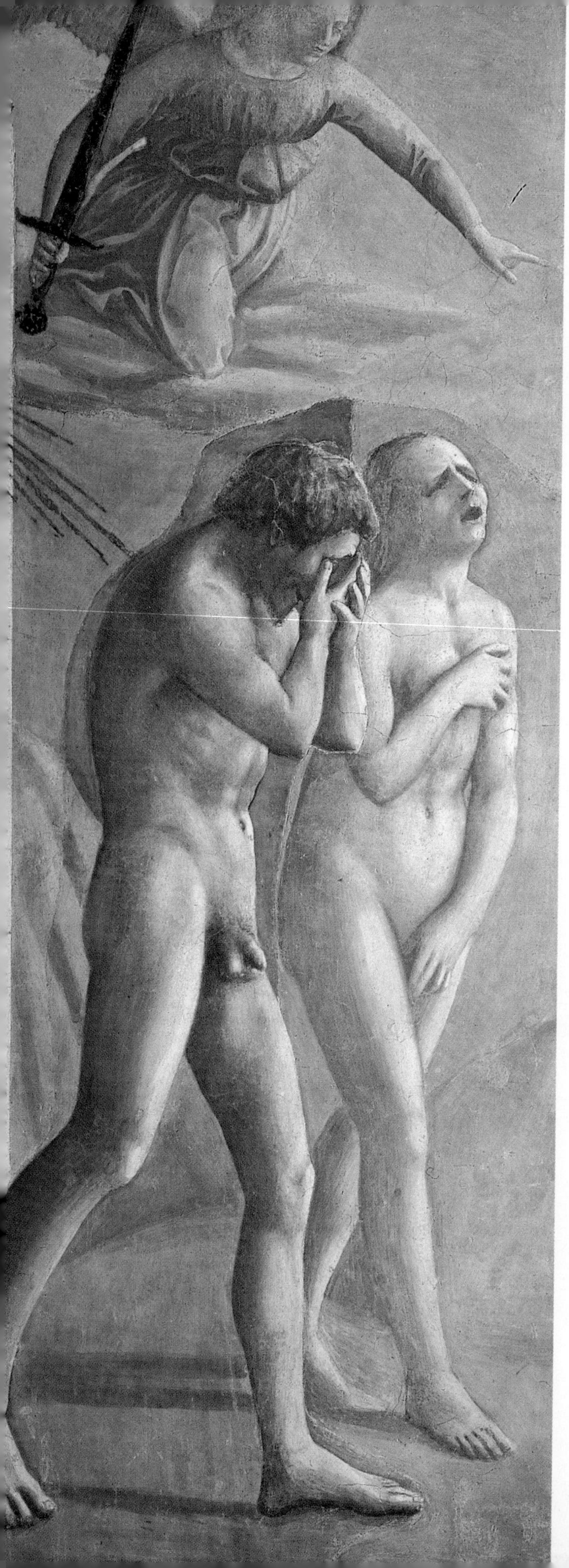

The expulsion of Adam and Eve (detail), by Tommaso Masaccio (fifteenth century).

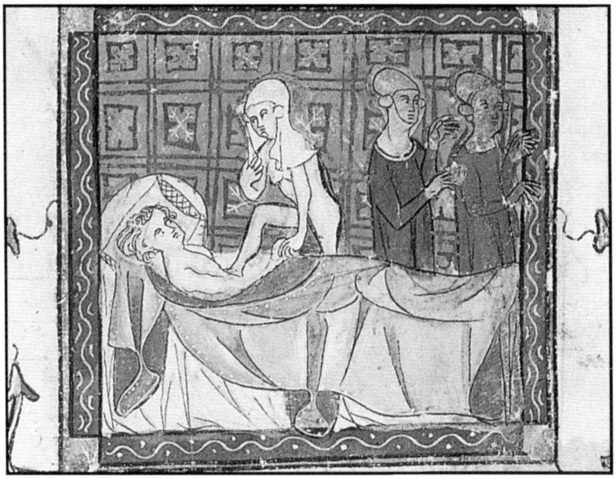

King Arthur's Wedding Night, from a fourteenth century French manuscript.

Lord. For him and his successors – even, or especially, those whose earlier life had been anything but celibate – sexual abstinence became a indicator of divine grace. Jerome, Tertullian and Ambrose, looking back, recognized that the sexual act had been repugnant, degrading, indecent, obscene.

There was an unspoken consensus that God might have found a more seemly way to ensure the perpetuation of the human race and it was St Augustine who, setting his mind to the problem, came up with an explanation. Sex in the Garden of Eden, if it had ever taken place, would have been cool and rarefied, a matter of utilizing the mechanical equipment supplied by the Creator to fulfil the requirements of the reproductive process. But Adam and Eve's fall into the sin of disobedience and lapse from grace were reflected in sudden and wilful activity on the part of their genitals.

Augustine believed that this explained the perversity of the human sexual organs, the intractable nature of the carnal impulse, and the shame aroused by intercourse. Lust and sex were integral to the doctrine of Original Sin, and every act of intercourse performed by Adam and Eve's descendants after the Fall carried the burden of the original evil.

Setting out to validate the Church Fathers' emotional revulsion against sex, Augustine succeeded in justifying it in a way that satisfied both faith and intellect. But by transforming every act of sex into a sin, he had an incalculable effect on the lives of future generations.

CHRISTIAN MARRIAGE

St Paul and St Augustine made chastity synonymous with virtue. If a priest, therefore, was to have moral authority over his flock, it was necessary for him to be chaste. Or, at least, celibate. The two words often were – and are – used interchangeably, but they do not mean quite the same thing.

The idea of celibacy – the unmarried state – did not, however, go down at all well with the early priesthood and the Germans swore they would rather give up their lives than their wives. It took almost six centuries for the Church to enforce its prohibition on clerical marriage. It never succeeded in enforcing chastity.

Modern churchmen sometimes speak of 'the family' as if it were a Christian invention, but their predecessors were more inclined to blame it on the devil. Seeing marriage as a series of concessions to human weakness, to the need for companionship, sex and children, the Church did what it could to undermine all three. One marriage was enough for anyone; second marriages were adultery, third fornication, and fourth nothing short of 'swinish'.

It also refused to consider sex as an integral part of marriage. After arguing about it for 500 years, it finally concluded that what marriage did was confer the right (not the duty) to indulge in sexual intercourse, a right that existed only within marriage. Further, continuing to hanker after chastity even within marriage, it refused to consider childlessness as a basis for divorce, although it had been acceptable as such in every society since the beginning of recorded history. However unintentionally, this gave unprecedented security of tenure to a large class of women who had previously suffered rejection for something that was as likely to be their husband's problem as their own.

Since sex and marriage had been interdependent since the days of the

Hebrews, it might seem as if not very much about sex within marriage had changed. But a number of new factors had been introduced. The Christian calendar included an inordinate number of holy days, and some theologians insisted on abstinence on all of them – on Thursdays in memory of Christ's arrest; on Fridays in memory of his death; Saturdays, in honour of the Virgin Mary; Sundays in honour of the Resurrection; Mondays in commemoration of the departed. Tuesdays and Wednesdays were largely accounted for by a ban on intercourse during fasts and festivals – the forty days before Easter, Pentecost, and Christmas; the seven, five or three days before Communion; and so on.

Such rules may regularly have been broken on the principle that no one would find out. But a priest, in his small parish, was perfectly capable of calculating nine months back from a new infant's date of birth, and if conception had taken place during Lent, for example, he was entitled to impose the penance of a year's fast on the child's parents.

For sexual, as for other sins, the priest had handbooks to guide him, the penitentials, which laid down the penances to be imposed on parishioners who strayed from the path of virtue. Penances included between three and fifteen years on bread and water for using contraceptive potions; from two to ten years for coitus interruptus; thirty days' fasting for a monk who masturbated in church; and so on.

The hypocritical clergy were often the subject of satire, such as in this seventeenth-century German engraving.

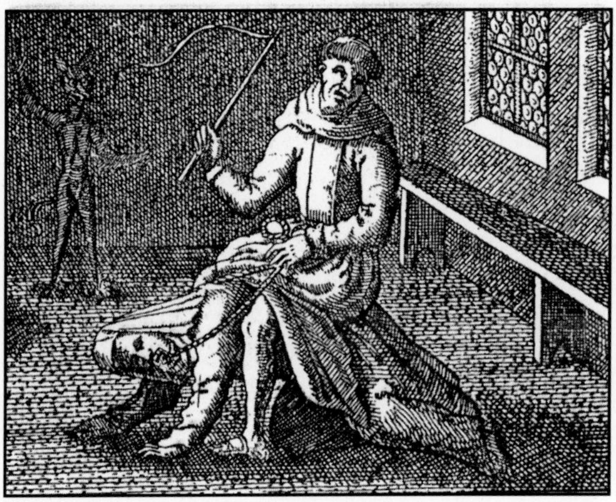

THE RISE OF WOMEN

With Judaism in its ancestry and the women of imperial Rome as an example of what could happen when women got out of hand, the early Church had no great opinion of the female sex. As St Paul pointed out, woman had been created for the benefit of man and ought to defer to him in all things; she was not to teach in church (a prohibition that remained in force in the Church of England until the early 1990s); should cultivate silence; and submit meekly to instruction, as became the daughter of Eve who had beguiled Adam into transgression. The Church Fathers added that she should take care to hide her charms, veil herself in church, and permanently abjure cosmetics; 'What', inquired St Jerome sarcastically, 'can a woman expect from Heaven when, in supplication, she lifts up a face that its Creator wouldn't recognize?' (St Jerome quoted in J. Coulson (ed.), The Saints, A Concise Bibliographical Dictionary *(1958) p.394)*

It was 800 years before things began to change. The period between the early twelfth and late sixteenth centuries was notable in the history of women, perhaps the most critical since the Neolithic era. Although at the end women were no better off legally, financially or physically than they had been at the beginning, their image had changed. Whereas once they had been despised not only by men but often by themselves, now they were respected, sometimes even admired. This reversal of attitude was to make possible all subsequent changes and improvements.

A number of factors were responsible. The departure of thousands of Western knights for the Crusades was perhaps the first; wives reluctantly entrusted with the management of their husbands' estates discovered that taxes, tithes and even politics were not beyond their understanding. When the Crusaders returned, too, they brought with them – among other souvenirs of their travels – the cult of the Virgin Mary, who had long been an object of devotion in Byzantium. Until then, the Western church had equated woman with Eve, the seductress, the architect of man's downfall. When Eve at last gave way to Mary, all women benefited.

But the most unpredictable influence was the strange game that evolved during the first half of the twelfth century, the game of 'Courtly Love'. It was class conscious and excruciatingly sentimental, an idealized affair between a highborn beauty and a romantic squire, and it had its origins in the Arab concept of 'pure love'. Adaptation to the Western situation was not easy. The whole point of the Muslim original was that the real woman was a mystery to the poet who worshiped her. In Europe, however, the unconsecrated spirituality of such a love was not at all easy to achieve when its object was not only visible and audible but, as far as it is possible to judge, willing and accessible too. In the end, the troubadour-poets were forced to endow their heroines not only with beauty and rank, but (whether the lady liked it or not) with unimpeachable virtue too. Virtue became the European harem.

The lady of Courtly Love might be a creature of the imagination, but the idea became so widespread and fashionable that it was enough to help inaugurate a new era. It also had an effect on the fleshly medieval ladies who acted as stand-ins for the image. With their reputations ennobled, they had little choice but to mend their manners. As men became more chivalrous, ladies became, if not necessarily more virtuous or chaste, at least more gracious.

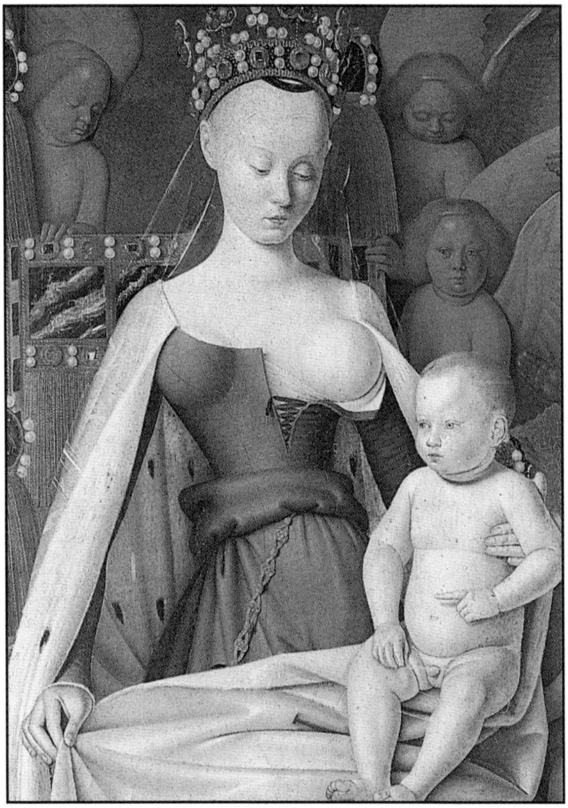

The Cult of the Virgin Mary, as depicted in this fifteenth century painting by Jean Fouquet (above).

The ideals of Courtly Love were promoted by medieval romances, as in this story of Sir Lancelot and Guinevere, from a fourteenth century manuscript (below).

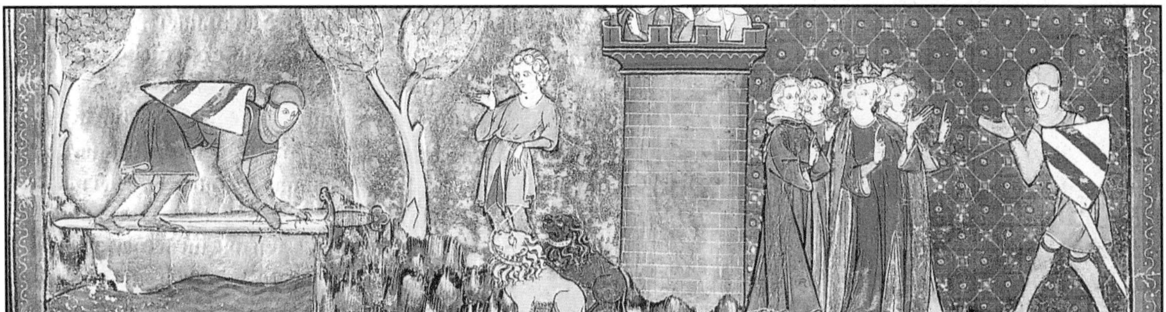

AFTER THE REFORMATION

An improvement in the position in the West received something of a setback at the beginning of the sixteenth century when the men of the Reformation, rebelling against Rome, swept away 1500 years of Catholic doctrine by going back to the scriptures and rediscovering (among other things) the 'good wife'.

They also, however, discovered that there was nothing in the Bible about celibacy being a virtue, wedlock a necessary evil, or divorce a sacramental impossibility. Indeed, according to Martin Luther, in Biblical terms virginity was undesirable, continence abnormal, chastity actively dangerous and marriage as necessary to the nature of man as eating and drinking. The desire to conceive was not the only legitimate justification for sex. Husband and wife might also have intercourse in order to 'avoid fornication, or to lighten and ease the cares and sadnesses of household affairs, or to endear each other' (Jeremy Taylor, *Holy Living* ii 3). The other face of this surprisingly open approach to sex in marriage was, however, an absolute and uncompromising disapproval of any kind of extramarital activity.

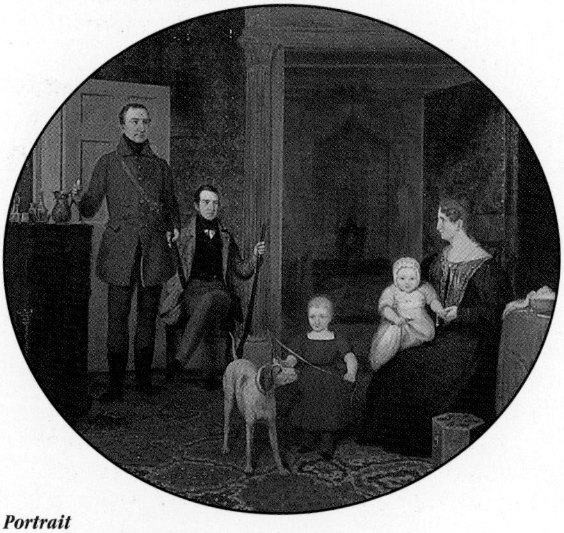

Portrait of the Van Cortland Family, by an anonymous nineteenth-century artist.

The Puritans who emigrated to North America a century later took the patriarchal household of the Old Testament with them, and also, for good measure, the traditional conviction that all God's creatures, even the Chosen, were born to an inheritance of sin. It was the duty of the strong in faith to help their weaker brethren to fight temptation, and they helped by flogging fornicators and adulterers; condemning the parents of a child born too soon after the wedding day to the pillory; and hanging the occasional adolescent boy for testing his uncertain masculinity on a mare or a goat.

Puritan morality was to have three direct effects on American society that still echo today. It produced a mental state of Victorianism a century before Victoria herself mounted the throne; it taught American women how to control their menfolk by being virtuous to the point of caricature (just like the lady of Courtly Love) while yet appearing to submit to them like good Old Testament wives; and it wove the public demonstration of family solidarity into the American ethos.

Although the resurrection of the 'good wife' put a temporary damper on the development of women as individuals, in the eighteenth century a scientific controversy blew up that proved, for the first time, that they had an independent importance in the general scheme of things. Although even the least observant must have recognized, during the course of 400 generations, that children as often resembled their mothers as their fathers, it had always been thought that woman was merely an incubator for the 'germinal particle' contained in man's seminal fluid; her ovaries were considered to be an unimportant female version of the testicles. But when the microscope was invented, scientists used it to discover, first, that the ovum was mobile, and then that seminal fluid was alive with miniature tadpole-like creatures. The full truth of how children were generated was not to be resolved until 1854, but long before that it had become accepted that, if God had endowed women with the right to contribute to the creation of their sons, they could not be as inferior as men had always thought.

THE AGE OF IMPERIALISM

Although Europe had come to give more thought to the 'sinfulness' of sex than to the perpetuation of the human race, there was a slight blip in the sixteenth century, when new worlds were discovered and imperial expansion began. If sexual intercourse, however sinful, could help guarantee new generations of Christians rather than new generations of pagans, the theory went...

Cortes with his mistress. Detail from a mural by José Clemente Orozco (sixteenth century).

It was a case of being wise after the event. Since the empire-builders did not, at first, take their women with them, they were naturally fascinated by the sexuality of newly discovered peoples, even if the first thing to strike them was something entirely different. This was what happened with the Spaniards in Mexico, so horrified by the ceremonial cannibalism of the Aztecs that they henceforth put the worst possible interpretation on everything else that fell under their gaze. When they discovered that the Maya – like the ancient Greeks – saw adolescent homosexuality as a perfectly normal phase of growing up, they promptly inflated it into a continent-wide addiction to sodomy although, in fact, both the Aztecs and the Inca were as dedicated to fertility as the early Hebrews had been and rewarded adult homosexuality with a very nasty death.

The Spanish conquest was to have a dire effect on the native populations of central and southern America. In addition to systematic slaughter, Spain had brought European diseases against which the peoples of the New World had no immunity. In Mexico and Yucatán before the conquest, there are believed to have been about twenty-five million people; little more than a century later only one-and-a-half million pure-blooded indigenes remained. But the Spaniards had been busy in other directions, too, enforcing the sexual and personal morality of the West while at the same time fathering children who, inheriting some of the characteristics of both parents, had a degree of immunity to European diseases. It was these so-called *mestizos*, part Indian, part Spanish, who were genetically equipped to survive, and it was they who founded the new hybrid races that inherited central and southern America.

It was the Portuguese, however, rather than the Spaniards, who saw interbreeding as a politically useful policy. When they captured Goa in the early sixteenth century – a tiny European foothold on the great landmass of Hindu India – the Portuguese saw no possibility of holding it by strength of arms and, instead, sought to induce loyalty to Portugal by simultaneously imposing Christianity and fostering a *mestiço* population. But, although the Goanese accepted the new religion, the experiment failed and the majority of the *mestiços* were reabsorbed into the Christianized Indian background.

It was different 200 years later when the British came to rule India. The Eurasians (or Anglo–Indians) were, in terms of Hinduism, outcasts who could not be reabsorbed into the Hindu Indian community. They were outsiders, forming an uneasy class of their own, and a class of which the British made calculated use. From the mid-nineteenth until the mid-twentieth centuries, the railways and the police could scarcely have functioned without them.

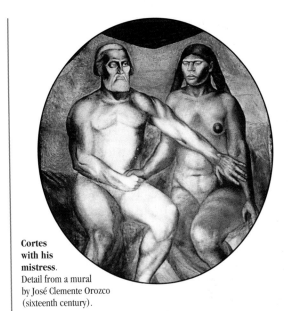

THE VICTORIAN ERA

Good wives, yes. Partners in the creation of sons, yes. But women as independent human beings? Not yet.

The frock-coated and increasingly bewhiskered Western gentlemen of the Victorian era, in the grip of acute nostalgia for the medieval period – so much more colourful than their own – cultivated a stilted and excessive courtesy toward 'the ladies' that they fondly believed to reflect the chivalric ideal. By doing so, they reduced them once more to the status of spectators at the tournament of life, giving them indulgence as a substitute for independence. Many women, of course, were happy to be indulged, cherished and treated as pure-minded angels to whom a man could turn for respite from the rough and demanding world of business.

Though not too often, in the sexual sense at least. There was a general belief that a man should not impose his animal desires on his wife any more than was absolutely necessary – once a month for preference, once a week if he was desperate, but never during menstrual periods or pregnancy. Men were encouraged, even by doctors, to feel that they were doing their wives a favour by taking their sexual demands elsewhere. Sex with a prostitute, where neither love nor passion was involved, was said to be 'generally attended with less derangement' than sex with a wife.

Prostitution, both amateur and professional, flourished as never before. There was an epidemic spread of venereal disease and a fashion for virgin prostitutes who, because this was their first experience of intercourse, could not be contagious; it took years for their clients to discover that, in some brothels, full-time virgins were patched up several times a week with the aid of a powerful astringent and a scrap of blood-soaked sponge.

As the nineteenth century progressed, the 'angel of the house' went on sitting in her ivory tower while her husband – whom she had been taught to regard as a cross between God and Sir Galahad – sought and was supplied with every conceivable outlet for his needs. Flagellation, boy brothels and masochistic pornography were particularly popular.

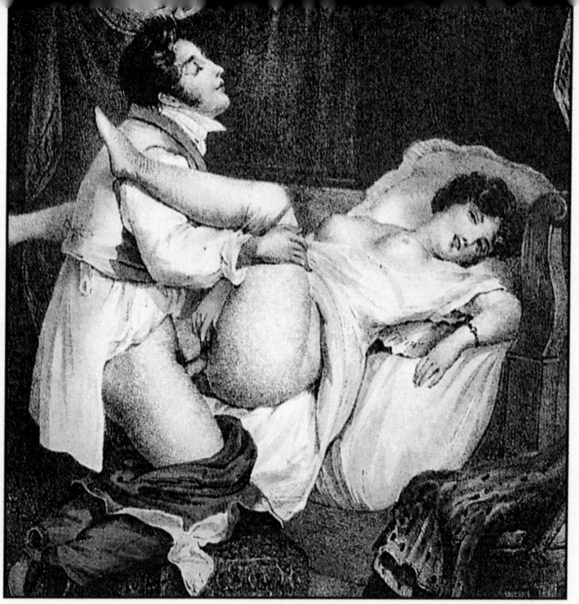

Prostitution flourished in the nineteenth century as men were encouraged to 'spare' their wives from the demands of their sexual appetites.

There was one surprising and beneficial consequence. In the Christian view, the only respectable form of contraception had always been abstention, which had meant that coitus interruptus, unreliable and unsatisfying for both partners, had always been the most commonly used method. By the 1880s, however, every man who had ever visited a prostitute was aware that, in making love to his wife, he ran the risk of infecting her. Condoms, available for over a century, had formerly been intolerably clumsy but recent developments in vulcanization had led to the development of a greatly improved crepe rubber type and men began using them in increasing numbers. Middle-class wives, innocently believing that it was to save them, not from venereal disease but from unwanted conception, found it more acceptable than coitus interruptus, and gradually began to take a more favourable view of the whole idea of artificial contraception – and also of intercourse itself. Marital relations began to improve.

But it was still the man who controlled conception.

INTO THE 20TH CENTURY

As the nineteenth century gave way to the twentieth, very little seemed to have changed in relations between the sexes. In 1893, New Zealand became the first country in the world to grant women the vote (thanks largely to a miscalculation on the government's part), but elsewhere the real battle had scarcely been joined. Both sides invoked women's 'special moral qualities'. The anti-suffrage lobby claimed that women should not have the vote because those qualities would be tarnished by contact with 'the ordinary machinery of political life'. The reformists argued that they should, that the dangerous experiment had already been tried of 'enfranchizing the vast proportion of crime, intemperance, immorality and dishonesty [i.e. men], and barring absolutely from the suffrage the great proportion of temperance, morality, religion and conscientiousness [i.e. women]' (Susan B. Anthony and Ida Husted Harper, The History of Woman Suffrage *(1902) p xxvi).*

It was a long battle, during which the 'angel of the house' gave way to the virago, Englishwomen tied themselves to railings and American women opposed racism, prohibitionism and self-righteousness. By the period between the wars, however, the battle had effectively been won, though even now enfranchisement of women is not worldwide.

Far more influential in changing women's lives was the new social freedom of the 1920s that enabled them to take real jobs and earn their own living. As G.K. Chesterton drily remarked, 'Twenty million young women rose to their feet with the cry, "We will not be dictated to" and promptly became stenographers.' But still, thanks largely to Hollywood, women saw romance as their birthright and marriage as their natural goal.

It was a vision that lingered even in the divorce-ridden decades after the Second World War. But, at the beginning of the 1960s, the revolution happened at last. Where permission to vote and permission to earn had failed to change women's view of themselves, a single medical development spectacularly succeeded. For thousands of years they had been swallowing powders and potions in the hope of controlling their fertility. For decades they had been struggling with diaphragms and Dutch caps. But the Pill, at last, was something that really worked and, since taking it was quite dissociated from the act of intercourse, it aroused none of the moral, political, social or aesthetic unease of other methods. For the first time, reliably and privately, women were in charge of their own reproductive capacity. It was from this transformation in their circumstances that the new feminists drew much of their strength.

The people of medieval Europe had twelve generations during which to adjust to the idea that women were worthy of respect, the Victorians three generations to accept that they were worthy of the vote. Many societies in the modern world have had to adapt to the idea of almost complete legal and sexual equality in a couple of decades – 5000 years of social and sexual tradition overturned in just a whisper of time. Predictably, the results have been chaotic – for women, for men and for moralists.

But it is not, of course, the end of the story. It never is, where life and sex are concerned.

Scenes from Woodstock in 1969 demonstrate the extent to which Western attitudes towards sexuality changed during the twentieth century.

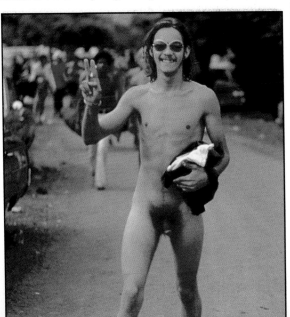

INTO THE MILLENNIUM

Greater knowledge of and public debate about sexuality during the late twentieth century has not only brought sexual enjoyment and fulfilment, but also division and confusion. Religious leaders, even within individual religions, remain divided about the acceptability of various sexual and moral behaviours. There is no universal consensus on what is 'normal' and 'permissible'.

Neighbouring countries – even neighbouring states in the USA – have differing laws about abortion, homosexuality, the age of consent and sexual practices. Many regimes world-wide have acted – and continue to act – repressively with regard to sexual issues. Some have been successfully challenged and have made adjustments to their laws and social codes, a good example being the changes that have taken place in post-reunification Germany. Further developments, in the wake of political change, are likely in the future.

The debate on abortion continues both undiminished and unresolved. The pro-choice movement insists on the rights of women, the anti-choice lobby labels abortion as murder – on occasion ironically resorting to violence itself to propound their views. Reconciliation seems unlikely. The reception and legalisation of the abortion drug RU486 in some countries has continued to fuel controversy.

HIV and AIDS has forced people to reconsider their attitudes towards sexual behaviour, even if vaccines or cures are developed. The World Health Organisation estimates that by the end of the century there will be thirty to forty million cases of HIV world-wide, mostly in Asia. In the USA, AIDS-related illnesses have risen to become the main cause of death in men, and the fourth major cause of death in women, aged twenty-five to forty-four. Chlamydia affects significant numbers of people in the USA, western and eastern Europe, Japan and China – and its incidence is growing.

Population increases of almost a hundred million people a year are unsustainable, forcing governments and individuals to look into measures to limit population growth. Long-standing views favouring large numbers of offspring are being challenged. Some religions – Roman Catholicism in particular – may have to address the issue of the use of artificial contraception. Many scientists believe that the resolution of the population issue is crucial if the planet is to survive.

The establishment of equal rights for lesbians and gay men will continue to be an important issue for the foreseeable future. Denmark has legalised homosexual marriages, and antihomosexual laws have been repealed in the Ukraine, Belarus, Latvia, Estonia and Lithuania. However, many countries, including the UK, still refuse to allow gay men or lesbians to serve in their armed forces and confusion still exists about the legal rights of same sex partners.

It is gradually being acknowledged that people with physical disabilities and learning difficulties are sexual beings whose needs and desires should be recognized and fulfiled. This area is one where, increasingly, self-advocacy is playing a vital role.

Pornography remains, and no doubt will remain, a controversial issue. Debates about what constitutes acceptable eroticism and what unhealthy pornography have raged for years. Clearly, what is eroticism to one person may be pornography to another, and vice versa. Some people see pornography as a violation of women's sexuality; others support sexual freedom of expression, believing that individuals have a right to express what they do and feel. Some find non-sexist erotic material for women more acceptable. The spread of 'pornographic' literature, films, television and art, causes concern amongst governments around the world. Although laws and attitudes may wax and wane in terms of how liberal or restrictive they are, it seems unlikely that a universal consensus on pornography will be achieved.

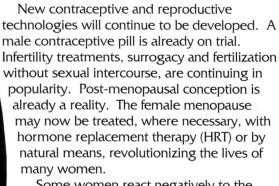

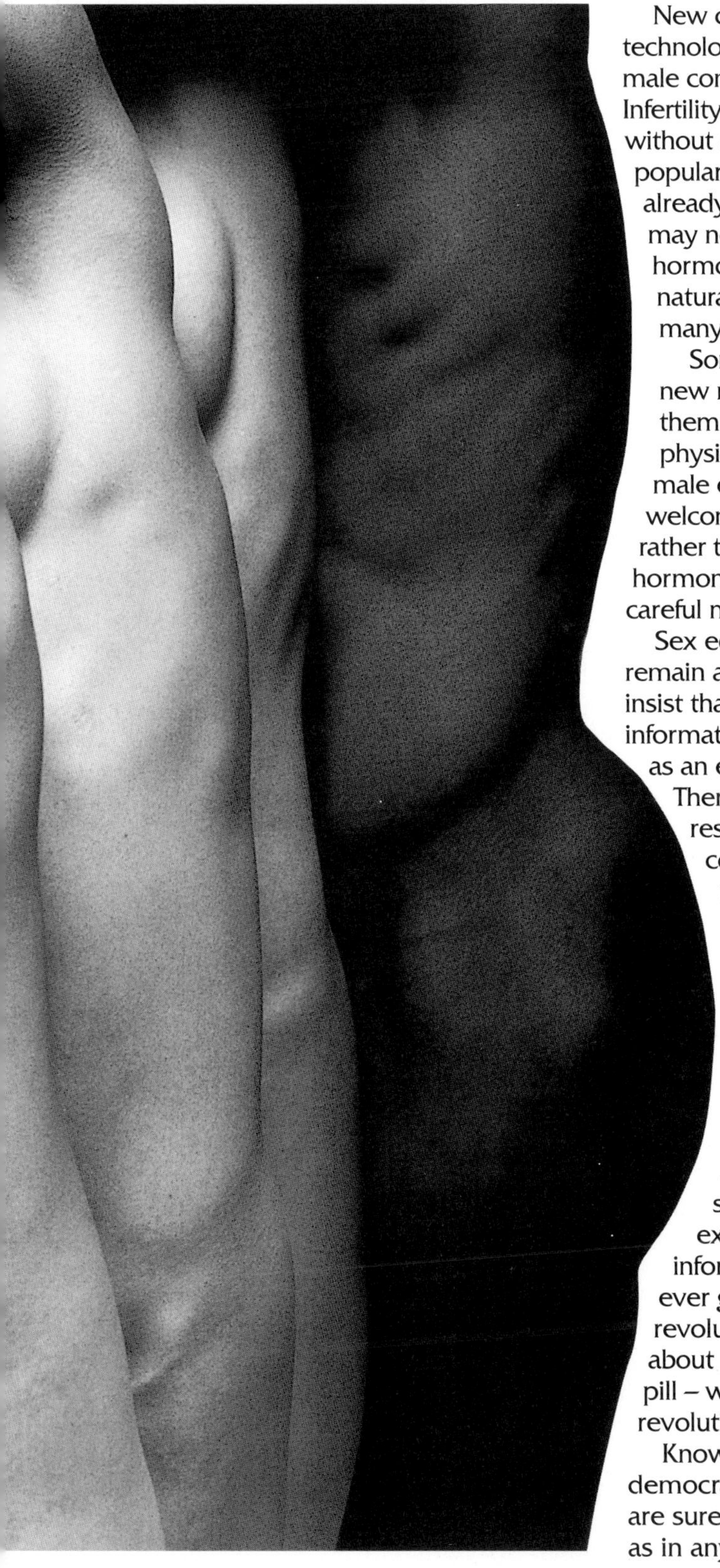

New contraceptive and reproductive technologies will continue to be developed. A male contraceptive pill is already on trial. Infertility treatments, surrogacy and fertilization without sexual intercourse, are continuing in popularity. Post-menopausal conception is already a reality. The female menopause may now be treated, where necessary, with hormone replacement therapy (HRT) or by natural means, revolutionizing the lives of many women.

Some women react negatively to the new reproductive technologies, regarding them as interference with women's physiology and psychology, by a chiefly male establishment. Most, however, welcome the increase in choice as liberating rather than repressive. All aspects of the new hormonal preparations nevertheless require careful monitoring and assessment.

Sex education for young people is likely to remain a source of conflict between those who insist that young people have a right to sexual information and those who see sex education as an encouragement to be promiscuous. There is an apparent need for dialogue and resolution in each society. Thanks to the courage and goodwill of representatives from different religious groups in the UK in discussing sex education, a good deal of mutual respect and agreement has been achieved.

These debates and concerns will be carried into the new millennium and it is likely that as some problems are resolved, others will emerge. What is clear, however, is that the amount of information about human sexuality can only increase. With the expanding communications industry, this information will become available to an ever growing world public. The 'sexual revolution' of the sixties – largely brought about by mass access to the contraceptive pill – will be continued in the information revolution of the late twentieth century.

Knowledge and understanding, which allow democratic discussion and individual choice, are surely as important goals in sexual matters as in any other area of human activity.

SEX & RELIGION

Every religion has its own perspective on sexual issues, drawn from traditions and specific teachings, often set out in written texts.

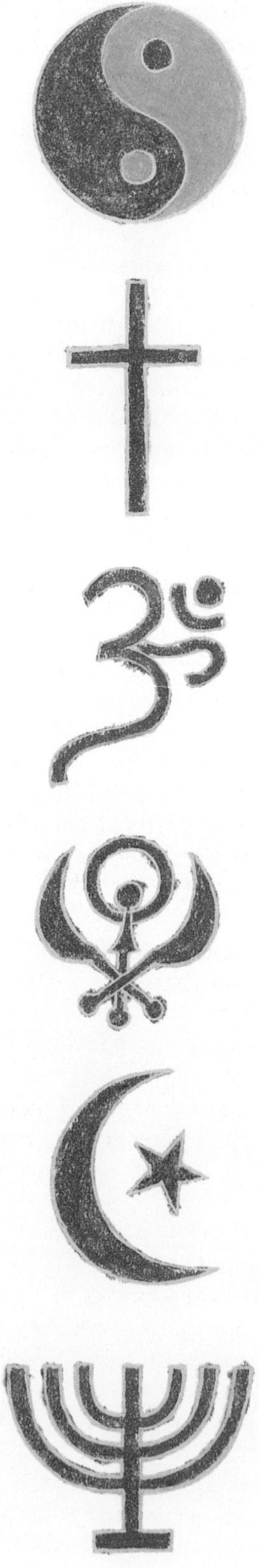

Buddhism
Buddhists are taught to define their own destiny according to their own understanding and interpretation of the world. They must avoid deliberate harm to living things and pursue acts of kindness (*metta*) and compassion (*karuna*) toward them.

While abortion clearly goes against basic Buddhist principles, other sexual decisions and behaviours, including the use of contraceptives, depend on the attitudes of the individual.

Christianity
The **Anglican Church's** view is that, ideally, sex should take place within the sacred, lifelong bond of marriage. Sexual relations within marriage are encouraged.

The Church acknowledges, but does not condone, homosexuality or masturbation. The predominant view concerning abortion is that a human being, formed in God's image, is created at conception and that, therefore, abortion is not justifiable. However, the Church allows for a wide range of views and these issues remain controversial.

According to **Roman Catholic** doctrine, sexuality is part of loving relationship within marriage. The primary purpose of sexual relationships is to produce children. The alternative is virginity or celibacy. Separation, in the case of marital breakdown, is allowed, but divorce is not recognized. Remarriage is only allowed in the case of annulment (where the marriage is deemed not to have existed) or dissolution (where it is considered invalid). Debates continue around the acceptability of premarital sex and divorce and around homosexuality and masturbation, in that both are non-procreative sexual acts.

Contraception is seen as part of non-procreative sex and therefore wrong;

See also:
contraception
masturbation
sexual orientation
circumcision
orgasm

however many Catholics in Western societies do use contraception. Natural family planning methods are allowed. Abortion is strictly forbidden as it is seen as counter to human dignity and rights. Life is considered to begin at the moment of conception.

Hinduism

Hinduism is a way of life, a code of values developed from many belief systems in which human sexuality is seen as a symbol of the creation of the universe. Hinduism centres on family life and favours reproduction. Many Hindus see the production of a son as a duty. Contraception is permitted, but not normally practised until after the birth of a son. Semen is considered the 'elixir of life' and partial sexual abstinence is recommended, particularly during religious festivals. Arranged marriages are preferred, as the marriage is considered to be between the two families. Divorce is allowed. There are no rules about masturbation or sex that does not have a reproductive purpose. Abortion is not specifically prohibited but neither is it entirely accepted as Hindus believe in the sanctity of life.

Sikhism

Marriage and family are important in Sikh life. Monogamy is seen as essential. Arranged marriages are not obligatory, but common. Divorce is strongly discouraged. Sex must take place within marriage. Girls are protected by the family from premarital sex and a girl who becomes pregnant before marriage brings dishonour to her family. Menstruation is considered an unclean time and women do not take part in religious ceremonies then; likewise they are considered 'unclean' until forty days after childbirth. Homosexuality and lesbianism are not allowed, but contraception is. Abortion is only approved under certain extreme circumstances, such as if the pregnancy threatens the health of the mother or if a girl is pregnant outside marriage.

Islam

In Islam, the sexes are seen as equal but different, although men are expected to treat women with respect. Marriage is a civil, rather than a religious, contract. Marriage and the love of husband and wife are 'signs of Allah'. A man is allowed to have four wives, and the woman's right to sexual satisfaction is recognized. A man has a duty to ensure that he does not abstain from sex with his wife for more than three months and a woman must not deny sex to her husband. Premarital sex is not allowed, but sex within marriage is seen as important both for satisfying sexual needs and bearing children. Contraception is permitted in certain circumstances. Abortion and vasectomy are forbidden. Female sterilization is only allowed if medical opinion states that the woman's life or mental health would be endangered. The husband is not allowed to practise the withdrawal method of contraception without his wife's permission. Islam disapproves of divorce, but it is allowed in certain circumstances. Homosexuality and lesbianism are strictly prohibited in Islam. Masturbation is discouraged as immoral.

Judaism

Marriage is encouraged, and marriages are sometimes arranged, but individual choice is taken into account. Sexual pleasure is seen as an important part of a relationship. Adultery is absolutely forbidden. Marriage breakdown is based on 'no fault' divorce. Premarital sex is not permitted. Sex is not allowed during menstruation. There are 'rites of passage' into adulthood – the Bar Mitzvah for boys and the Bat Mitzvah for girls. Boys are circumcised as soon as possible after birth.

Masturbation is forbidden, as are homosexuality and lesbianism. Contraception is allowed, the Pill is the most acceptable form of contraception, the condom the least. Jewish law states that a man should not use contraception. Abortion is not generally allowed but if the mother's health is in danger or there is the likelihood of congenital disease, it may be permissible.

SEXUAL PIONEERS

Eroticism had manifested itself for centuries in the literature, art and sexual practices of the non-Christian world before studies of sexuality and the promotion of sexual liberation began in the West at the end of the nineteenth century.

The early pioneers were influenced by new knowledge of the Eastern world as travellers and scholars brought back information on erotica. They were also influenced by the political, legal and medical context in which they lived and worked. Since then, their work has been challenged as being biased and patriarchal. They were, however, the precursors of modern sexology and sex therapy and presented fundamental challenges to the sexual thinking of the time.

More recently, feminist thinkers and sociologists who have been concerned with sexual revolution have pointed to an essential de-medicalizing of sex, and to the need for sexual relationships to be reinterpreted and redefined in the context of differing kinds of sexuality, rather than in the context of the mechanics of sex. Such thinking was not alien to nineteenth- and early twentieth-century sexual reformers, nor was campaigning for sexual rights. They were often, however, forced to work in isolation. The world has, since that time, become more of a global village and more challenged and challenging. As the British sociologist, Jeffrey Weeks states, 'The object of sexological study is notoriously shifting and unstable, and sexology is bound, by countless delicate strands to the preoccupations of its age'. The limitations and methodologies of the early pioneers, the most influential of whom are discussed here, need to be seen in this light.

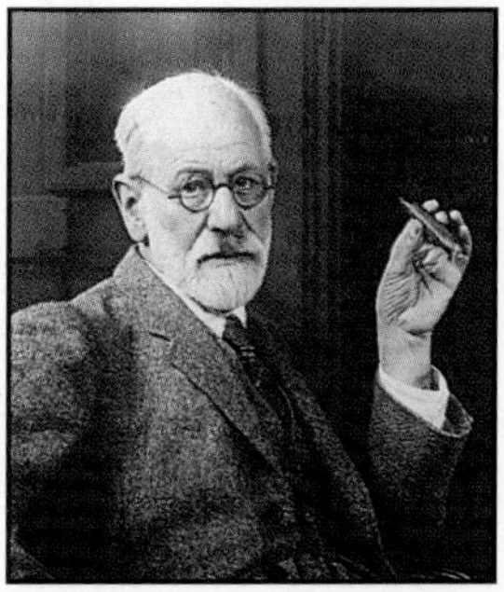

Sigmund Freud

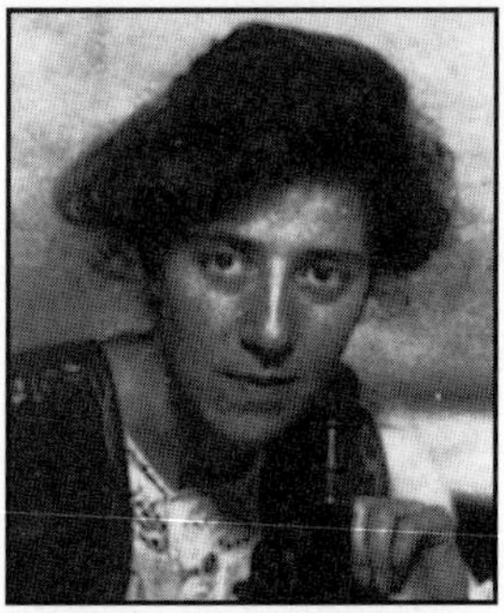

Marie Stopes

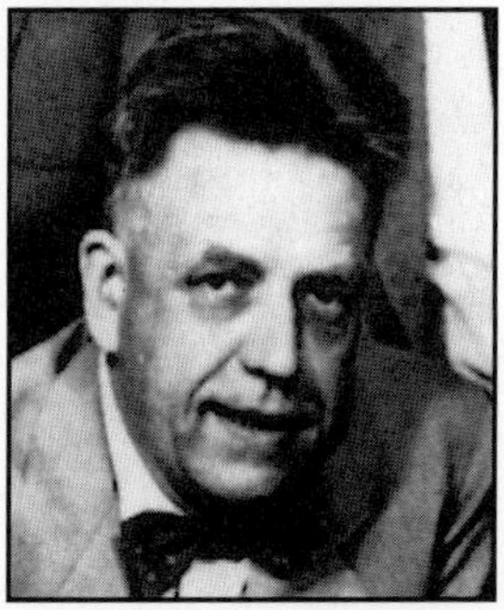

Alfred Kinsey

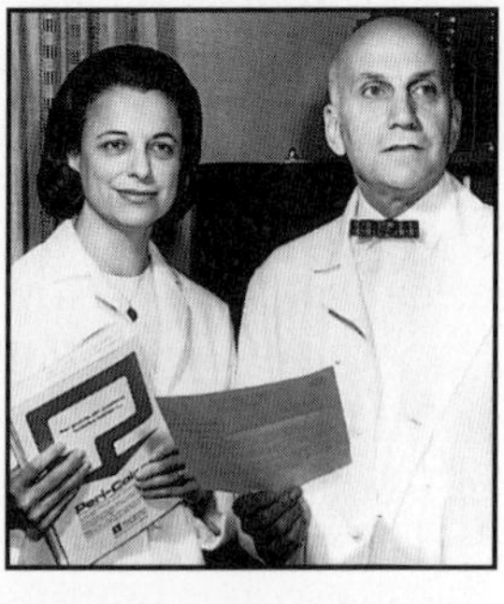

Masters and Johnson

See also:
sexual awareness in children
masturbation
sexual orientation
transvestism
transsexuality
hormone

Sir Richard Burton (British, 1821–90)
Burton was a diplomat, an oriental and Arabic scholar and an explorer, who was interested in sexology. He wrote about the sexual practices of the countries in which he travelled, including India, Arabia and Somalia.

He translated the *Kama Sutra* (1883) and *The Perfumed Garden* (1886), in addition to *The Arabian Nights*, in seventeen volumes, between 1884 and 1886. This latter, with its footnotes on sexual practices, encouraged the perceptions of debauchery and unusual sexual license in the East prevalent in sexually ambivalent Victorian England and Europe.

On his death his wife destroyed many of his more erotic writings.

Edward Carpenter (British, 1844–1929)
Carpenter was an upper-class Englishman who influenced British socialism at the end of the nineteenth century. He was homosexual and lived together with his partner, George Merrill, in Derbyshire for thirty years. He wrote of homosexual and lesbian love as being on the highest plane of love in *The Intermediate Sex* (1908). He also wrote *Love's Coming of Age* (1896).

Henry Havelock Ellis (British, 1859–1939)
Ellis was trained as a doctor, and became a prolific writer and editor of works of science, literature and sociology. He was married to to the lesbian writer Edith Lees and pursued a romantic correspondence with Olive Schreiner.

He was an unusual Victorian in that he openly advocated sex as an important element in life. He put forward the notion of sexual practices, including sadomasochism, coprophilia, necrophilia, transvestism and inversion, being on a continuum of behaviour. He also mooted that every child has tendencies which are both heterosexual and homosexual.

Sexual Inversion, the first volume of his *Studies in the Psychology of Sex* (1897–1910), in which he sets out the view that homosexuality is not a disease, but inborn, was prosecuted in England but published in the USA.

He was a supporter of rights for women and strongly advocated their right to the enjoyment of sex, although it would be more passive than in men. He felt, however, that motherhood and menstruation made them dependent on men. In addition he campaigned for sex education and the right to express one's individual sexuality without fear.

Michel Foucault (French, 1926–84)
Foucault is best known for his *History of Sexuality* (1976) in three volumes – volumes four and five were unfinished. He was a radical thinker who challenged the medicalization of sex and placed it at the centre of 'discourse'. He identified power structures as dominating sexuality and included psychoanalysis as part of these structures.

He has been an important figure in defining sexuality and sexual identity, including that of women, gays and lesbians, as socially and historically constructed, rather than a medical phenomenon.

Sigmund Freud (Austrian 1856–1939)
Freud left Vienna for London after the annexation of Austria by Germany in 1938. His middle-class Jewish family came from Moravia.

Freud was the founder of psychoanalysis, based on his work with patients suffering from 'hysteria' who were encouraged to 'free associate'. His first work on this, co-authored with Josef Breuer, was *Studies in Hysteria* (1895).

His theories on the Oedipus complex postulated that children felt a sexual desire for their parent of the opposite sex and jealousy of their same-sex parent. In boys, this would be destroyed by the castration complex; in girls, the castration complex would make the Oedipus complex reality. His later work explored the concepts of the id, ego and super ego divisions of the mind.

He had a profound interest in culture and religion, in addition to sexuality. His explorations of the inter-relationships of sexuality, the influences on the developing character and mental life were original and highly influential.

Magnus Hirschfeld (German, 1868–1935)
Hirschfeld founded the first institute of sexology in Berlin and later became eminent in the World League for Sexual Reform. The Institute of Sexology delivered sex education and marriage guidance. He wrote about transvestism and, more famously, about homosexuality in *Homosexuality of Man and Woman* (1925) and *Sexual Anomalies and Perversions* (1938), the summary of his writings.

He was, as a Jew, persecuted by the Nazis and his books burned in public in 1933. After this, he lived in the USA and later in France.

He rejected the popular views that homosexuality was a disease, insisting that it was another inherent sexuality. He pioneered the view that hormones governed sexual behaviour. He campaigned for the rights of homosexuals and lesbians and, in 1897, founded the Scientific–Humanitarian Committee, which sought to abolish German laws against sodomy. He was also involved in the making of films that were a plea for enlightenment in sexual matters.

Richard Freiherr von Krafft-Ebing (German, 1840–1902)
Krafft-Ebing was a psychiatrist who worked in the courts of Austria and Germany. He was appointed Professor of Psychiatry at the University of Strasbourg in 1869 and was Professor of Psychiatry at the University of Vienna from 1892 until his death.

He attacked Freud's work as fantasy. He saw 'degeneracy' as the vital factor in sexual deviance, and masturbation as a manifestation of degeneracy. He described the dire consequences of masturbation as insanity, disease and hereditary complications. He saw homosexuality as a disease.

In 1886, he published *Psychopathia Sexualis*, a text based on case studies of psychotic behaviour. Although now challenged, and originally written to be read by doctors only, at the time it was an immensely popular and influential work. In 1897 he supported moves to make male homosexuality legal in Germany, but with reservations.

Alfred Charles Kinsey (American, 1894–1956)
Kinsey is best known for his ground-breaking reports, *Sexual Behaviour in the Human Male* (1948), written with Wardell Pomeroy and Clyde Martin, and *Sexual Behaviour in the Human Female* (1953). The reports were based on thousands of interviews with American men and women, describing their sexual behaviour.

The interviews were largely with white, middle-class Americans, and spectacularly increased knowledge of sexual practices. They revealed an enormous diversity, including premarital and extramarital sex, oral sex, masturbation and homosexuality. This latter (that thirty-seven per cent of American males had had at least one homosexual experience) caused outcry and disbelief. Kinsey suggested a sexual continuum with seven points from exclusively heterosexual activity to exclusively homosexual activity, with bisexuality as the average.

He also put forward theories of sexuality linked to the different brain functionings of men and women to account for the 'submissiveness' of women and the 'aggressiveness' of men. He also, however, discussed social conditioning and hormonal influences on sexuality.

Heterosexuality, married sex and vaginal intercourse were considered to be the norms for Kinsey. He did, nevertheless, challenge current sexual thinking, and strongly influenced later developments. He founded the Institute for Sex Research at the University of Indiana in 1942, still renowned for its research into sexuality.

Jacques Lacan (French, 1901–81)
Lacan was a follower of Freud. He reinterpreted Freud and the theory of the Oedipus complex as being primarily to do with patriarchy and the importance of the phallus, which is a linguistic and symbolic term, unlike penis which is a biological term.

He put forward the theory of love being not a simple two-way, but a five-way, exchange – the subject, the object, the idea that the subject has of the object, the image that the object has of the subject and the Other (the sexual relationship controlled by the law of the Oedipus complex).

William H. Masters (American, born 1915) and Virginia E. Johnson (American, born 1925)
Masters and Johnson researched sexual responses, rather than sexual behaviours. They carried out hundreds of case studies on sexual intercourse, including observing couples, and recorded their findings. They studied the stages and changes during arousal and orgasm and measured the effects on heart rate, breathing and blood pressure. They found that men and women had similar sexual responses in arousal and orgasm and that the clitoris was the important factor in female orgasm. They also showed that women could have multiple orgasms. The results of this work were published in 1966 in *Human Sexual Response*.

They developed, based on their work, a two-week treatment for sexual problems and published *Human Sexual Inadequacy* in 1970. This created huge interest and encouraged training in sexual therapy.

Their later work has been challenged and criticized – their theories on homosexuality proposed that homosexuality, while not a disease, could be cured and that homosexual and heterosexual sexual responses were similar. These views are recorded in *Homosexuality in Perspective* (1979). They have also been criticized for writing about AIDS in a sensationalist manner.

Ivan Petrovich Pavlov (Russian 1849–1936)
Just before the turn of the century, Pavlov, a Russian psychologist, discovered 'conditioned reflexes', and the way they could be manipulated, during his famous experimental work with dogs. One application of his work has been in 'reconditioning' sexual tastes through aversion therapy. Sex therapists, including Masters and Johnson, have also used his work to treat problems such as premature ejaculation, frigidity and impotence.

Margaret Sanger (American, 1880–1966)
Sanger took up the challenge set out by earlier American campaigners for women's rights to contraception, notably Frances Wright in the 1820s and Elizabeth Cady Stanton in the 1880s.

She worked with Emma Goldman, who also advocated women's rights to enjoy sex. In 1914, Sanger first published *The Woman Rebel*, and the pamphlet on contraceptive usage, *Family Limitation*, for which she was arrested. She then left the USA for Britain. The case against her was dropped and she returned to the USA to open the first birth control clinic in New York. The clinic was popular with women, but closed by the police and its staff jailed.

She founded the American Birth Control League in 1921 to lobby those with power and influence and monitor and research issues relevant to birth control. Contraception was legalized in the USA in 1965, an event to which Sanger's work had made an enormous contribution.

Marie Stopes (British, 1880–1958)
Stopes was an important campaigner for sexual and reproductive rights for women. Her first marriage was unconsummated, a fact which encouraged her to research sexuality by reading comprehensively what was available at the time. As a result of this, she published, in 1918, the books *Wise Parenthood* and *Married Love*. The latter was revolutionary in that it encouraged women to enjoy sex, even during pregnancy, and to take control of their fertility.

Women wrote to her for advice (some of these letters were published in *Dear Dr Stopes*, edited by Ruth Hall in 1978) in great numbers and she responded with radical suggestions on how to improve their sex lives. She opened the first British birth control clinic, staffed entirely by women, in 1920 in London. This clinic, The Marie Stopes Clinic, still exists.

She was condemned by the Roman Catholic Church and by the British establishment and fought long battles for her beliefs.

5 DICTIONARY OF SEX & SEXUAL TERMS

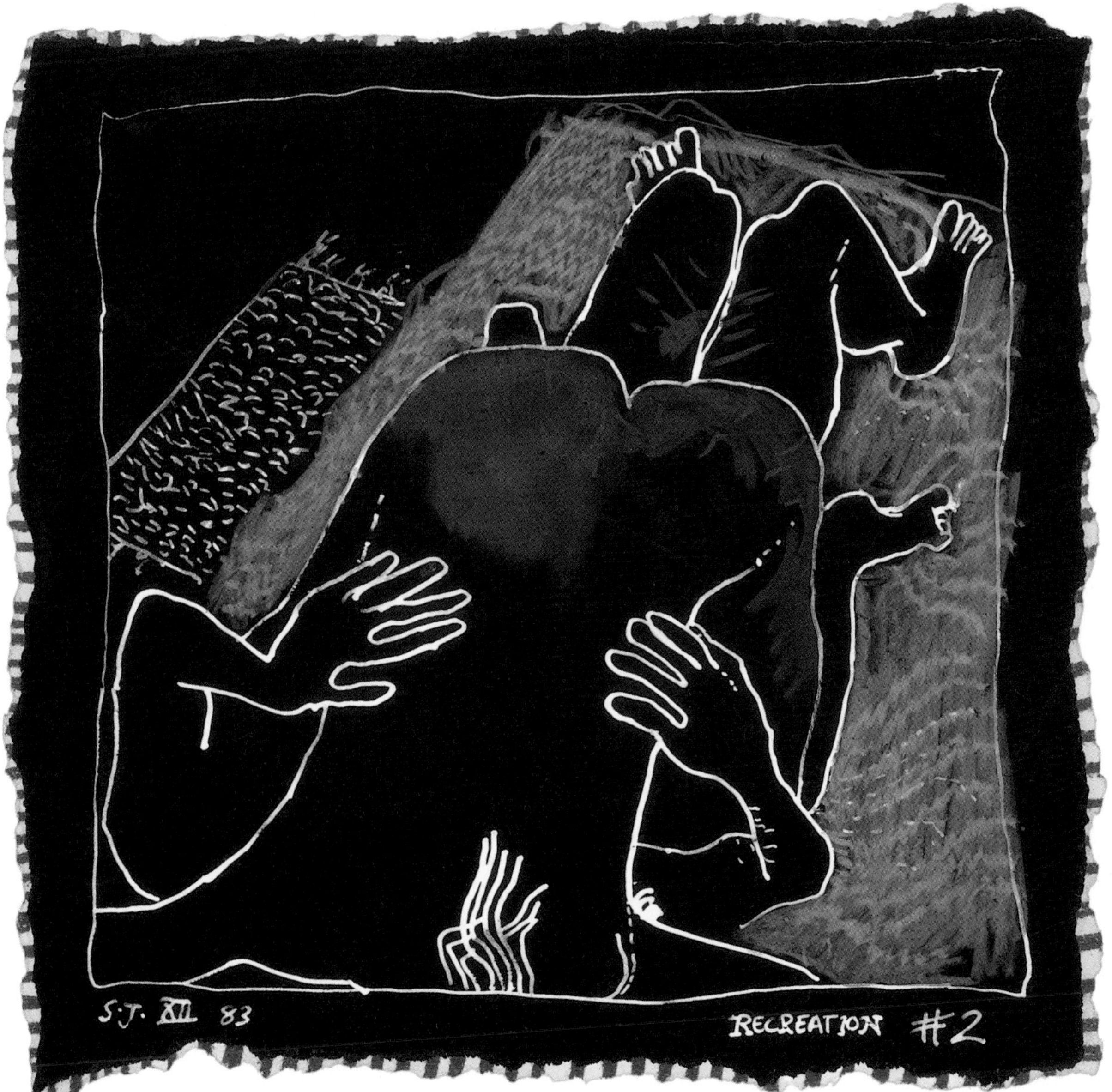
S.J. XII 83
RECREATION #2

Abortion Premature termination of pregnancy, either natural and spontaneous, or induced. Deliberately induced abortion is most commonly by means of a short surgical operation, or by medical means, through the administration of certain drugs and/or prostaglandins. The most common causes of natural abortion include accident and infection.

Abstinence Refraining from sexual activity for personal, moral or religious reasons. Abstinence can also be practised as a contraceptive measure. *See* Celibacy.

Adolescence The stage of development between childhood and adulthood, beginning with puberty. In the course of adolescence, the young person becomes physically and sexually mature. It is also a time of significant psychological and emotional development, affecting personal and sexual identity.

Adultery Sexual intercourse where one or both of the partners involved is married to, or in a similarly committed relationship with, another person.

Adulthood The stage of development when an individual has reached maturity and full physiological development.

Afterplay Term (now rarely used) to refer to intimacies and sexual interactions that take place after the climax of sexual activity. *See* Foreplay.

Age of consent The age at which individuals can legally engage in sexual contact with other people. This varies from one culture to another.

AID (Artificial Insemination by Donor) Also called Donor Insemination, the procedure by which the semen of an anonymous donor is inserted mechanically into a woman's vagina close to the cervix in order to achieve a pregnancy.

AIDS (Acquired Immune Deficiency Syndrome) The syndrome that can represent the last phase of HIV infection, sometimes known as 'full-blown AIDS'. It occurs when the immune system has broken down to the point where cancers and opportunistic infections can take hold. The disease is not fully understood but it appears that up to ten years or more may pass from initial infection to the development of AIDS and, in some cases, AIDS may not develop at all. *See* HIV, Kaposi's sarcoma.

Amenorrhoea Absence of periods. The term primary amenorrhoea is used when menstruation has not started by the age of sixteen; secondary amenorrhoea is when periods stop for six months or longer. Causes of secondary amenorrhoea include pregnancy and rapid weight loss.

Ampallang Rod inserted horizontally through the glans of the penis as a form of genital piercing. It functions as body decoration and may heighten sexual arousal for the man's partner. *See* Piercing.

Anal intercourse Sexual intercourse in which the man's penis is inserted into his partner's anus. *See* Sodomy.

Anal stimulators Devices used to stimulate the anus, such as Thai beads, butt plugs or anal vibrators.

Androgyne Person that has both male and female sexual characteristics. Also known as a hermaphrodite.

Anilingus Applying the mouth or tongue to a partner's anus to give it erotic stimulation. Also know as rimming. *See* Rimming, Dental dam.

Anus The orifice at the base of the rectum. The anal area is an erogenous zone for many people; the anus itself may be used for penetrative intercourse, between heterosexual or male homosexual couples, in which the penis is inserted into the partner's anus.

Apadravya Rod inserted vertically into the glans of the penis as a form of genital piercing. It functions as body decoration and may heighten sexual arousal both for the man and his partner. *See* Piercing.

Aphrodisiac Anything (substance, smell, words, music etc) believed to increase sexual desire or performance. The word is derived from the ancient Greek word *aphrodisios*, meaning belonging to Aphrodite, the Greek goddess of love.

Arab straps Straps that are fastened around the penis. Like other similar devices – cock and ball straps, cock rings, Gates of Hell – they are usually made of rubber or leather, and help produce and maintain a man's erection by trapping blood in the penis. Sometimes they are used therapeutically in cases of erection failure. Some people also find their appearance arousing and they may also provide physical stimulation for the wearer's partner.

ARC (AIDS-Related Complex) HIV-related illness; the stage before 'full-blown' AIDS. *See* AIDS.

Areola Area of pigmented skin surrounding the human nipple that swells a little during sexual arousal.

Armpits The armpits are erogenous zones for many people, particularly women. Axillary intercourse, in which a man's penis is gripped in his partner's armpit while he thrusts, is a common form of non-penetrative intercourse. The strong body odours produced in this area also give it a fetishistic appeal for many.

Arousal Physiological and mental changes that occur to the body in response to sexual stimuli and which prepare it for sexual interaction or intercourse.

Auto-eroticism Term for masturbation.

Axillary sex *See* Armpit.

AZT (Azidothymidine) The first drug admitted by Western governments for use in the treatment of HIV and AIDS.

Bacterial vaginosis Infection caused by overgrowth of bacteria that occur naturally within the vagina. Symptoms may include a watery, grey vaginal discharge with a 'fishy' odour.

Balanitis Inflammation of the glans of the penis or clitoris, usually caused by an infection. Irritation may also occur.

Barrier contraception Contraceptive methods that act as a physical barrier to prevent the male sperm from coming into contact with the female ovum. Barrier methods, especially the condom and other methods used in conjunction with spermicides, can give some protection against sexually transmitted diseases. *See* Cervical cap, Condom, Diaphragm.

Bartholin's gland A gland located near the vaginal opening. During sexual arousal it produces secretions which provide some lubrication. Some have believed it to be responsible for reported cases of female ejaculation at orgasm but this is more likely to be the Skene glands. *See* Ejaculation.

Bathhouses Sometimes used as meeting places for sexual encounters for gay men, and sometimes lesbians, since Roman times.

Ben-wa-balls *See* Love balls.

Bestiality Sexual activity with animals involving intercourse, masturbation or oral stimulation. Pleasure may also be derived from watching animals engage in sexual activity, or a fetishistic attachment to animal skins or furs.

Bigamy The practice of having more than one spouse. While illegal in some cultures or religions, it is traditional in others.

Birth control Limitation and/or planning of pregnancies by means of contraception.

Bisexuality Sexual attraction to and/or activity with people of both sexes.

Blastocyst A small sphere of cells that enters the uterus from the fallopian tube and develops a cavity within itself as it implants in the lining of the uterus. The inner cell mass of the blastocyst develops into the embryo, an early stage in human prenatal development.

Blue movie A pornographic film or video. The term is derived from the blue pencil originally used to censor material considered unsuitable for general viewing.

Body hairdressing The style in which the body hair is fashioned. Many women shave their underarms and legs; some men shave their chest hair. Hair around the genital area can be dyed, plaited, shaved into shapes and patterns, or removed completely.

Body language Movements and gestures of the body that convey signals or messages, often at an unconscious level, to other individuals.

Body rubbing *See* Tribadism.

Bondage A sexual practice in which pleasure is gained by one partner being physically restrained by being tied up or bound. It can be a way of defining active and passive sexual roles and is also sometimes part of dominant or sadomasochistic sexual practices.

Bottom As well as the human posterior or rump, the term is used for the passive partner during dominant/submissive sex play, particularly where sadomasochistic practices are involved.

Breasts The fleshy female mammary glands that provide milk for offspring. In humans they are associated with sexual signals and are also an erogenous zone producing strong sexual arousal in some women.

Buggery A common term for anal intercourse. *See* Anal intercourse.

Butch A type of lesbian identity involving a rejection of conventional femininity for the adoption of masculine characteristics. *See* Femme.

Buttocks Fleshy muscular tissue, which constitutes the human rump. The buttocks are a source of attractiveness and/or an erogenous zone for many people.

Butt-plugs Solid tapering blocks, usually made of latex or rubber, for use in the anus and rectum. Most are between 15 to 18 cm long and about 25 cm in girth. They may be used to dilate the sphincter, or muscles surrounding the anus, prior to anal sex or as anal stimulators.

Calendar method A method for working out which days a woman is most likely to be ovulating by keeping an exact record of the timing of her menstrual cycle. *See* Natural methods.

Camp An expression used in reference to male homosexual subculture. It is characterized by exaggeratedly effeminate styles of speech, dress or movement.

Candaulism The practice of a spouse watching their partner having sex with another person.

Candida albicans An infection, sometimes known as thrush, caused by a type of yeast. It is a common organism, occurring naturally in the gut and on the skin, that can cause symptoms if there is excessive growth. These may include irritation and soreness around the genital area and a thick, white, yeasty discharge from the vagina or penis. It can be spread by sexual contact and sexual partners can reinfect one another.

Castration The removal of the testicles, scrotum, penis, clitoris or ovaries.

Casual sex Short-term sexual relations. It usually involves an emphasis on the physical rather than the emotional side of sex.

Catamite A boy kept for the purposes of homosexual intercourse.

Celibacy A commitment to refrain from sexual activity or intercourse, for personal, moral or religious reasons.

Cervical cap A barrier method of contraception, consisting of a circular dome of thin rubber which is placed over the cervix and is held in place by suction.

Cervical mucus method A method for working out which days a woman is most likely to be ovulating by observing the regular changes in vaginal discharge, which becomes more copious, slippery and clear near the time of ovulation. Also known as the mucus method. *See* Natural methods.

Cervix The neck of the uterus, which extends into the top of the vagina. It forms the passageway between the vagina and uterus. *See* Vagina, Uterus.

Chancroid A bacterial infection that usually occurs only in tropical or sub-tropical regions. The symptoms include ulcers and sometimes abscesses that appear around the genitals.

Change of life A term for the menopause or climacteric, the period in a woman's life during which the menstrual cycle ceases. *See* Climacteric, Menopause.

Chastity Abstaining from sexual intercourse, especially before marriage.

Child sexual abuse Sexual activity involving children, against their will or without their understanding, usually by an older person.

Childhood The stage of development from birth to the onset of puberty.

Chlamydia Sexually transmitted disease caused by a bacterial infection. Initially symptoms may include some pain and discharge, or there may be no symptoms at all. However, if untreated, the infection can cause pelvic inflammatory disease in women and urethritis in men.

Chromosomes Units found in every living cell of the body, responsible for the transmission of hereditary characteristics. Chromosomes are arranged in pairs consisting of two identical parts, except in the case of the pair that determine gender. This consists of two 'X' chromosomes for a female and an 'X' and a 'Y' for a male. Any other combinations of X and Y chromosomes can result in gender anomalies, as in Klinefelter's Syndrome where an XXY combination produces a person with male outward appearance but underdeveloped testes and penis, who will be infertile. *See* Genes.

Cicatrization The deliberate scarring of the body, originally practised in certain African tribes as signs of fertility, accomplishment or bravery, and in other cultures for other reasons, such as body decoration, sexual arousal and ritualistic purposes.

Circumcision For males, the removal of the foreskin of the penis, often performed for religious reasons or, increasingly, for reasons of hygiene. For females it involves an incision into, or complete removal of the clitoris and sometimes infibulation (sewing together) of the outer labia.

Climacteric The period of time during which there is a gradual decline in the production of sex hormones. In women it is marked by the end of menstruation, when the ovaries cease to be active, which usually occurs between the ages of forty-five and fifty-six. In men it is less pronounced but generally the production of testosterone begins to decline from about the age of forty, with a corresponding drop in sex drive. *See* Menopause.

Climax The height of arousal during sexual activity, usually the point at which orgasm is reached. It is characterized by involuntary muscle spasms and waves of intense pleasure through the body. *See* Orgasm.

Clitoral stimulator A rubber, latex or plastic ring, sometimes with a variety of knobs, bumps and soft projections, that is placed around the base of the penis and rubs against the clitoris during intercourse. It may also provide extra sensation to the vaginal opening and vaginal wall.

Clitoridectomy The surgical removal of the clitoris in female circumcision. In certain cultural groups – including some African societies and Islamic groups – it is a male-imposed practice, performed as a social or initiation rite, to reduce the woman's enjoyment of sex in order to discourage the woman from adultery. It may also be performed to keep orgasm as a male prerogative. In Western societies it has been used as a means of discouraging juvenile sexual activity. In some cases. it may be performed for medical reasons.

Clitoris Female erectile organ, situated above the vaginal opening where the inner labia meet. It develops from the same tissue in the embryo as the penis in the male and, while small (usually no more than 2 to 3 cm long), it is highly sensitive. It contains muscular tissue and many nerve endings, as well as erectile tissue arranged in two columns, the corpora cavernosa. In the course of sexual arousal it thickens and may lengthen as it becomes engorged with blood, and the glans or head emerges from beneath the prepuce or hood formed by the inner labia, making it more exposed and sensitive. Just before orgasm it withdraws beneath the prepuce but remains sensitive. The sole function of the clitoris is sexual arousal and pleasure, where it plays a key role in the stimulation leading up to a woman's orgasm.

Cock and ball straps Straps that are fastened around the base of the testicles and penis, usually made of rubber or leather. *See* Arab straps.

Cock ring Ring fastened around the base of the penis to help produce and maintain a man's erection. It should be an easily removable device made from rubber or leather, never metal or hard plastic. *See* Arab straps.

Coitus Sexual intercourse. The term is most commonly used to refer to the penetration of the vagina with the penis, but also used to describe other kinds of intercourse (see below).

Coitus analis Latin term for anal intercourse.

Coitus in axilla Sexual intercourse in which the man's penis is inserted into the armpit of his partner. *See* Armpit.

Coitus inter femora Sexual intercourse in which the man's penis is gripped between his partner's thighs, without penetrating the vagina or anus.

Coitus interruptus Also known as withdrawal, it involves withdrawing the penis during intercourse, before ejaculation occurs.

Combined pill A contraceptive pill that contains both oestrogen and progestogen. It is usually taken for twenty-one consecutive days with a seven-day break before recommencing the cycle.

Come Verb meaning to reach orgasm. It is also used as a noun meaning semen, when it is more commonly spelt cum.

Come out An abbreviation of the expression 'to come out of the closet', meaning to openly declare homosexual or bisexual orientation.

Computer sex Sexually explicit material – text, pictures, videos – exchanged by means of computer networks and the Internet. Bulletin boards may be set up and correspondences may develop.

Conception Fertilization of an ovum by a sperm, resulting in the start of a new life. The union of the two cells usually occurs in the fallopian tubes. About a day later the fertilized cell starts to divide, and the growing ball of cells passes down the fallopian tubes to the uterus where it continues to develop.

Concubine In polygamous societies this is a secondary wife, usually of lower social rank. In other societies it simply means a woman who cohabits with a man.

Condom The male condom is a thin latex sheath, which is placed over an erect penis before intercourse. It functions chiefly as a barrier form of contraception, by preventing sperm from being released into the vagina, and as a means of preventing the spread of sexually transmissible diseases. Coloured, textured, flavoured and even padded condoms are also available for use as sex aids/toys. The female condom, made of polyurethane, is a tube closed at one end with a flexible ring at each end, one of which is inserted into the vagina, behind the pubic bone, while the other lies flat against the vulva. It has the same function as the male condom. *See* Sex aids, Sex toys.

Contraception Any means of preventing conception from occurring as a result of sexual intercourse. The range of options include natural, mechanical and hormonal methods.

Coprolalia The use of sexually arousing language during sex. Also known as 'talking dirty'.

Coprophilia Sexual arousal from practices involving faeces and/or the process of defecation. *See* Scat.

Copulation Sexual intercourse or coitus.

Cowper's gland Gland located below the prostate gland in the male, possessing ducts which lead into the urethra. It produces a mucus substance that is important in lubricating the penis and that neutralizes any acidity caused by urine, which could kill sperm. This substance also forms part of the seminal fluid.

Crabs *See* Pubic lice.

Cremaster One of the two sets of muscles that support the testes and are attached to the testes themselves. *See* Dartos.

Cross-dressing Dressing in the clothing, under clothing and sometimes make-up associated with the opposite sex. *See* Transvestism.

Crotch The area between the legs, where the torso ends and the legs begin. The term is often used to refer specifically to the genital area.

Croupade Any rear-entry position taken during intercourse, in which the man penetrates squarely from behind, that is without either partner having one leg between that of the other's. *See* Cuissade.

Cruise To actively seek a sexual partner. The term is most commonly used with reference to looking for a homosexual partner.

Cuissade A half-rear entry position during sexual intercourse in which the woman has one of her legs between those of her partner.

Cunnilingus Oral sex in which the mouth or tongue is used to stimulate the vulva and clitoris of a woman.

Cutting The activity of cutting the body with razors or knives, which may form part of sadomasochistic practices.

Cystitis Inflammation of the bladder. Causes include certain bacterial and non-bacterial infections, allergic reactions to toiletries and friction during intercourse. Symptoms typically include a burning sensation when passing urine, a need to pass urine more often, and cloudy urine or blood in the urine.

Daisy Chain A group sex practice that involves a circle of people, each engaged in sexual interaction with the person in front of them. It can involve oral, vaginal and/or anal sex.

Dartos One of the two sets of muscles that support the testes, attached to the inside of the scrotum. *See* Cremaster.

Deep-throat A form of fellatio that involves accommodating the whole length of the penis in the mouth and throat. In order to do this the person performing fellatio needs to overcome the 'gagging' reflex.

Dental dam A square of latex rubber which is placed over the vagina or anus to avoid risk of the transmission of sexually transmissible infections and diseases during cunnilingus and/or anilingus.

Detumescence The subsidence of a swelling, in particular the return of the penis to its original flaccid state, following erection.

Diaphragm A barrier method of contraception consisting of a circular dome of thin rubber, kept in shape by a pliable circular spring. It should be used in conjunction with a spermicide. The diaphragm is inserted into the vagina and sits behind the pubic bone, covering the entrance to the cervix. Previously known as the Dutch Cap.

Dildo An artificial erect penis – usually made out of plastic or rubber and available in various sizes and shapes – that may be used in masturbation or as a sex-aid for couples.

Dom Abbreviation of the term dominant, used to refer to an active partner in practices involving bondage and sadomasochism. The term 'top' is also used.

Donor insemination *See* AID.

Drag Women's clothes worn by a man, sometimes with theatrical effect.

Dutch cap *See* Diaphragm.

Dydo A piercing through the edge of the glans of the penis. *See* Ampallang.

Dysmenorrhoea Particularly painful menstruation, typically involving nausea, cramps and headaches.

Ectopic pregnancy A type of pregnancy in which the fertilized egg becomes embedded and starts to grow outside the uterus, usually in one of the fallopian tubes.

Egg or **egg cell** *See* Ovum.

Ejaculation The release of seminal fluid from a man's penis at orgasm. Ejaculation has also been observed in females where fluids are released from the Skene glands either side of the urethra, usually following stimulation of the G-spot. *See* Bartholin's gland.

Emergency contraception Contraceptive measures, including a hormonal pill combining oestrogen and progestogen (effective up to seventy-two hours after intercourse) or the insertion of an intrauterine device (IUD) within five days of the expected ovulation date. These can be used by women who have had unprotected sexual intercourse or who suspect their method of contraception may have failed.

Endometrium The lining of the uterus, made up of cells and blood, that is shed once a month in the process of menstruation if no fertilized egg is implanted. If an egg is fertilized it is passed along the fallopian tube until it reaches the uterus, where it becomes implanted in the endometrium. *See* Menstrual cycle.

Enema The introduction of liquid into the anus to clean or clear out the bowels. It is sometimes performed for sexual stimulation or as preparation for other sexual practices.

Eonism Term for transvestism, introduced by Havelock Ellis.

Epididymis Tube through which sperm is passed from the testes, where sperm cells mature and are stored before being passed into the vas deferens prior to ejaculation.

Erection The stiffening and swelling of the penis, clitoris or nipples following engorgement with blood as a result of sexual arousal.

Erogenous zone Any part of the body that is particularly sensitive to sexual stimulation. Erogenous zones vary from one person to another and can include the breasts, mouth, ears, nose and any other part of the body, as well as the genitals.

Erotic Sexually arousing and exciting.

Erotophobia The fear of sex and sexuality.

Eunuch A man whose testes have been removed in castration.

EveryDay pill A contraceptive pill, either progestogen-only or combined, that is produced in packs containing – as well as the twenty-one active pills – seven inactive pills that are taken in the seven-day break. It is often taken by women who find it difficult to remember to start taking the pill again after the seven-day break. *See* Combined pill.

Exhibitionism Pleasure derived from displaying oneself sexually, especially in public. *See* Flasher.

Fallopian tubes Two tubes, each about 10 cm long, that extend from either side of the uterus. The ends lie near to the ovaries and are bell-shaped, with finger-like structures (fimbriae) that help to catch the ovum as it is released from the ovary. The tubes are lined with hairlike cilia that help to carry the ovum down the tube towards the uterus. Fertilization of an ovum usually occurs within a fallopian tube.

Family planning Planning and controlling the timing, frequency and/or number of pregnancies by means of contraceptive measures. *See* Birth control, Contraception.

Family planning clinic A special clinic that provides information and advice about family planning and contraception and provides the contraceptives themselves where necessary.

Fantasy (sexual) Imagining sexual situations, involving real or imaginary places and people, as a sexual stimulus.

Fellatio Oral sex, involving the tongue or mouth in the stimulation of the penis.

Female sterilization A surgical operation in which the fallopian tubes are clipped or cut and tied, so that the ovum cannot travel to the uterus or the sperm travel to meet the ovum. *See* Sterilization.

Femme Term sometimes used to describe a feminine – as opposed to butch – lesbian. *See* Butch.

Fertilization The penetration of an ovum by a sperm and the fusion of their genetic material. *See* Conception.

Fetishism An attachment to a particular object, material or part of the body other than the genitals, which enhances sexual arousal.

Fisting The insertion of the whole hand into the anus or vagina.

Flaccid Lacking firmness, therefore limp and soft. In the sexual context this usually refers to a penis that is not erect.

Flagellation The act of whipping or flogging for sexual arousal. It is often a sadomasochistic or dominant/submissive sexual practice.

Flanquette Any of the half-facing group of sexual postures in which the woman lies facing her partner with one of her legs between his.

Flasher A man who displays his genitals in public places. *See* Exhibitionism.

Foreplay Term (now rarely used) to describe sexual activity that takes place in the early stages of arousal. *See* Afterplay.

Foreskin The retractable fold of thin, hairless skin that covers the head or glans of the penis. This is sometimes removed in part or whole in the practice of circumcision. *See* Prepuce, Circumcision.

Fornication Archaic term for sexual intercourse between unmarried people.

Fourchette The delicate area of skin about 2 to 3 cm above the anus, where the inner labia join at the back of the vaginal opening in the female.

French kissing A kiss with one or both partners' tongues inserted into the other's mouth.

Frenulum or **frenum** The bridge of particularly sensitive skin at the back of the glans of the penis in the male, between the glans and the skin of the shaft.

Frigidity A psychological block preventing a person from being able to become completely involved in or to enjoy sexual intercourse.

Frottage Sex play that involves rubbing the penis between a partner's thighs, armpits or chest, without penetration. *See* Coitus in axilla, Coitus inter femora, Gluteal sex.

Frotteur The practice of rubbing up against another person's clothed body – with or without their consent – for sexual excitement.

Furtling The use of fingers inserted into cut-outs in the genital areas of photographs, for sexual arousal. This was particularly popular in Britain in the Victorian age.

Gang-bang Sexual practice where a woman has vaginal intercourse with several men in succession; also used to refer to group rape.

Gardnerella *See* Bacterial vaginosis.

Gates of Hell Rings, usually made of metal or leather, that are placed around the penis. *See* Arab straps.

Gay Term commonly used to refer to homosexual behaviour, people, culture etc. The word lesbian is used more commonly to refer to women who prefer sex with women.

Gender The state of being biologically male or female.

Gender identity The individual's conscious sense of being male or female, as determined by biological, psychological and social influences.

Gender reassignment The process undergone by some transsexuals, to bring their physical sex characteristics into line with their gender identity. The process includes living for a period of time as the desired sex, a course of the appropriate male or female hormones, surgery to remove or enlarge the breasts, and surgery on the reproductive organs and external genitals.

Gender role The pattern of behavioural characteristics associated with being male or female in a particular culture. It is the outward expression of gender identity, often related to socially-ascribed roles. *See* Chromosomes.

Genes The units that make up chromosomes, which are found in each body cell. Genes are made up of DNA, which is responsible for the transmission of inheritable characteristics. See Chromosomes.

Genital herpes *See* Herpes.

Genitals The external sex organs; in a male, the penis and testicles; in a female, the vagina, clitoris and labia.

Genital warts Small warts or growths caused by the human papilloma virus. They are found on or around the genitals and can be transmitted through sexual intercourse.

Gerontophilia Sexual interest in and attraction to older people.

Gigolo A man who receives money from women for escorting them and/or having sex with them.

Glans The rounded, highly sensitive head of the penis or clitoris, which has a high concentration of nerve endings and is therefore very responsive to touch. *See* Frenulum.

Gluteal sex Sexual practice where a man's penis is stimulated by being moved between the buttocks of his partner.

Gonads The organs that produce the reproductive cells and the sex hormones: the ovaries of a woman or the testes of a man. Male and female gonads develop from the same tissue in the embryo, before sexual differentiation takes place in the ninth week of pregnancy. Also known as the sex glands.

Gonorrhoea Sexually transmitted disease caused by the bacteria gonococcus. It can affect the urethra, cervix, rectum and occasionally the throat if it is passed by oral-genital contact. It attacks the mucous membranes, causing inflammation and the production of pus. Characteristic symptoms include a discharge of white or yellow fluid from the penis or vagina and pain when urinating, but these are usually more obvious in men. If untreated, gonorrhoea can lead to sterility.

Grope suit Tight underwear made for women, to produce sexual excitement and orgasm. Usually consists of a tight rubber G-string and a bra, each with protuberances on the inside to stimulate the vagina, G-spot, clitoris and nipples.

G-spot A specific area that is particularly and intensely responsive to sexual stimulation in some men and women. Also known as the Grafenberg spot after Dr Ernst Grafenberg who first described it. The male G-spot has been identified as the prostate gland: the female as a small area on the front wall of the vagina, although opinions still vary with regard to the nature of the G-spot and – in the case of the female – even its existence. For some people stimulation of the G-spot is the key to reaching orgasm, for others it serves to intensify the sensations of orgasm, while for others it has little or no effect.

Guiche A piercing in the ridge of flesh behind the scrotum. *See* Ampallang.

Hafada A piercing made through the scrotal sac. It can be made at the side, so that it is visible from the front, or from underneath and behind, running in a line down the centre seam of the scrotum. *See* Ampallang.

Hard on The state of male sexual arousal resulting in the erection and hardening of the penis.

Hepatitis B A virus present in the blood and other bodily fluids of an infected person, causing inflammation of the liver. It is passed on through contact with infected body fluids and can therefore be transmitted sexually.

Hermaphrodite A person that has both male and female sexual characteristics.

Herpes A viral infection, the most common form of which is the herpes simplex virus. Type I affects the mouth and occasionally the genitals and type II just the genital and anal areas. It is characterized by the formation of small watery blisters on, in or around the genitals and cold sores on the mouth, although it may be asymptomatic. It can be passed through genital and oral-genital contact.

Heterophobia The fear and/or hatred of heterosexuality.

Heterosexism Term for the prejudice experienced by lesbians and gay men from some heterosexual people.

Heterosexuality Sexual attraction to and/or activity with members of the opposite sex.

HIV The Human Immunodeficiency Virus, which if contracted prevents the immune system from working as it normally should, by attacking the 'CD4 cells', which coordinate the fight against infections. This leaves the body defenceless to both infection and disease. HIV can be transmitted through sexual activity. *See* AIDS, Kaposi's sarcoma, ARC.

Homoeroticism Any material that suggests lesbian or gay sexuality and/or love.

Homophile Term for homosexual. The Greek root 'philos', to love, means that the word literally means love of the same sex.

Homophobia Fear and/or hatred of homosexuality.

Homosexuality Sexual attraction to and/or activity with members of the same sex. Current estimates suggest that between five and ten per cent of men and a smaller percentage of women are exclusively homosexual throughout their lives. However, Kinsey's studies suggested that about thirty-seven per cent of males and thirteen per cent of females had some overt homosexual experience in adult life and more recent estimates are higher than this. It is also known that homo-erotic fantasy is common amongst people of all sexual orientations.

Hormonal methods of contraception Methods of preventing conception involving the use of synthetic hormones similar to those produced naturally by the body. Taken either by pill, injection or implant, they have been one of the most popular female contraceptives since the 1960s. Research and trials continue on hormonal contraceptives for use by men. *See* Natural methods, Mechanical methods, Pill (contraceptive).

Hormone One of several types of natural, chemical substances produced by endocrine glands in the body and which regulate bodily processes such as growth, metabolism and reproduction. The sex hormones, including oestrogen, progesterone and testosterone, play a major role in the sexual and reproductive functions of the body.

Hormone Replacement Therapy (HRT) The treatment in tablet, patch or gel implant form, for menopausal symptoms in women. It involves the administration of natural oestrogen and/or synthetic progesterone, which the ovaries have ceased to produce.

Hymen A thin membrane that partially covers the entrance to the vagina in young girls. It may be broken by physical exercise, by using tampons or at first intercourse.

Hysterectomy The surgical removal of the female uterus, usually because of infection, disease, prolapse or excessive bleeding.

Impotence A sexual dysfunction in males that involves an inability to achieve or maintain an erection sufficient to perform sexual intercourse. The cause may be physiological or psychological: among the most common causes are anxiety, stress and emotional conflicts.

Incest Sexual relations between individuals who are members of the same family.

Inner labia *See* Labia minora.

Intercourse Common term for coitus, involving the insertion of the man's erect penis into his partner's vagina or anus, followed by rhythmic thrusting that usually involves climax in orgasm. *See* Coitus.

Intrafemoral sex Coitus inter femora, or sexual intercourse in which the man's penis is gripped between his partner's thighs, without penetrating the vagina or anus.

Inversion A term for homosexuality used at the turn of the century and employed by sex researchers of that time.

IUD (Intrauterine Device) A method of contraception consisting of a copper or copper and silver device, the first designs of which released progestogen. The device is professionally inserted into a woman's uterus. It prevents fertilization and/or implantation of a fertilized ovum. May also be used as emergency contraception. *See* IUS.

IUS (Intrauterine System) An intrauterine device known as Mirena that releases progestogen. It can be left in place for five years.

IVF (Invitro Fertilization) The fertilization of an ovum, by a sperm, which occurs 'artificially' outside the body, often in a test-tube under laboratory conditions.

Kakila Term used in the *Kama Sutra* to describe the sexual practice now known as the sixty-nine position, which involves two people simultaneously performing oral sex on one another.

Kama Sutra Possibly the world's first sex manual, also seen by many as a literary classic. It describes the sensual pleasure to be derived from music and poetry as well as giving a great variety of advice and information on the enjoyment of sex. It was written by Vatsyana in the fourth to fifth centuries AD, but was based on earlier sources.

Kaposi's sarcoma (KS) A form of skin cancer that is particularly associated with HIV infection and the development of AIDS. It causes a growth of the blood vessel walls resulting in red and purple lesions on the skin. The condition is named after Moritz Kohn Kaposi (1837-1902), an Australian dermatologist who first described the condition. *See* HIV, AIDS.

Kinsey Six Slang term for a homosexual. The term refers to a scale of sexual orientation devised by the pioneering sex researcher, Alfred Kinsey, where a six was reserved for those who had no interest at all in heterosexual activity. *See* Homosexuality.

Kissing Touching or caressing with the lips and tongue as an expression of love, friendship, desire or respect. *See* French kissing.

Klinefelter's syndrome An XXY combination of chromosomes. *See* Chromosomes.

KY Jelly The brand name of a popular water-based lubricant, used widely to facilitate penetration.

Labia majora or **Outer labia** The two 'lips' that surround the vaginal opening, usually lying close together to protect it. At the front they join at the mons pubis; at the back they join at the perineum. They are plump enough to act as a cushion during intercourse. They contain sweat- and odour-producing glands, which keep the smooth inner part moistened and give the vulva its highly individual sexual odour.

Labia minora or **Inner labia** the smaller, hairless 'lips' or folds of skin within the outer labia, immediately around the vaginal opening. At the front they join to form the hood of the clitoris and at the back they form the fourchette. They contain sebaceous glands on their outer side and sweat glands on the inner parts which help with lubrication. During sexual arousal they become engorged with blood (in a similar manner to the penis), which makes them darken in colour and swell to two or three times their normal size. *See* Fourchette.

Latex love Term for safer sex practices where condoms (usually made of latex) or dental dams are used. *See* Condoms, Dental dams.

Lesbian A woman who is sexually attracted to other women. The word is derived from the island of Lesbos, which was the dwelling place of the Greek lesbian poet Sappho (610-580 BC).

Libido The term coined by Sigmund Freud to refer to human sexual motivation. Now understood as sex drive, sexual desire or urge. *See* Sex drive.

Littre's glands Small mucus glands that open into the urethra in men and women. In the male they are similar to the Cowper's glands, in that they release a pre-ejaculatory, lubricating fluid.

Love Arguably the most powerful human emotion, love is a very strong feeling of affection, care, attachment or desire for someone or something.

Love balls, love eggs Two hollow balls, sometimes containing small weights inside them, joined by a cord. They are placed inside a woman's vagina, where the weights cause them to move around as the woman moves. They may keep her in a state of constant arousal or bring her to climax. They are also useful in exercising the pelvic floor muscles.

Lubricants Oils, creams, gels or other substances, which are used to add moisture to the genital area or any other part of the body, to reduce uncomfortable friction during sex play. *See* KY Jelly.

Lust Strong sexual desire or drive.

Maidenhead A term sometimes used to refer to the hymen, or to female virginity.

Make love Euphemism for having sexual intercourse and/or engaging in other forms of sexual activity, sometimes used to differentiate sex with emotional involvement from mechanical sex.

Masochism A form of sexual behaviour in which a person derives sexual pleasure from feeling pain, or having humiliation or domination inflicted on them. The word is derived from Sacher-Masoch (1836-1886), who wrote several books celebrating his own sexual fantasies involving physical abuse. See Sadism, Sadomasochism.

Massage Rubbing, stroking or kneading a person's body, sometimes with oil, sometimes for sensual or sexual pleasure or to relieve stress, pain or stiffness.

Masturbation Sexual stimulation of one's own or another's sexual organs, usually with the hands, but also with other parts of the body or with objects.

Mechanical methods of contraception Means of preventing conception while allowing full penile-vaginal intercourse to occur, by using a device which functions as a barrier preventing sperm and ovum from meeting. Mechanical methods include the condom, the diaphragm and the IUS and IUD. *See* Natural and Hormonal methods of contraception.

Ménage à trois Three people engaging in sexual activity together, often involving a couple and an outside lover. *See* Troilism.

Menarche The first occurrence of menstruation in a woman's life, usually in the course of puberty.

Menopause Precisely, the last occurrence of menstruation in a woman's life. However the term is more commonly used to refer to the whole of the climacteric. *See* Climacteric.

Menstrual cycle The hormonal cycle, lasting approximately twenty-eight days, by which the female reproductive system is maintained. It ensures that each month an ovum is matured and released (ovulation) and the lining of the uterus is prepared for the possibility of a pregnancy. If conception does not occur, this lining is shed in menstruation, so that a new lining can be prepared during the following cycle.

Menstruation Sometimes called 'a period'. *See* Menstrual cycle.

Mini-pill *See* Progestogen-only pill.

Missionary position A position during sexual intercourse where the man is on top of the woman and lying between her legs.

Monogamy The state or practice of having only one sexual partner over a specific period of time.

Mons pubis Fatty cushion-like tissue that covers the upper part of the pubic bone in females. In males it is a layer of fatty tissue found over the junction of the pubic bones. Also known as the mons veneris.

Mons veneris *See* Mons pubis.

Morning-after pill Inaccurate term for the emergency contraceptive pill. It is in fact effective up to seventy-two hours after intercourse.

Mucus Slippery, protective secretion produced from the mucous membranes and glands. Mucus produced in the genital area can provide extra lubrication during intercourse.

Mucus method *See* Cervical mucus method.

Multiple orgasm Several orgasms experienced in rapid succession, without any refractory period between each one. Usually, only women are physically capable of having multiple orgasms, but, by practising and developing ejaculatory control, some men may also be able to have more than one orgasmic peak in quick succession. In most cases not all will involve ejaculation. *See* Refractory period.

Natural methods of contraception Avoiding conception by making sure that the man does not ejaculate inside the woman's vagina during the period when she is at her most fertile. This includes coitus interruptus, but also various methods – sometimes known as rhythm methods – of judging when ovulation is most likely to occur, such as the calendar method, the cervical mucus method and the temperature method.

Necrophilia Sexual attraction to and/or sexual activity with dead bodies.

Nipple The tip of the breast. It is an important erogenous zone and becomes erect during sexual arousal. In women it contains the outlet of the milk ducts.

Nocturnal emission Involuntary ejaculation during sleep, in particular during a sexually arousing dream; also known as a wet dream. Nocturnal emissions occur in some eighty per cent of young males.

NGU or **non-gonococcal urethritis** Inflammation of a man's urethra, caused by a number of different types of bacteria other than the gonococcus (the bacterium which causes gonorrhoea). It is usually passed on through sexual contact. Characteristic symptoms include discharge from the penis and pain or difficulty in urinating. If untreated, the inflammation can spread to the prostate and sometimes to the testes.

Nonoxynol-9 The chemical present in most spermicides. In laboratory conditions it has been shown to destroy HIV. However, it is not reliable in destroying HIV during sexual practices.

NSU or **non-specific urethritis** Essentially the same as non-gonococcal urethritis. *See* NGU.

Nymphomania A neurotic condition experienced by women who feel a compulsion to have sex with as many men as possible.

Oestrogen A steroid hormone produced in the ovaries and other glands in the female. The counterpart to testosterone, it is often considered an exclusively 'female' hormone, but is in fact produced in both males and females. It is also produced by the placenta during pregnancy. Oestrogen stimulates changes in a woman's reproductive organs during her monthly cycle and promotes female primary and secondary sexual characteristics at all stages of development. *See* Testosterone.

Onanism Any sexual activity that does not put sperm to procreative use, for example in masturbation.

It is derived from Onan, Judah's son (Book of Genesis), who 'sinned' by ejaculating onto the ground.

Opportunistic infections A general term for infections or diseases that take hold when the immune system has been damaged by HIV. *See* HIV, ARC.

Oral contraception Hormonal pills taken by mouth for contraceptive purposes. *See* Pill (contraceptive).

Oral sex The use of the mouth, lips and tongue to arouse and stimulate the genitals of another. It includes fellatio and cunnilingus and is also known as oral-genital sex.

Oral-genital sex *See* Oral sex.

Orchitis Inflammation of one or both of the testicles.

Orgasm The climax of sexual excitement, usually involving rhythmic contractions of the pelvic and genital muscles, which produces highly pleasurable sensations throughout the body. In the male it is usually accompanied by ejaculation as well. These contractions occur at intervals of 0.8 seconds in both male and female and usually last less than one minute. Blood pressure, pulse and breathing rates all increase.

Outer labia *See* Labia majora.

Outing The term given to the practice of publicly exposing people's homosexuality against their will.

Ovaries The two female sex glands or gonads, located on either side of the uterus, that produce the female sexual hormones oestrogen and progesterone and the reproductive cells the ova. Each ovary stores as many as half a million ova. In the mature female, one ovum is matured and released into a fallopian tube every month, alternating between the two ovaries, in the process of ovulation. The ovaries are equivalent to the testes in the male.

Ovulation The cyclic release of an ovum from an ovary into one of the fallopian tubes. *See* Menstrual cycle.

Ovum The female reproductive cell. Usually, in a mature female, one ovum is produced each month in one of the ovaries. *See* Ovaries.

Paedophilia Sexual attraction to, or sexual activity with, children.

Pederasty (1) The act of penetration in anal sex. (2) Homosexual activity between men and young boys.

Peeping Tom A person who derives sexual excitement from watching others undress or engage in sexual activity. Also known as a voyeur.

Pelvic inflammatory disease (PID) Inflammation of the uterine lining and fallopian tubes in the female. Causes include bacterial infections including chlamydia and gonorrhoea, and long term use of IUDs. Symptoms include chronic pain and fever. If untreated, it can lead to infertility. *See* Chlamydia, Gonorrhoea.

Penetration The insertion of a man's erect penis into the vagina or anus of his partner in sexual intercourse.

Penile implants Flexible or inflatable rods inserted by surgical operation into the penis to replace the cavernous tissue and thus create a mechanical form of achieving and maintaining an erection.

Penile injections Used to treat erectile problems by self-injecting a drug into the cavernous tissue of the penis to create an erection.

Penis The primary male sex organ. The penis is akin to the clitoris in the female, developing from the same tissue in the embryo. It is made up of erectile and muscular tissue, supplied with many sensory nerves. The erectile tissue lies in three columns, two on the back forming the corpora cavernosa, and one on the front forming the corpus spongiosum and extending to form the glans or head. This tissue is arranged in a honeycomb structure. In the course of sexual arousal the muscle fibres that make up the honeycomb relax to allow blood to fill the structures, causing the penis to become erect. The urethra – through which urine is passed out of the body from the bladder and semen is passed on ejaculation – passes along the length of the penis through the corpus spongiosum, to its opening in the tip of the glans. The penis is covered with loosely-attached, fatless skin, which folds back on itself at the tip to make up the prepuce or foreskin in an uncircumcised male. At the back of the glans is a highly sensitive bridge of skin, the frenulum.

Penis corsets Lace-up coverings for the penis, made of leather or rubber, used to help achieve and maintain an erection or for show. *See* Arab straps.

Perineum In men, the area between the scrotum and the anus; in women, the area between the vagina and the anus.

Period *See* Menstruation.

Pervert A person who enjoys certain sexual activities that other people consider offensive.

Pessary (1) A medical tablet that is inserted into the vagina, where it dissolves and releases medication. Some spermicides are in pessary form. (2) The ring pessary is a device inserted into the vagina for women who have a prolapse of the vaginal walls and who do not want, or cannot have, an operation to repair the vagina.

Petting Old-fashioned term for sexual activities such as caressing parts of the body, either as a prelude to, or instead of, intercourse.

Phallus (1) A word for the erect penis. (2) Image of the male sexual organ, especially one associated with symbols of reproductive power.

Pheromones Chemical substances emitted by the body into the air, some of which are reputed to stimulate sexual attraction or desire in members of the opposite sex.

Phimosis Abnormal tightness of the foreskin that prevents it from being pulled back over the tip of the penis. The condition can often be corrected by gentle stretching, but in more severe cases circumcision may be necessary.

PID *See* Pelvic Inflammatory Disease.

Piercing Sexual body piercing typically involves piercing of the nipples or parts of the genitals such as the foreskin, scrotum, clitoris or labia. *See* Ampallang, Apadravya, Prince Albert.

Pill (contraceptive) A pill, taken daily, which contains synthetic hormones, usually oestrogen and/or progestogen. It works by modifying the level of these hormones within the female body in order to prevent pregnancy from occurring. *See* Combined pill, Progestogen-only pill, EveryDay pill. A male equivalent has yet to become available. *See* Hormonal methods of contraception.

Pimp Person who inducts and manages sex workers (formerly referred to as prostitutes). *See* Sex worker, Prostitution.

Platonic love Term used to describe love and admiration for another/others that does not involve sexual feelings or activity. The word is derived from a passage written by Plato in the *Symposium*.

Polyandry The practice of having more than one husband at the same time.

Polygamy The practice of having more than one wife or husband at the same time.

Polygyny The practice of having more than one wife at the same time.

Pornography Any material, such as writing, books, films and photographs designed to produce sexual arousal. Unlike eroticism, the term pornography has come to be associated with material that is violent or exploitative.

Posthitis Inflammation of the foreskin.

Pre-come or **Pre-cum** Fluids produced by certain glands, passed out of the penis prior to ejaculation. It consists mainly of lubricating secretions but may contain some sperm. *See* Cowper's Gland and Littre's Gland.

Premarital sex Sexual intercourse that takes place before either of the partners is married.

Premature ejaculation A sexual dysfunction where a man involuntarily ejaculates early in the course of sexual activity.

Prepuce Retractable fold of thin, hairless skin that covers the glans of the penis in the male (also known as the foreskin) and the clitoris in the female. It is sometimes removed in the traditional practice of circumcision. *See* Circumcision.

Priapism Prolonged, painful erection of the penis due to obstruction of the blood vessels in the penis.

Primary sexual characteristics Related to the sexual organs directly involved in sexual activity and reproduction, namely the ovaries and vagina in the female and testes and penis in the male. These develop in the embryo and mature at puberty.

Prince Albert A ring for genital piercing which is passed through the glans of the penis into the urethra, just above the frenum. *See* Ampallang, Piercing.

Proctitis Inflammation of the rectum.

Progestogen An artificial form of the natural hormone progesterone.

Progestogen-only pill (POP) A contraceptive pill that contains only progestogen. These pills are not widely used.

Progesterone A natural female hormone that is secreted chiefly from the ovaries. It prepares the uterus to receive and sustain a fertilized ovum.

Promiscuous Pejorative description of a person who has several different sexual partners over a relatively short period of time.

Prostate gland The male gland that surrounds the neck of the bladder and the urethra. It produces one of the major constituents of semen and has also been identified as the male G-spot. Stimulating it (using a finger inserted in the anus) can bring some men to orgasm.

Prostitution The practice of engaging in sexual activities in exchange for money or favours. A person who engages in such activity is known as a prostitute or, more commonly, a sex worker. *See* Pimp, Sex worker.

Puberty The stage of development at the beginning of adolescence when the sexual organs mature and secondary sexual characteristics emerge. This usually occurs from the age of ten in girls and from eleven in boys. *See* Adolescence, Secondary sexual characteristics.

Pubic bone Bone located at the front of the pelvis.

Pubic hair Hair that grows in the region just above and around the external genital organs.

Pubic lice Small wingless, parasitic insects that infest the hair in the pubic area and occasionally on other parts of the body. They feed on blood by biting into the skin. This may cause irritation. They are usually passed through close bodily contact. Also known as crabs.

Pudendum or **Pudenda** A collective term used to describe the external genitals, especially those of a woman.

Queen A popular term used to describe gay men. It is derived from the old English word *quaen* meaning a female prostitute.

Queer A term used to describe a lesbian or a gay man. Its usage has been documented in Britain as early as the 1920s.

Radical sex Sexual practices that are considered unconventional.

Rainbow 1960s term for group sex involving people of different skin colours.

Rainbow flag A symbol for the lesbian and gay movement that has been used since 1978. The artist Gilbert Baker produced the first prototypes, which consisted of eight strips in pink, red, orange, yellow, green, turquoise, indigo and violet.

Ramayana An Indian literary classic written by Valmiki, which includes descriptions of lesbian sexual activities.

Rape To force a person to have sexual intercourse against their will. Victims of rape can be male or female, of any age or social background. Rapists are almost always male, although cases of sexual assault by women have also been reported. Their relationship to the victim may be as stranger, acquaintance, friend, family member, date, lover or long term partner or spouse. It is estimated that at least fifty per cent of rapists know their victims.

Rear entry Various positions for sexual intercourse in which the man penetrates his partner from behind.

Rectum The lowest part of the alimentary canal whose opening is the anus. *See* Anus.

Refractory period The period of time following orgasm, during which the male sexual response to arousal is temporarily impossible. *See* Multiple orgasm.

Rent boy A male sex worker, often young, who provides gay sexual services.

Reproductive organs The organs that are involved in the processes of reproduction, including the production of reproductive cells (sperm and ova), sexual intercourse enabling sperm and ovum to meet, and the nurturing of the foetus should conception occur. They include the ovaries, fallopian tubes, uterus and vagina in the female, and the testes, epididymis and penis in the male.

Rhythm method A natural method of contraception. *See* Natural methods.

Rimming The practice of licking or sucking the anus of a partner. *See* Anilingus, Dental dam.

Row boat Sexual practice where a woman has intercourse with one man in the 'on top' position, while giving fellatio to two other men, one standing on each side of her.

Sadism A form of sexual practice in which a person gains pleasure from inflicting pain on another. The word is derived from the Marquis de Sade (1740-1814), whose writings featured descriptions of such practices. *See* Masochism, Sadomasochism.

Sadomasochism (SM or S&M) A form of sexual practice in which pleasure is gained from a combination of sadism and masochism.

Safe period The stage of a woman's menstrual cycle when she is least likely to be able to conceive. *See* Natural methods.

Safer sex Any form of sex that does not involve the exchange of body fluids, including non-penetrative sex, penetrative sex with the use of a condom, or the use of dental dams.

Salpingitis Inflammation of the fallopian tubes caused by an infection such as gonorrhoea or tuberculosis, or a reaction to an IUD. Symptoms include pain on one or both sides, fever and increased menstrual flow. *See* Gonorrhoea.

Sapphist Term for lesbian. The word is derived from the Greek, lesbian poet Sappho (610-580 BC). *See* Lesbian.

Sapphism Lesbianism. *See* Sapphist.

Scabies An infestation of parasitic mites, which burrow into the skin where they lay eggs, usually on the hairy parts of the body. Their saliva and droppings cause acute irritation. They are spread by close contact, including sexual contact, and poor hygiene.

Scat Any sexual practice that involves faeces. *See* Coprophilia.

Scissors (1) Term referring to lesbian sex practice involving manually stimulating a partner's anus and clitoris simultaneously. (2) Sexual position where the partners' legs are between one another's and their torsos are at right angles.

Scrotal sac *See* Scrotum.

Scrotum The sac of loose, wrinkled skin that contains a man's testicles. Also known as the scrotal sac.

Sebum An oily substance that is first produced at puberty. It is released from the sebaceous glands of the skin and makes the skin and hair more greasy.

Secondary sexual characteristics The physical characteristics, excluding the reproductive organs, that develop during puberty and distinguish male and female. They include men's greater facial hair and women's greater body fat.

Semen A mixture of seminal fluid and sperm, ejaculated from the penis at the point of orgasm.

Seminal fluid One of the two main constituents of semen, produced chiefly in the prostrate gland. It functions as the medium in which the sperm is carried and nourished.

Seminal vessicles Small sacs, at the back of a man's prostrate gland, which discharge seminal fluid into the urethra just before ejaculation.

Seminiferous tubules Tightly coiled tubes in the testes where the sperm are produced. Each testis contains as many as 800 tubules, each of which may be 40 cm or more in length.

Sex aids Any object used to generate or enhance sexual arousal and/or orgasm. Some of the most common are dildoes, vibrators, clitoral stimulators, extension condoms, vaginal balls and various 'stay longer' creams and lotions. *See* Sex toys.

Sex change *See* Gender reassignment.

Sex drive The urge or desire to have sex; also the amount or frequency of sexual activity which an individual requires in order to be sexually satisfied.

Sex hormone The hormones that determine the development of the sexual organs and secondary sexual characteristics and that also maintain and regulate the reproductive system and sexual feelings. The extent of their role in psychological and emotional changes is not yet fully understood. The principal sex hormones in women are oestrogen and progesterone; in men it is testosterone. *See* Oestrogen, Progesterone, Testosterone.

Sex toys Objects used to enhance sexual arousal. *See* Sex aids.

Sexual abuse Any form of unwanted sexual advance or use of sex to intimidate or threaten. This can range from verbal harassment to sexual assault and rape. *See* Rape.

Sexual arousal Feelings of sexual excitement, accompanied by mental and physical changes. Physical signs of arousal include erection of the penis and tightening of the scrotal sac in the male, and swelling of the areolae and clitoris together with increased vaginal lubrication in the female. Both men and women experience increased pulse and breathing rates. *See* Erection.

Sexual harassment The use of sex to threaten or intimidate; in particular, unwanted, offensive and/or repetitious sexual advances.

Sexual intercourse *See* Intercourse.

Sexual inversion or **Inversion** Term used at the beginning of the twentieth century to refer to homosexuality.

Sexual orientation An individual's pattern of sexual interest and attraction. This may be towards people of the same sex, the opposite sex, or both sexes.

Sexual response *See* Sexual arousal.

Sexual satisfaction Deep feelings of contentment and well-being experienced after sexual activity, particularly after orgasm.

Sexually transmitted disease (STD) Any illness that can be transmitted through sexual contact.

Sex worker Term developed in the 1980s as a substitute for the word prostitute.

Shaft The main part of the length of the penis (from the base to below the glans) or clitoris. *See* Penis, Glans, Clitoris.

Sheath *See* Condom.

Shrimping The practice of sucking the toes for sexual arousal.

Shudo Japanese term for pederasty. *See* Pederasty.

Sixty-nine Form of oral sex in which two people perform oral sex on each other at the same time. It is so-called because the positions adopted by the couple while performing this practice resemble the figure 69 when viewed from the side. The French translation, *soixante-neuf*, is also used.

Sleep with someone Euphemism meaning to have sexual intercourse with someone.

Smegma Sebum-based substance that can accumulate under the foreskin of the penis or the hood of the clitoris.

Sodomy Anal intercourse. The word is derived from the 'sinful' biblical city of Sodom. *See* Anal intercourse.

Soixante-neuf *See* Sixty-nine.

Solicit To offer sexual services in return for money, especially in a public place. *See* Pimp, Prostitution.

Spanish fly Powder made from dried Lytta vesicatoria beetles. It contains an active ingredient, cantharidin, which inflames the urethra. It is sometimes taken as an aphrodisiac. It can be fatal.

Spanking The practice of smacking or hitting a partner for sexual excitement.

Sperm The male reproductive cell, produced constantly in the testes of the mature male, and released through the penis at ejaculation. *See* Testes, Semen.

Spermatic cord The cord that passes from each of the male testes through the inguinal canal in the groin. It contains the vas deferens which conveys sperm to the ejaculatory duct.

Spermicide Any substance, usually a gel or cream, designed to kill sperm. It may be injected into the vagina prior to intercourse or used in conjunction with other forms of contraception. *See* Contraception.

Sponge A barrier form of contraceptive that consists of a small, round sponge soaked in spermicide, placed inside the vagina over the cervix. It is less reliable than other forms of contraception.

Squeeze technique A technique for delaying ejaculation or developing ejaculatory control, in which the head of the penis is squeezed just before the point when ejaculation becomes inevitable.

'Stay longer' creams and sprays Products designed to help a man to delay ejaculation, usually by reducing penile sensitivity with small amounts of local anaesthetic. *See* Sex aids.

STD *See* Sexually transmitted disease.

Sterilization A surgical operation that renders an individual unable to conceive a child (woman) or cause impregnation (man). *See* Vasectomy, Female sterilization.

Straight Slang term for heterosexuals. It may also be used as an expression for conservatism, while its use in drug-taking circles refers to someone who is either not under the influence of a mind-expanding drug or who does not consume such substances.

Sub Abbreviation of the term submissive, used to refer to a passive partner in practices involving bondage and sadomasochism. The term bottom is also used. *See* Bondage, Bottom.

Sub-dom Sexual practices in which partners take defined dominant and submissive roles. Sub-dom practices may or may not involve bondage, role-playing and sadomasochism.

Swinging Partner-swapping and sharing within groups of friends or associates. Swinging may involve singles or couples having sex play in pairs or groups, in front of each other or in private, with mutual consent and usually at the same venue. It may be arranged through swinging clubs or parties, through friends or through advertisements in specialized magazines.

Sympto-thermal method *See* Temperature method.

Syphilis Sexually transmitted disease caused by the treponema bacterium. It enters the body through tiny cracks in the skin and lives and multiplies in the blood and other body fluids of an infected person. It is passed on by the fluid secreted from the characteristic sores or chancres. These develop wherever the bacteria enters the body – usually on or near the penis or vagina, or sometimes in the anus or mouth. If untreated the bacteria can affect other parts of the body including the brain. In very severe cases disfigurement or death may result.

Temperature method A method of predicting when ovulation occurs by taking a woman's body temperature at the same time each day. Ovulation has occurred when body temperature has risen slightly for three days. *See* Natural methods.

Termination *See* Abortion.

Testes or **testicles** The two male sex glands or gonads located in the scrotum, which produce the male sex hormone testosterone and the reproductive cells, the sperm. Sperm are produced, matured and nourished in the long, narrow, tightly coiled seminiferous tubules within each testis, before being released into the epididymis where they are matured further and stored until needed. Sperm production is constant throughout most of the male's mature life. The testes are equivalent to the ovaries in the female. *See* Seminiferous Tubules, Sperm.

Testosterone A steroid hormone produced in the testes in the male and in other glands. Often described as a 'male' hormone, it is in fact produced in both males and females. In males, it causes the development of the sex organs in the foetus. At puberty it is responsible for the maturation of the sex organs and the development of the secondary sexual characteristics. In the adult it influences male and female sexual desire and male sexual performance. *See* Oestrogen.

Thai Beads Sex aid consisting of plastic beads threaded onto a string or rod, inserted into the anus and moved in and out to enhance sexual arousal. *See* Sex aids, Sex toys.

Thrush *See* Candida albicans.

Ticklers Rubber or latex sheaths for the penis, which have bumps and knobs on them, either down the shaft or at the tip, to stimulate the clitoris, vagina and/or cervix. Ticklers are produced as sex aids, not contraceptives. *See* Clitoral stimulator.

Transgendered A term used to describe a transsexual who has had a gender reassignment operation. *See* Gender reassignment.

Transsexualism Condition where gender identity does not follow biological gender. *See* Gender identity, Gender reassignment.

Transvestism Desired or habitual dressing in the clothing and/or under clothing associated with the opposite sex, sometimes with the appropriate make-up and accessories as well. Transvestites may be male or female and are usually heterosexual. In most cases the motivation behind transvestism is a form of fetishistic attraction to the clothing and accoutrements of the opposite sex, but it may also have to do with an attraction to the gender role of the opposite sex, symbolised by their clothes.

Tribadism A primarily lesbian sexual practice in which one partner lies on top of the other and both move together to stimulate each other's clitoris.

Trichomoniasis A sexually transmitted disease caused by a small parasite that infects the vagina, causing inflammation and irritation. It can also spread to the cervix. Men are only rarely infected, in the urethra, where it can cause NGU.

Tricking (1) Enjoyment of casual sex; a trick refers either to the casual encounter itself or to the partner in such an encounter. (2) Paid encounter secured by sex worker.

Troilism Term used to describe three people having sex together, in any combination of male and female. *See* Ménage à trois.

Uncut Term used to describe an uncircumcised penis.

Unprotected sex Sexual activity that does not involve safer sex practices. These may lead to pregnancy or infection. *See* Condom, Contraception.

Urethra The tube through which urine passes from the bladder; in men the urethra also carries semen during ejaculation. *See* Penis.

Urethritis Inflammation of the urethra, usually caused by bacterial infection. *See* NGU.

Urolagnia *See* Water sports.

Uterus or **womb** The female reproductive organ in which an embryo grows, matures and is nourished. The uterus lies between the bladder and the rectum, where it is held in place by various ligaments. The main part of its wall is made up of muscle. The two fallopian tubes are attached on either side, linking it with the ovaries, while the cervix or neck of the uterus provides the passageway between the uterus and the vagina. The lining of the uterus is known as the endometrium, and is prepared each month for the implantation of a fertilized ovum as part of the menstrual cycle. *See* Menstrual Cycle, Cervix, Vagina.

Vacuum device A sex aid designed to help a man achieve and maintain an erection. It is placed over the penis; air is pumped out and the vacuum created causes an erection. A tight band is placed around the base of the penis to maintain the erection and the device is removed.

Vagina The passage between the vulva and the cervix. It is a fibro-muscular structure covered with a thin mucous membrane. The various layers of muscle – together with the numerous folds of skin by which they are covered – give the vagina great capacity for expansion and contraction. The smooth muscle within the vaginal wall is not under voluntary control and relaxes and stretches as necessary during sexual arousal, penile penetration and childbirth without conscious effort, while the muscle fibres surrounding the outer third of the vagina can usually be tensed and relaxed voluntarily. In the course of sexual arousal the vagina dilates and 'sweats' a lubricating substance from its walls. As the woman approaches orgasm the upper part of the vagina balloons and the outer part swells to form what is sometimes known as the 'orgasmic platform', on which the rhythmic muscle contractions of orgasm are focused.

Vaginismus Condition in which the muscles around the outer third of the vagina contract very tightly making penetration painful, difficult or impossible.

Vaginitis Inflammation of the vagina, caused by infection, injury or atrophy.

Vas deferens The tube that conveys sperm from the testes to the penis, as part of the spermatic cord. *See* Testes.

Vasectomy Surgical operation in which the vasa deferentia are cut and tied so that sperm cannot be passed along them and are therefore not released in the ejaculate. *See* Sterilization.

Vasocongestion The process of tissue becoming engorged with blood, as when the penis becomes erect.

Venereal Disease (VD) Any disease that can be transmitted by sexual contact, now more commonly termed Sexually Transmitted Diseases (STDs).

Vestibule The area between a woman's inner labia where the vaginal opening and the urethral opening are situated.

Vibrator Sex aid, powered by mains electricity or batteries, that vibrates rhythmically to produce sensual pleasure. Vibrators are made in a great variety of shapes but the most common are those shaped as erect penises. Some have attachments for simultaneous stimulation of the clitoris, others for use in the anus; anal vibrators are also available. Vibrators are also made in the shape of vaginas. Vibrating devices are most frequently used for masturbation on or around the genitals but they may be used to stimulate any part of the body.

Virgin Person who has never experienced sexual intercourse.

Voyeur A person who enjoys and becomes sexually aroused by watching others undress or engage in sexual activities. *See* Peeping Tom.

Vulva The external female genitalia.

Watersports (WS) Sexual acts that involve one partner urinating over (golden shower) or into (golden screw) their partner.

Wet dream *See* Nocturnal emission.

Wide-on The state of advanced female sexual arousal that results in a relaxation of the vaginal muscles. It is analogous with the male hard-on.

Withdrawal *See* Coitus interruptus.

Womb *See* Uterus.

PICTURE CREDITS

Thanks to Condomania and Sh! Erotic Emporium for Women for supplying props

All Image Bank photographs are posed by models.

SEXUAL FACTS

Opener: Simon Jennings
12. (bottom) Ann Summers Ltd.
13. (top right) Joe Bulaitis (bottom) Simon Jennings
14. (bottom) Musée d'Orsay, Paris
15. Simon Jennings
16. (top, diagram) Ian Seaton
17. (bottom) Marshall Cavendish
20. (left) Marshall Cavendish
21. (top) Reproduced with kind permission from *The Collected Drawings of Aubrey Beardsley* by Bruce Harris (ed.), Crown Publishing inc.
(bottom) Simon Jennings
22. (bottom) Science Photo Library
23. (top) Science Photo Library (bottom) Hugo Boss Ltd.
26. (left) Stapleton Collection
28, 29. Science Photo Library
30. (top) Image Bank; (bottom) Image Bank
31. Image Bank
32, 33. (background and inset right) Image Bank; (inset centre) Science Photo Library
34, 35. Joe Bulaitis/Ian Seaton
36, 37. Joe Bulaitis/Ian Seaton
39. (bottom, left and right) Science Photo Library
40, 41. Image Bank
42. (top) Mark Pennington
43. Mark Pennington
44. (bottom left) Mark Pennington
45. Mark Pennington, Chartex Ltd. (femidom)
46. Mark Pennington
47. (right) Mark Pennington
48. Image Bank
49. (top) Zefa; (bottom) Stapleton Collection
50. United Colours of Benetton
51. (top) Mansell Collection
51. (bottom) Liba Taylor/Panos Pictures
52. (top, middle) Mark Pennington
54. Science Photo Library
60. (top) Science Photo Library; (bottom) Tim Nunn/Panos Pictures
61. Bill Cooper
62. Smithsonian Institution/Jeff Tinsley
63. (top) Image Bank; (bottom) United Colours of Benetton
64. The Rape of the Sabines by Peter Paul Rubens (1577–1640) National Gallery, London/ Bridgeman Art Library, London

SEXUAL FEELINGS & BEHAVIOUR

66, 67. Simon Jennings
68, 69. (background) Ian Seaton
68. (left) Renate Hillermann; (top) Image Bank; (bottom) Zefa
69. Mark Pennington
70. Seated Woman with Bent Knee, 1917 by Egon Schiele (1890–1918) Narodni Galerie, Prague/Bridgeman Art Library, London
71. (bottom) Reproduced with kind permission from *The Collected Drawings of Aubrey Beardsley* by Bruce Harris (ed.), Crown Publishing inc.
72. (top) Reproduced with kind permission from *The Collected Drawings of Aubrey Beardsley* by Bruce Harris (ed.), Crown Publishing inc.; (bottom) Stapleton Collection
74, 75. Image Bank
76. (top) Rex Features; (bottom) Rex Features
77. (top) Rex Features; (bottom) Simon Jennings
78. (top) Mary Evans; (bottom) Rex Features
79. 3 Over 1 Design
80. (top) Rex Features; (middle) InterAction Stock/Milton Diamond; (bottom) Marshall Cavendish
81. Marshall Cavendish
82. InterAction Stock/Milton Diamond
83. (top) Zefa; (bottom) Rex Features
85. (top) Image Bank; (bottom) Rex Features
87. (top) InterAction Stock/Milton Diamond; (bottom) Image Bank
89. Zefa
90. Rex Features
91. Ann Summers
92. Image Bank
93. Zefa
95. La Belle Dame Sans Merci by Sir Frank Dicksee (1853–1928) City of Bristol Museum and Art Gallery/ Bridgeman Art Library, London
96. (top) Beatriz Reis; (bottom) Image Bank
97. Image Bank
99. Image Bank
100, 101. Marshall Cavendish
102. Lovers, 1911 by Egon Schiele (1890–1918) Private Collection/Bridgeman Art Library, London
103. Marshall Cavendish
107. (top left) Image Bank; (middle left) Image Bank; (middle left) Marshall Cavendish; (top right) Marshall Cavendish; (middle right) Marshall Cavendish
108. Tuppy Owens
109. (top) InterAction Stock/Milton Diamond; (bottom) Image Bank
111. (middle) Marshall Cavendish
122, 123. Photographs by Robert Taylor from *Safer Sexy: The Guide to Gay Sex Safely* by Peter Tatchell (Cassell 1994)
123. (top right) 3 Over 1 Design
124, 125. Laurence Jaugey-Paget
126. (bottom) Simon Jennings
129. Stapleton Collection
130. (left) Rainer Wick
(top) Simon Jennings; (bottom) Inklink
131. (top) Inklink; (bottom) Rainer Wick
132. (top) Marshall Cavendish
133. (top) Inklink

134. (top) Stapleton Collection
135. (top) Stapleton Collection; (bottom) Photograph by Robert Taylor from *Safer Sexy: The Guide to Gay Sex Safely* by Peter Tatchell (Cassell 1994)
137. (left) Stapleton Collection; (right) Reproduced with kind permission from *The Collected Works of Aubrey Beardsley* by Bruce Harris (ed.), Crown Publishing inc.
138, 139. Image Bank
140. (left) Laurence Jaugey-Paget; (right) Marshall Cavendish
141. (left) Marshall Cavendish
142. (left) Marshall Cavendish; (right top and bottom) Ann Summers Ltd.
143. (bottom) Marshall Cavendish
144. (top) Proserpine, 1874 by Dante Gabriel Rossetti (1828–82) Tate Gallery, London/Bridgeman Art Library, London; (bottom) Marshall Cavendish
145. (bottom) Marshall Cavendish
146, 147. (background) Mark Pennington
146. (left) Image Bank
147. (top) Tuppy Owens
147. (bottom left and right) InterAction Stock/Milton Diamond
148. (left) Image Bank
150. Rex Features
152. Mark Pennington
155. (left) Ann Summers Ltd.
156. Image Bank
157. Rex Features
158. Michele Martinoli
159. (top) Rex Features
159. (bottom) InterAction Stock/Milton Diamond
160. (top) Tuppy Owens; (bottom left) InterAction Stock/Milton Diamond; (bottom right) Reproduced courtesy of Macmillam General Books
161. Zefa; (inset) Rex Features
162. (left) Stapleton Collection (right) Tuppy Owens
164. (top) Reproduced with kind permission from *The Collected Works of Aubrey Beardsley* by Bruce Harris (ed.), Crown Publishing inc.; (bottom) Marshall Cavendish
165. (top, bottom) Tuppy Owens; (middle) Ann Summers Ltd.
166. (left) Gisbert Bauer; (right) Tuppy Owens
167. Stapleton Collection
168. (top) The Swing, 1767 by Jean-Honore Fragonard (1732–1806) Wallace Collection, London/Bridgeman Art Library, London; (bottom) Marshall Cavendish
169. (top) Tuppy Owens
170. Rex Features
171. Rex Features
172. Liz Boggis
173. (top) Ronald Grant Archive/Allied Entertainment; (bottom) Image Bank
174. (left) Stapleton Collection; (top right) Image Bank; (bottom right) Marshall Cavendish
176. Marshall Cavendish
177. Marshall Cavendish

SEX & YOU

179. Simon Jennings
180. Deborah Samuel/Special Photographers Library
184. Tansy Spinks/Special Photographers Library
186. Tansy Spinks/Special Photographers Library
192. Ewan Fraser/Special Photographers Library

SEX & CULTURE

199. Simon Jennings
200. (top to bottom) Werner Forman Archive; InterAction Stock/Milton Diamond; Private Collection, New York; Private Collection, New York; Gisbert Bauer
201. Dorset County Council Archaeology Service
202. Mansell Collection
203. The Daughters of Judah in Babylon by Schmalz, Herbert Gustave (1856–1935) Christie's, London/Bridgeman Art Library, London
204. Musee du Louvre, Paris: copyright photo RMN – Chuzeville
205. Werner Forman Archive
206, 207. AKG/Erich Lessing
208. Reproduced from *Erotic Art of the Masters, 18th, 19th and 20th Centuries* by Bradley Smith (Gemini-Smith)
209. Humay and Murayun, lovers surrounded by attendants, from the 'Shahnama', 1396 Persian Literary Texts, British Library, London/Bridgeman Art Library, London
210. Gisbert Bauer
211. A Prince involved in united intercourse, described by Vatsyayana in his 'Kama Sutra', Bundi, Rajasthan, Rajput School, c.1800 Private Collection/ Bridgeman Art Library, London
212. Adam and Eve banished from Paradise by Tommaso Masaccio (1401–28) Brancacci Chapel, Santa Maris del Carmine, Florence/Bridgeman Art Library, London
213. King Arthur's Wedding Night, French, 14th century (manuscript) Bibliotheque Inguimbertine, Carpentras/ Bridgeman Art Library, London
215. Virgin and Child by Jean Fouquet (c. 1425–80) Koninklijk Museum voor Schone Kunsten, Antwerp/Bridgeman Art Library, London; Lancelot proves his love of Guinevere, Roman de Lancelot du Lac (1344) Pierpont Morgan Library, New York/Bridgeman Art Library, London
216. Portrait of the Van Cortland Family, c.1830 by Anonymous, American Museum, Bath/ Bridgeman Art Library, London
217. Mary Evans
218. Stapleton Collection
219. Rex Features
221. Eikoh Hosoe
224. (top to bottom) Mary Evans/Sigmund Freud, copyright courtesy of W.E. Freud; Marie Stopes International; Corbis – Bettman/UPI; Topham

INDEX

Q

R

S